Familial Endocrine Cancer Syndromes

Fady Hannah-Shmouni

Editor

Familial Endocrine Cancer Syndromes

Navigating the Transition of Care for Pediatric and Adolescent Patients

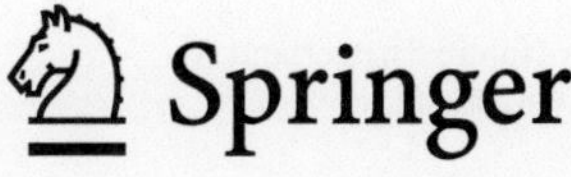 Springer

Editor
Fady Hannah-Shmouni
Division of Endocrinology
University of British Columbia
Vancouver, BC, Canada

ISBN 978-3-031-37277-3   ISBN 978-3-031-37275-9   (eBook)
https://doi.org/10.1007/978-3-031-37275-9

This Springer imprint is published by the registered company Springer Nature Switzerland AG
The registered company address is: Gewerbestrasse 11, 6330 Cham, Switzerland
Paper in this product is recyclable.

Preface

Benign and malignant endocrine neoplasms in childhood and adolescence form a widely heterogeneous group of disorders often presenting with subtle clinical or biochemical features that are often missed or misdiagnosed during a clinical encounter. Endocrine neoplasias developing in young patients are quite characteristic for certain familial endocrine cancer syndromes that are usually inherited. A wide spectrum of non-malignant and malignant tumors within each syndrome exists, with poor genotype-to-phenotype correlation. Thus, experienced clinicians working in established centers of excellence are generally required to care for at-risk or affected individuals with these syndromes.

Advancements in medical treatment and technology have increased the life expectancy of children with special healthcare needs, the majority of whom are now living into adulthood. Therefore, there is an increased need for planned programs with extensive resources for transition of youth with special healthcare needs from the pediatric system to adult health services. Currently, there is limited literature that defines and identifies transition practices that produce positive outcomes. However, there is a significant amount of qualitative data available on the patient, parent, and healthcare provider perceptions of barriers to successful transition.

There is an increased need for direction, resources, and education in the development of transition of care programs and guidelines for pediatric and adolescent patients with familial endocrine syndromes. The transition of care from the pediatric system to adult health services currently presents various emerging concerns and barriers that ultimately leads to inefficient, delayed, and broken care; medical errors; and psychosocial impact on the individual. Most healthcare providers are not equipped with the necessary resources, skillset, and education to holistically care for the individual during this critical period of their life and disease management. These limitations lead to poor transfer experiences and changes in healthcare environments to the patients.

To address these issues, we have compiled 13 informative chapters written by world-renowned healthcare providers and researchers in the fields of endocrinology, pharmacy, radiology, infertility, pediatrics, internal medicine, psychology, and genetics. From topics covering psychosocial impacts to pharmacokinetic and homecare resources, the intent of this book is to provide guiding principles for a safe and informative transition of care for pediatric and adolescent patients with various familial endocrine cancer syndromes that are transitioning from pediatric to adult health care. Transition research is growing and numerous models of implementation and evaluation are emerging. Through this comprehensive work, we hope to provide resources, time, expertise, and research for our patients, their families, and their healthcare providers.

Vancouver, BC, Canada   Fady Hannah-Shmouni

About the Editor

Fady Hannah-Shmouni, MD ABIM FRCPC is an Iraqi-Canadian physician-investor who brings a wealth of expertise in endocrinology, hypertension, and genomic medicine. He is a clinical professor of medicine, and endocrinologist, at the University of British Columbia, with over 10 years of clinical and business experience in early-stage investments, advisory, and academic research. He is deeply committed to empowering consumers with access to cutting-edge technologies in precision medicine like artificial intelligence, genomic medicine, and healthspan advancements.

He serves as the Managing Partner and Founder of FHS Capital (fhscapital.io), a privately held early-stage investment fund, focusing on real estate, sustainable express car wash services, biotechnology and digital assets. He managed seed financing for Ovenue, Flyby, Healthspan Digital, and GeneSeq, and serves as a medical advisor for venture-backed companies like Eli Health and Science & Humans. He is the Founder/CEO of Healthspan Digital, a Smart Precision Medicine (Predictive, Preventative, Personalized, Participatory) and direct-to-consumer operating system and clinical service based on Longevity Biomarkers.

Dr Hannah-Shmouni is active in clinical practice, retains a staff physician and professor position at Vancouver General Hospital (UBC), and a fellow with the Royal College of Physicians and Surgeons of Canada. He completed clinical training in internal medicine at Yale School of Medicine, adult endocrinology at the National Institutes of Health, and clinical biochemical genetics at the University of Toronto. He is a board-certified physician in internal medicine and endocrinology by the American Board of Internal Medicine and the Royal College of Physician and Surgeons of Canada, and in clinical hypertension by the American Society of Hypertension.

His research career started as a physician-scientist in endocrinology and genetics at the NIH under the mentorship of esteemed geneticist Dr. Constantine A. Stratakis (Bethesda, Maryland: 2015-2021). During his time there, he served as the Head of Graduate Medical Education, Associate Program Director of Endocrinology Fellowship Program and Principal Investigator on several adrenal protocols. He has authored over 100 original articles, book chapters, and reviews on endocrine-genetic conditions, and was the founding member and first Editor-in-Chief of the medical journal Endocrine and Metabolic Science (Elsevier). Dr Hannah-Shmouni's business and academic passion is to offer guidance, build relationships, and provide resources to support innovative businesses and entrepreneurs.

Contents

Chapter 1
The Psychosocial Impact of Familial Endocrine Cancer Syndromes (FECS) on the Patient and Caregiver

Kate Hetherington, Jacqueline D. Hunter, Robin Lockridge, Meera Warby, Margarita Raygadam, Claire E. Wakefield, and Lori Wiener

Introduction

Familial endocrine cancer syndromes (FECS) encompass a breadth of heritable conditions with varying risks of developing cancer. A genetic diagnosis may provide important diagnostic, prognostic, and therapeutic benefits [1]. Offering genetic testing to patients with a clinical suspicion of having an endocrine cancer syndrome (either through single-gene or panel analysis), aims to identify a germline pathogenic variant(s) in a known inherited endocrine cancer syndrome [2].

K. Hetherington · J. D. Hunter · C. E. Wakefield
Discipline of Paediatrics and Child Health, School of Clinical Medicine, Faculty of Medicine and Health, UNSW Sydney, Sydney, Australia

Behavioural Sciences Unit, Kids Cancer Centre, Sydney Children's Hospital, Sydney, Australia
e-mail: k.hetherington@unsw.edu.au; jacqueline.hunter@unsw.edu.au; c.wakefield@unsw.edu.au

R. Lockridge
Clinical Research Directorate (CRD), Frederick National Library for Cancer Research, Frederick, MD, USA
e-mail: robin.lockridge@nih.gov

M. Warby
Hereditary Cancer Centre, Department of Medical Oncology, Prince of Wales Hospital, Sydney, Australia

Prince of Wales Clinical School, UNSW Sydney, Sydney, Australia
e-mail: meera.warby@health.nsw.gov.au

M. Raygadam · L. Wiener (✉)
Pediatric Oncology Branch, Center for Cancer Research, National Cancer Institute, National Institute of Health, Bethesda, MD, USA
e-mail: raygadam@mail.nih.gov; wienerl@mail.nih.gov

F. Hannah-Shmouni (ed.), *Familial Endocrine Cancer Syndromes*,
https://doi.org/10.1007/978-3-031-37275-9_1

""

Establishing a genetic diagnosis can be beneficial to the patient. Enabling predictive testing in at-risk relatives can also have potential health implications for family members. With increased breadth and availability, cost reduction and overall faster turn-around-time of genetic testing, individuals and their families are now experiencing unprecedented exposure to information about their genetic risks and health [3]. Family members identified as being at increased risk can receive appropriate screening and management, while relatives not harboring the variant can be reassured. Predictive testing in childhood is endorsed by multiple advisory bodies when testing in childhood would provide immediate benefit to their healthcare [1, 4]. Despite the benefits of knowing one's risk, there may be a significant psychological impact associated with receiving a genetic diagnosis as well as practical implications.

To address the complex issues associated with predictive testing, families undergoing genetic testing will typically see a genetic counselor as part of the process. Genetic counseling aims to increase a family's understanding of testing options, deliver education on screening and management, and provide an environment for exploration of the psychosocial impact of the information [5].

FECS require lifelong management and surveillance: understanding the implications of FECS may be particularly challenging when the information is received in early childhood. As many cancer endocrine syndromes are transmitted in an autosomal dominant fashion, it is important for risks for future offspring to be addressed, including a discussion regarding reproductive options, such as pre-implantation genetic diagnosis, prenatal diagnosis, and testing of children after birth [6]. Revisiting genetic counseling in the mid- to late teenage years and again at the time of family planning is also vital to ensure that patients understand their diagnosis, medical management recommendations, and reproductive risks and options [5].

The identification of a FECS is the beginning of a lifelong relationship with genetic services that can assist with patient management and surveillance as well as facilitating predictive testing in relatives. Throughout this journey, it is critical to provide age-appropriate information at important developmental stages to help children and their families navigate their options and to provide psychosocial support [5].

In this chapter, we begin by reviewing research relevant to understanding the impact of FECS on the wellbeing and quality of life of child and adolescent patients and their families. We discuss common FECS including multiple endocrine neoplasia (MEN) types 1, 2A, 2B, von Hippel-Lindau disorder (VHL), and hereditary pheochromocytoma and paragangliomas linked to succinate dehydrogenase (SDH). Next, the chapter describes implications associated with genetic testing, surveillance, and reproductive considerations. This is followed by ethical issues that arise in genetic counseling regarding FECS in children and adolescents. Throughout the chapter, recommendations for future work in this area are presented. Of note, due to the lack of research exploring the psychosocial impact of FECS on children and adolescents we have at times relied on what we can learn about the impact of these conditions from adults. At times we have also drawn from studies including young people affected by Li Fraumeni syndrome (LFS). While LFS is not considered an endocrine cancer syndrome, it shares some characteristics with FECS, and in the absence of FECS specific data may provide useful insights into the experiences of children and adolescents affected by FECS.

Psychosocial Impact of Living with a Familial Endocrine Cancer Syndrome on Patients and Their Caregivers

Studies examining quality of life and overall wellbeing of persons living with hereditary cancer syndromes are still quite limited, especially in pediatric and adolescent populations. Despite recent advances in the diagnosis and management of FECS, data suggests that the diagnosis of a chronic complex syndrome such as MEN1, MEN2, Von Hippel-Lindau disease or the diagnosis of SDH related paragangliomas can have a negative impact on an individual's quality of life, and psychological wellbeing. In this section, we review published findings on patients and caregivers, by condition. Given the lack of data exploring the experiences of pediatric and adolescent patients we have included relevant adult data to provide an indication of the possible psychosocial impacts. In examining the impact on caregivers, we have drawn on data from parents of young people with, or at-risk of, FECS as well as caregivers of adults with a FECS (including partners). Given the hereditary nature of these syndromes, some affected children and adolescents will have a parent/caregiver with a FECS, while others will not. Table 1.1 provides an overview of the studies described below.

Table 1.1 Overview of studies examining the psychosocial impact of FECS on patients and parents or caregivers

References	FECS	Design	Sample	Measures	Findings
Lockridge et al. [7]	MEN2 and MTC	Cross sectional	Adults	Structured psychosocial interview	Approximately half of all participants reported that pain interferes with their daily life and their mood.
			15 pediatric (<12 years)	The Distress Thermometer/Problem Checklist	Pediatric patients frequently reported experiencing attention challenges and difficulty concentrating. Parents reported mood shifts and became upset easily. The most frequent need for services included education about MTC, treatment and research participation, and the opportunity to meet others with MTC
			31 pediatric (12–17) years)		
			17 adults (≥18 years)		
Van Engelen et al. [8]	CPS	Semi-structured interviews	20 interviewers (11 parents and 9 adolescents; 12–18 years)	Semi-structured interviews coded using thematic analysis of interview transcripts	Themes included: challenges of surveillance, factors influencing the surveillance experience, parental experience of having a child with CPS, positive factors that help families navigate surveillance-related worries, and adolescent understanding of their condition of report of impact on daily life.
					Parents and adolescents both reports worry associated with surveillance of CPS.

Martins and Carvalho [9]	SDH	Cross-sectional national survey	103 SDH pathogenic variant carriers	Multidimensional Impact of Cancer Risk Assessment (MICRA)	Participants who developed pheochromocytomas and paragangliomas (PPGL) displayed significant increases in testing-related distress and global suffering as compared to unaffected carriers. On the MICRA, no other significant differences were observed.
			Adults (mean age/SD: 44.25 ± 16.84)	36-item Short Form Health Survey (SF36)	For parents, having PPGL was significantly correlated with guilt about passing on the disease, and worry about the child getting cancer.
				HADS	Distress, uncertainty, and global suffering (due to test result) increased with age and decreased with education level.
					Sample mean for anxiety and depression fell below cutoffs for a mood disorder (assessed with HADS).
					Affected pathogenic variant carriers presented lower global quality of life and higher anxiety and depression levels than healthy carriers (SF36).
Mongelli et al. [10]	MEN2A	Cross-sectional	45 adults (≥18 years) with MEN2A	Patient-Reported Outcomes Measurement Information System (PROMIS)	MEN2A patients reported worse anxiety, depression fatigue, pain interference, sleep disturbance, and lower physical functioning as compared with US normative data.
					MEN2A patients reported greater fatigue than patients with different types of cancer.

(continued)

Table 1.1 (continued)

References	FECS	Design	Sample	Measures	Findings
Peipert et al. [11]	MEN1	Cross-sectional survey	153 adults (≥18) who self-reported physician diagnosis of MEN1	PROMIS	Patients with MEN-1 reported worse anxiety, depression, fatigue, pain interference, sleep disturbance, physical functioning, and social functioning compared to normative data and greater anxiety, depression, fatigue, and pain interference than patients with different types of cancer.
Goswami et al. [12]	MEN1	Cross-sectional survey	207 adults (≥18) with a diagnosis of MEN1	PROMIS-29	Individuals with MEN1 reported worse anxiety, depression, fatigue, pain interference, sleep disturbance, physical function, and social function scores compared with US normative data.
Rodrigues et al. [13]	MEN2	Cross-sectional (qualitative and quantitative assessment)	43 adults (≥18 years) with clinical and genetic MEN2 diagnosis and long-term follow-up	Hospital Anxiety and Depression scale (HADS)	Anxiety and/or depression observed in 46% of cases.
				European Organization for Research and Treatment of Cancer Quality of Life Questionnaire C30 (EORTC QLQ C30)	Generally, patients reported a satisfactory global state of health.
				Scale of Mental Adjustment to Cancer (MINI-MAC)	Patients who transmitted RET pathogenic variants had higher scores for discouragement/anxious preoccupation.
				Semi-structured interviews	Patients who were well-informed about disease had lower mean score values for depression and anxiety.

Kasparian et al. [14]	VHL	Cross-sectional (qualitative semi-structured interviews)	23 participants (15 patients ages ≥18 years, 8 caregivers)	Semi-structured telephone interviews	A diverse range of experiences were reported. Challenges included uncertainty about the future, frustration, financial and caregiver burden, perceived isolation, and limited career opportunities. Resiliency was also reported.
				Impact of Events Scale (IES)	
				HADS	
				Carer Burden Scale	
van Hulsteijn et al. [15, 16]	SDH	Cross-sectional	174 paraganglioma patients and 100 controls	HADS	Paraganglioma patients reported a significantly impaired QoL on the HADS, MFI-20, and SF-36 compared controls and the literature. No difference between anxiety and the literature was found between patients and controls (HADS).
			Adults (mean age/SD: 52.2 ± 13.5)	Multidimensional Fatigue Index 20 (MFI-20)	Compared with age-adjusted reference values, paraganglioma patients' anxiety and total HADS score was impaired.
				SF-36	Asymptomatic carriers and the general population did not differ with regard to QOL.
					41 patients completed 5-year evaluations; all domains remain unchanged with the exception of an increased score on the MFI-20 corresponding to reduced activity.

(continued)

Table 1.1 (continued)

References	FECS	Design	Sample	Measures	Findings
Lammens et al. [17]	VHL and Li Fraumeni syndrome (LFS)	Cross-sectional	50 adult partners of individuals diagnosed with or at high risk of LFS or VHL.	Impact of Events Scale (IES)	Levels of distress and worries of partners and their high-risk spouses were significantly correlated.
				Cancer Worry Scale (CWS)	Younger age and lack of social support were associated with increased distress and worry.
				Health-related Quality of Life (HRQL)	
Lammens et al. [18]	VHL	Cross-sectional	171 family members from 43 families (VHL pathogenic variant carriers and 50% at-risk non-carriers) ages > 16 years	Impact of Events Scale (IES) (VHL-specific distress)	Participants reported moderate to severe distress. Loss of first-degree relative to VHL significantly related to distress. Frequent concerns about the possibility of developing additional tumor and surgery. HRQL was comparable to the general population, with the exception of "general health" scale.
				Cancer Worry Scale (CWS) (VHL-specific worries)	
				Health-related Quality of Life (HRQL)	

Havekes et al. [19]	Head and neck paragangliomas	Case-control study	82 adult patients recruited from an outpatient endocrinology clinic. 54 of the patients had undergone genetic testing, resulting in 45 testing positive for an SDHD pathogenic variant.	HADS	Paraganglioma patients had significantly reduced QoL in 12 out of 21 scales compared with their own controls, and 18 out of 21 scales compared with age and sex matched values from previous studies.
				MFI-20	Patients reported higher fatigue scores across domains, poorer health scores on the NHP and SF-36.
				Nottingham Health Profile (NHP)	Paraganglioma patients did not report worse anxiety and depression compared with their own controls, but did report increased scores compared with age and sex matched values from previous studies.
				SF-36	
Grosfeld et al. [20, 21]	MEN2		47 parents from 13 families (22 couples, 3 single parents) who had children that underwent testing MEN2. Children ($n = 40$) were <16 years. Pathogenic variants were found in 20 children.	IES	Mean baseline scores between two groups (those with children who were positive for MEN2 pathogenic variants and those who were not) were not significant.
				State-Trait Anxiety Inventory (STAI)	Parents with a carrier-child experienced a significant increase in anxiety after disclosure of results.
				The Symptom Checklist 90 (SCL90)	After disclosure, parents with a carrier-child had higher scores on IES and STI than those of non-carrier children.
					Parents with no secondary education had higher scores on all measures of distress.
					Parent disease history did not correlate with scores on measures of distress.

(continued)

Table 1.1 (continued)

References	FECS	Design	Sample	Measures	Findings
Grosfeld et al. [20, 21]	MEN2		Two groups; Group 1 comprised of persons ≥16 requesting genetic testing for themselves ($n = 71$) and Group 2 comprised of parents requesting testing for their children <16 ($n = 23$). Partners were also included in the groups.	STAI	On average, mean STAI and GSI scores were consistent with the general population.
				Zung Self-Rating Depression Scale	Participants in Group 1 reported more psychological complaints and preoccupation with test results than those in Group 2.
				Utrecht Coping List (UCL)	
				IES	
				General Severity Index (GSI) of Symptom Checklist 90 (SCL90)	

Multiple Endocrine Neoplasia (MEN)

Multiple Endocrine Neoplasia, Type 1 (MEN1)

More than 1300 different pathogenic variants in the *MEN1* gene have been found to cause MEN1 [22]. This condition is characterized by an increased predisposition to the development of benign and malignant tumors in the endocrine glands including the parathyroid glands, pituitary glands, and pancreas [23]. While there do not appear to be any pediatric or adolescent specific studies, several studies have examined health-related quality of life and emotional wellbeing in adults living with MEN1 and compared scores with population norms.

Berglund et al. examined psychosocial outcomes in 29 adults with MEN1 who were recruited during a hospital stay and then followed them up 6 months later when at home [24]. The study found lower quality of life scores in the general health and social functioning domains of MEN1 patients compared to population-based norm values [24]. There were no significant differences on measures of anxiety, intrusion, and avoidance between assessments in hospital and 6 months later at home. Depression scores increased between these time points only for those MEN1 patients categorized as having a high burden of disease and treatment. The authors also found optimism, assessed at the hospital, was a predictor of good mental health 6 months later.

Two recent studies have assessed quality of life in adults living with MEN1 using the Patient-Reported Outcomes Measurement Information System (PROMIS) 29-item profile and compared responses with US population norms [11, 12]. In the larger of these studies, Goswami et al. [12] found adults living with MEN1 ($N = 207$) reported worse quality of life compared with US normative data in all domains. Persistent hypercalcemia after parathyroid surgery was associated with higher levels of anxiety, depression, fatigue, and decreased social functioning. Patients less than 45 years of age at diagnosis reported worse physical and social functioning. Being older was associated with worse pain interference. Persistent hyperparathyroidism, traveling a considerable distance to attend doctor's appointments, and high frequency of doctor's appointments were all associated with worse quality of life.

Peipert et al. [11] recruited 153 adult patients from an MEN1 support group and found similar results to Goswami et al. Adult patients living with MEN1 reported worse quality of life in the domains of depression, anxiety, fatigue, pain interference and sleep disturbance compared with the US general population. Adults with MEN1 also reported higher levels of anxiety, depression, and fatigue compared with many other chronic conditions such as cancer, primary hyperparathyroidism, and rheumatoid arthritis.

Aside from Berglund's et al. [24] study that included a second time point, each of the studies with persons living with MEN1 were limited by a cross-sectional design. Future studies should include biological markers (for example, PTH and calcium levels) to determine whether symptoms could be part of neurocognitive symptoms seen in primary hyperparathyroidism. Fifty percent of persons living with MEN1 have a parent with the same condition, however, we do not yet understand the role this plays in the heightened anxiety found in these studies. There is also a need for studies examining the impact of MEN1 in children and adolescents, to determine whether they experience similar issues to those seen in adults.

Multiple Endocrine Neoplasia, Type 2 (MEN2)

MEN2 is caused by pathogenic variants in the *RET* gene which lead to a moderate to high risk of developing medullary thyroid cancer and other specific tumors affecting the endocrine system [25]. MEN2 can be broken down into two further subtypes with differing clinical characteristics; MEN2A and MEN2B [25]. Persons living with MEN2A have certain disease manifestations that are not experienced by patients with MEN2B (e.g., primary hyperparathyroidism and cutaneous lichen amyloidosis) whereas persons living with MEN2B more often experience gastrointestinal or musculoskeletal manifestations [25]. A recent review of the literature [26] illustrates how MEN2 can impact all areas of familial, social, financial, and psychological wellbeing.

While research exploring MEN2 in pediatric or adolescent populations is limited to interim analyses from a natural history study currently underway at the National Cancer Institute [7, 27], a small number of studies have examined MEN2 in adult populations. In a cross-sectional study, using semi-directed interviews, psychological assessment measures, and review and analysis of medical records, Rodrigues et al. [13] investigated disease-related issues and psychological distress that affects quality of life in adults living with MEN2. The study included 43 adults, all of whom had medullary thyroid carcinoma. Other disease manifestations included pheochromocytoma (42%), postoperative hypoparathyroidism, and adrenal insufficiency after bilateral adrenalectomy (28%). Overall distress was present in 46% of the patients, with 26% reporting symptoms of depression and 42% reporting symptoms of anxiety. One quarter of the patients required individual psychotherapy. Those who were better informed about the disease presented with lower mean score values for depression and anxiety and higher scores on scales reflecting cognitive and emotional functioning and ability to do usual activities. Rodrigues et al. [13] also identified feelings of guilt in 35% of respondents with MEN2-positive children. Parents who had transmitted MEN2 to child experienced higher levels of anxiety and guilt than parents who had not. Guilt associated with the transmission of a genetic condition to offspring, also known as transmission guilt, was a consistent theme among parents with FECS in multiple studies [13, 14, 26].

In the first study to use the PROMIS-29 to compare patient-reported outcomes between MEN2A as a population distinct from MEN2B and other chronic conditions, Mongelli et al. [10] recruited 45 adult patients with MEN2A. Compared with the general US population, the MEN2A group reported worse quality of life in the domains of anxiety, depression, fatigue, pain, physical functioning, sleep disturbance, and ability to participate in social roles. Those with MEN2A also reported physical functioning scores similar to those of patients with MEN1, major depressive disorder, and neuroendocrine tumors. Aside from reporting greater fatigue, those with MEN2A reported better physical functioning compared with patients with congestive heart failure, chronic obstructive pulmonary disease, and rheumatoid arthritis.

As part of an MEN natural history study underway at the National Cancer Institute, psychosocial data is being collected from pediatric and adult patients with MEN2B and Medullary Thyroid Carcinoma and/or their caregivers [7, 27]. Participants in this study are administered a structured psychosocial assessment, an adapted Pediatric Distress Thermometer (DT) and a problem checklist. Interim analysis including 87 participants aged 2–41 (*mean age of* 14.4 years) indicates that more than half of youth respondents and nearly three quarters of adult patients reported worry. Pain was commonly endorsed by participants, with approximately half of the individuals surveyed indicating that pain interfered with their life. Nearly two-thirds of adult patients also reported fatigue and only 18% reported their health was "very good" to "excellent." In comparison, more than 50% of youth reported their health was "very good" to "excellent." This suggests that medullary thyroid carcinoma may be more difficult to live and cope with as individuals age. The majority of youth and just over half of adult patients reported they had sought out mental health treatment. There was variability among caregivers, youth, and adults regarding preferred services; for example, whereas caregivers commonly reported a desire for support groups, far fewer youth and adult patients endorsed a preference for this service. Yet, 80% of youth and their caregivers endorsed a desire to connect with others living with their same condition. Participants described the hardest parts of living with medullary thyroid carcinoma and MEN2B as being the treatment and general disease burden, uncertainty of the future, impact on social life, and impact on physical wellbeing [27].

Von Hippel-Lindau Disease (VHL)

Von Hippel-Lindau disease (VHL), a hereditary tumor susceptibility syndrome, predisposes individuals to be at increased risk of developing multiple benign and malignant tumors at various sites and at different ages throughout the lifespan [28]. There are limited preventive options [28]. No studies have examined the psychosocial impact of living with VHL in children and adolescents specifically, however, a small number of studies have been done including adult patients and caregivers. To assess the prevalence of distress among VHL affected families and factors associated with distress, Lammens et al. [18] invited 48 families with VHL in the Netherlands to participate in a study. Seventy-two percent of the families approached completed a self-report questionnaire, resulting in 123 participants over 16 years of age (mean age 40.6 years). A considerable proportion of participants reported clinically relevant levels of distress, including 50% of family members living with VHL, 40% of those who were carriers, and 36% of the non-carriers. Heightened levels of distress were significantly associated with having lost a first degree relative due to

VHL during adolescence. These findings suggest the importance of screening for distress in VHL clinics and paying special attention to those who have experienced the death of a close relative to VHL, particularly during adolescence.

Lammens et al. [17] also conducted a cross-sectional study of distress in partners of individuals diagnosed with or at high risk of VHL or Li Fraumeni syndrome (LFS). While LFS is not a FECS, it is another rare hereditary tumor syndrome characterized by a high risk of developing multiple tumors at various sites or age [29]. Participants completed a self-report questionnaire assessing distress, worries, and quality of life. Fifty-eight percent of individuals with a partner consented to having their partner approached for the study. Of the 50 partners (91%) who completed the questionnaire ($n = 33$, 66% with/at-risk of VHL; $n = 17$, 34% with/at-risk of LFS), 28% reported clinically relevant levels of syndrome-related distress. Partners' levels of distress and worries were significantly correlated with those of their high-risk spouse. Younger age and a lack of social support were also associated with heightened levels of distress and worries. The majority of partners (76%) believed that professional psychosocial support should be routinely offered to them. This study also explored partners' perspectives on the impact of VHL and LFS on their relationship, identifying both positive and negative impacts. Those who reported a positive impact (52%) described how the condition taught them to appreciate life and their partner more, bringing them closer together. Fourteen percent of partners indicated that the condition had negatively impacted their relationship, and described challenges including difficulty discussing the condition, anxiety and stress associated with test results, arguments related to adherence to screening, and practical issues over frequent hospitalization.

In 2015, Kasparian et al. conducted an exploratory study of the lived experiences of families with VHL [14]. Purposive sampling was used to recruit patients with VHL from a range of age groups and life stages and their caregivers. In total, 23 participants over 18 years of age ($n = 15$ patients, $n = 8$ caregivers) were recruited and invited to participate in semi-structured telephone interviews aimed at understanding the psychosocial impacts of VHL across several life domains. Participants in the study described psychological challenges associated with VHL including sustained uncertainty about future tumor development, frustration regarding the need for lifelong medical screening, and feelings of isolation, particularly among patients who were the first to be diagnosed with FECS in the family. Patients and caregivers described career limitations, financial impacts and difficulties accessing expert medical and psychosocial care and connecting with others affected by the disease. Examples of psychological growth and resilience, and efforts to improve supportive care services, were also voiced by patients living with VHL. The authors suggested that more sophisticated systems for connecting VHL patients and their families with holistic, empathic, and person-centered medical and psychosocial care were needed.

Consistent with Lammens et al. [17] study, Kasparian et al. identified positive and negative ways in which VHL can impact relationships. Some participants described how VHL placed strain on family relationships, such as finding it difficult to talk to unaffected siblings about the condition. As one participant put it, "I avoid talking about [VHL] with my siblings, because I know they don't understand or don't want to" (woman with VHL, 41 years). Other participants described how VHL had been positive for familial relationships, strengthening bonds with parents and siblings. This strengthening appeared particularly prevalent between family members who shared the condition in common, with affected siblings describing how they found it easier to talk to other siblings who had the condition, compared with those who did not. One participant described a sense of immense appreciation for the dedication of their parents in managing their health needs, commenting "Mum is the reason I'm probably still here, because mum keeps track of everything" (man with VHL 23 years).

Caregivers in [14] study (including $n = 3$ partners, and $n = 5$ parents) reported little reprieve from caregiving responsibilities, difficulties balancing the needs of VHL affected and unaffected family members, fears about the future, and, for some, guilt regarding the onset of tumors in their children. Parents also described struggling to negotiate the disparate needs of their affected and unaffected children, and the internal conflict they faced over this [14]. In particular, parents described difficulties associated with ensuring they were able to adequately support and provide for their affected children, without unfairly treating or neglecting their other children [14].

SDH-Related Paraganglioma and Pheochromocytoma Syndrome

While paragangliomas are usually slow growing, they can cause a wide variety of symptoms. These include cranial nerve impairment and (paroxysmal) hypertension, palpitations, sweating, and headache due to the high levels of catecholamines produced by pheochromocytomas [30]. Hereditary Pheochromocytoma and Paraganglioma syndrome is caused primarily by pathogenic variants in the SDH genes (*SDHA, SDHAF2, SDHB, SDHC, SDHD*) [30]. Penetrance is variable and gene specific. High levels of catecholamines can cause anxiety, worry, and distress [16]. While there were no studies exploring the psychosocial impacts of SDH-related paraganglioma and pheochromocytoma syndrome on children and adolescents, a small number of studies have examined this syndrome in adult samples.

Van Hulsteijn et al. [16] examined quality of life and coping styles in 174 adults living with paraganglioma, most of whom had pathogenic variants in succinate dehydrogenase (SDH) sub-unit genes (including n = 25 *SDHB*, n = 2 *SDHC*, n = 122 *SDHD*, n = 25 without an *SDH* pathogenic variant). One hundred peers were enrolled as controls and participants were also compared with age-adjusted reference populations. Participants completed three validated quality of life questionnaires: the Hospital Anxiety and Depression Scale, the Multidimensional Fatigue Index, and the Short Form 36, as well as a questionnaire describing possible signs and symptoms associated with paragangliomas.

Study participants reported significantly impaired quality of life compared with their peer controls, mainly on the fatigue and physical condition subscales. They also had significantly impaired scores on physical, psychological, and social subscales compared with age-adjusted reference populations and reported greater seeking of social support compared with other patient groups (patients with chronic pain, patients with pituitary adenoma, and vestibular schwannoma patients). Increased scores on the Hospital Anxiety and Depression Scale and decreased quality of life appeared to be mainly related to head and neck paraganglioma associated complaints (i.e., hearing loss, tinnitus, hoarseness, and problems in swallowing). There was no difference in quality of life between carriers of pathogenic SDH-related variants and paraganglioma patients without an identified SDH-related pathogenic variant. The quality of life of asymptomatic carriers did not differ from the general population. The study investigators were able to follow-up with 41 patients, 5 years later, at which point quality of life scores remained lower than the reference population but were stable over time.

The authors also explored coping styles using the Utrecht Coping List as well as illness and risk perceptions, and disease-related worry [15]. The study cohort was compared with a control group and data derived from the literature. No significant differences were found in coping styles between various categories of SDH-related pathogenic variant carriers or paraganglioma patients without an SDH-related pathogenic variant. Illness perceptions, risk perception and disease-related worry were strongly correlated. Pathogenic variant carriers with manifest disease reported more negative illness perceptions and a higher perceived risk of developing subsequent tumors than asymptomatic carriers.

An earlier study by Havekes et al. [19] assessed quality of life with persons living with head-and-neck paraganglioma. A total of 105 patients were invited to participate in the study, with 82 returning questionnaires. Of these 82 patients 54 had undergone genetic testing, with 45 (83%) found to have an *SDHD* pathogenic variant. Participants reported reductions in energy and increased social isolation compared with controls. Patients also reported experiencing problems in physical and social functioning and role limitations due to physical problems.

Key Points
- There is limited research exploring the psychosocial impact of FECS on children and adolescents.
- Research on adults with FECS suggests that while the psychosocial impact varies between syndromes these conditions result in significant psychosocial burden and worsened quality of life.
- There is some data to suggest that the burden of disease and treatment is associated with poorer quality of life.
- Along with the challenges, positive impacts reported by adults with FECS include strengthening of relationships with parents and siblings, emotional growth, and resilience.

- Research including caregivers of adults with a FECS suggests a proportion experience clinically relevant levels of syndrome related distress, correlated with the distress experienced by their affected partner.
- Partners and parents report anxiety and distress over their loved one's condition, as well as caregiving responsibilities and relationship challenges.
- Studies of caregivers of adults with MEN2 and VHL indicate some parents who transmit a FECS to their child experience guilt and anxiety, in some cases leading to strained relationships.

Genetic Testing Experiences

Families affected by hereditary cancer syndromes must decide whether to pursue diagnostic testing for at-risk children. For child-onset conditions parents often act as surrogate decision makers for their child, a role that some parents experience as challenging. When arranging testing for a child, informed consent needs to be obtained from parent(s)/guardian(s). In these situations, active age-appropriate participation should be sought from the child and maximized in developmentally appropriate ways. Despite concerns about potentially exacerbating parental and patient anxiety, genetic counseling has been found to empower families by providing information and facilitating proactive surveillance programs [31–33]. Genetic testing has been viewed by young people as a positive experience, although this may be dependent on the family's experience with cancer.

A small number of studies have explored families' experiences of genetic testing for FECS via studies of adults, including parents. No studies have focused specifically on the experiences of children and young people affected by these syndromes. In the following section we first describe published studies exploring the experiences of young people from families affected by Li-Fraumeni syndrome (LFS), before going on to describe studies of adult patients and parents of at-risk children seeking genetic testing for a FECS, presented by condition. Table 1.1 provides an overview of the FECS focused studies described below. While LFS is not considered an endocrine cancer syndrome, it shares some characteristics with FECS. In the absence of FECS specific data, research on LFS may provide useful insights into the issues faced by at-risk young people considering genetic testing.

Data from Adolescents At-Risk of Li-Fraumeni Syndrome (LFS)

Alderfer et al. [34] interviewed 12 adolescents and emerging young adults (aged 12–25) in families affected by LFS to obtain their perspectives on offering genetic testing to young people. All the young people from LFS affected families believed genetic testing should be offered for children, and all thought children should be involved in the decision about whether to pursue testing. However, participants qualified these perspectives suggesting that genetic testing should be optional, need parent approval and that in some circumstances it was ok for parents to make the decision to have a child tested without involving their child. Most young people felt that the age of a child was an important consideration in determining their role in decision making, with a consensus that children under 6 years did not need to be involved, and children aged 10–15 should have some say. Young people perceived the advantages of testing to be to learn about risk status, enable disease prevention, reduce uncertainty and associated anxiety, and imbue a sense of empowerment. Perceived disadvantages included the experience of negative emotions associated with a positive result and physically undergoing the required blood test. Among the participants in the study who were aware of having undergone testing ($n = 7$) most indicated they did not appreciate the seriousness and lifelong impact of a positive result until after testing when they began to understand details of the surveillance process. Most indicated that undergoing testing and receiving results had no impact on their family relationships and had either no impact or resulted in a positive change to their outlook. All the participants who had undergone genetic testing said they would do the testing again.

Multiple Endocrine Neoplasia (MEN)

Research by Grosfeld et al. [20, 21] provides valuable insight into the experiences of parents pursuing genetic testing for MEN2 or familial medullary thyroid carcinoma for their child. Demographic, personality characteristics, attitudes, and distress were examined in a sample of parents applying for testing of their at-risk child (aged <16), adults (>16 years) applying for testing for themselves, along with applicants' partners [21]. In a separate study they then investigated the psychological reactions of 22 parent couples and 3 single parents following disclosure of their child's genetic test results [20].

In their study exploring pre-disclosure experiences, the most common reason parents gave for pursuing testing was the desire for certainty (85% of parents), with 39% reporting feeling ambivalent about testing. With regards to expectations of testing, roughly half of parents in the study expected their children to return a positive genetic test result indicating presence of MEN2. Parents expected that if their child was found to have MEN2 that they would react with resignation, confirming what they thought would happen. Parents felt reassured by the knowledge that children identified as MEN2 positive would receive preventative treatment. Parents anticipated that if their child was found not to have the condition, they would feel relief, tempered by disbelief and confusion. Parents from MEN2A families anticipated finding it difficult to accept a favorable result for their children more than those from familial medullary thyroid carcinoma families. On average parents did not appear to experience significant psychological distress, with mean anxiety and psychological complaints no higher than those in the general population, and mild to moderate test-related anxiety. Participants in the sample of adults seeking testing for themselves (and their partners) reported greater psychological distress than parents seeking testing for their child (and their partners).

While the authors did not report results by age for adults (>16 years) seeking testing for themselves, they reported that two-thirds of the 14 participants reporting high levels of distress in the sample were young adults (aged 15–20 years). Compared with older adults, these younger participants had higher risk perception, higher tendency towards depression, and a greater tendency to use avoidant coping.

Grosfeld et al.'s follow-up study involved 47 parents ($n = 22$ couples, $n = 3$ singles) from 13 families requesting testing for 40 children (<16 years, mean age of 6.2 years) [20]. Most parents in the study were applying to have one child tested (56%), with the remainder applying to have 2 or more children tested ($n = 11$). Parents received genetic counseling involving a clinical geneticist and social worker or psychologist during the testing process and waited an average of 3 months after applying for testing to receive their child's results. Pathogenic variants in the *RET* gene associated with MEN2 were found in 20 out of the 40 tested children. The authors describe parents as experiencing "opposing reactions" after results were disclosed, including feeling relief to have some certainty along with concern for their child's health. Parents who were told their child was found to have MEN2 responded with resignation, moderate to high levels of test-related and general anxiety, but few psychological complaints such as depressive mood and sleep disturbance (measured using the Symptom Checklist 90). These parents reported limited disruption to their future perspective apart from some increased concerns for carrier children and some socioeconomic disadvantage. Forty-three per cent of parents whose children tested positive also reported disruption in their daily activities. Parents whose child tested negative for MEN2 showed significantly less anxiety and no disturbances in their daily activities, although 55% of parents reported feelings of guilt towards siblings who were found to have the condition.

Von Hippel-Lindau Disease (VHL)

Rasmussen et al. [35] explored the uptake of presymptomatic genetic testing for VHL in 157 at-risk relatives from 12 families. All at-risk relatives were invited to attend a genetic counseling session to learn more about VHL and consider options for testing and surveillance. Ninety-two individuals (including $n = 43$ children less than 18 years) attended a genetic counseling appointment, all of whom then went on to have genetic testing. The remaining 65 at-risk relatives did not follow-up the invitation for genetic counseling, receiving information about VHL and options for testing/surveillance through family members. None of these individuals pursued genetic testing.

Studies of VHL affected families indicate that parents are very motivated to have their children tested early. Qualitative data from a study by Kasparian et al. [14] including 23 VHL affected adults (including $n = 15$ patients and $n = 8$ carers) indicated that most wanted their children to undergo genetic testing either before the age of ten ($n = 10$) or at birth ($n = 3$). Of the eight patients in this study who had children, six had already requested testing for their children (with the remaining two having undergone Pre-implantation Genetic Diagnosis (PGD) to ensure they had unaffected children) [14].

These findings are consistent with those of an earlier study of 41 adults with VHL ($n = 24$ women, $n = 17$ men) including 14 patients with children, that asked parents about their attitudes towards presymptomatic genetic testing in their children [36]. Most parents had either already had their children tested or indicated a willingness to do so as soon as possible (11 yes, 3 undecided, 0 no). In 6 of these families, 9 children (aged between 3 and 18 years) had already been clinically tested. The authors noted an interesting discrepancy between parents' willingness to test their children and their attitudes towards getting tested themselves such that 3 of 10 patients who became aware of their own diagnosis after age 20 indicated they would not have appreciated knowing this earlier, with another 3 indicating they were unsure.

SDH-Related Paraganglioma and Pheochromocytoma Syndrome

Martins and Carvalho [9] recently conducted a study examining the psychological impact of genetic testing for pathogenic variants in SDH-related genes in individuals with and without pheochromocytoma/paraganglioma. Their study aimed to explore the psychological impact of genetic testing for patients affected and unaffected by tumors, as well as the association between demographic, clinical, and personality factors and testing-related distress, uncertainty, and global suffering (measured using the Multidimensional Impact of Cancer Risk Assessment). This study included 103 participants who had received their genetic diagnosis an average of 2.76 years earlier. Almost half of the participants had not developed pheochromocytoma/paraganglioma. The sample's mean global suffering score was 27.32, below the cut-off for high scores (≥ 32), although almost 30% of the sample scored on or above 32.

Tumor affected carriers of pathogenic variants in SDH-related genes reported higher testing-related distress, uncertainty, and global suffering and lower global quality of life than unaffected carriers. Among participants with tumors, most felt that finding out they had a pathogenic variant did not make it harder to cope with their cancer, and more than half felt the genetic test result made it easier to cope with their cancer. Feeling like the genetic test result made it easier to cope with cancer was more often reported by individuals whose tumor was identified through presymptomatic screening than those whose tumors were identified due to disease symptoms.

Seventy-one percent ($n = 69$) of the sample had children. Among these participants, receiving a positive genetic test result led to most (88.4%) worrying about the possibility of their children getting cancer, and almost half (46.4%) feeling guilty about the possibility of passing the disease risk onto their children. There was an interaction between having tumors, having children and higher distress, such that participants who developed tumors and had children were more distressed than participants who developed tumors but did not have children, or participants who did not develop tumors (with or without children). Negative psychological impacts of testing were associated with increased age, decreased education, and having children. Testing-related distress and uncertainty were also positively correlated with the personality characteristic of neuroticism and negatively correlated with extroversion.

An earlier study looked at presymptomatic genetic testing in children and adolescents at risk of paraganglioma and pheochromocytoma [37]. While the aim of this study was to describe the genetic testing procedure with a view to developing quality criteria, the results provide some insights into families' emotional experiences. The authors report on genetic testing of 23 children and adolescents (mean age of 9.22) resulting in 16 positive cases (including $n = 10$ *SDHB*, $n = 4$ *SDHD*, $n = 3$ *VHL*, $n = 4$ *RET*, $n = 2$ *AIP*) and 7 negative cases. The authors categorized families' emotional reactions to receiving results as either calm or tense, based on the emotional atmosphere accompanying the announcement of the result. A family's reaction was categorized as calm if no major negative emotional reaction was observed in the young person or parents and tense if an uncontrolled emotional reaction was observed in the young person or parents. Emotional reactions to results were categorized as calm in 18/23 (78.3%) cases and tense in 5/23 (21.7%). The authors then looked at the association between adherence to four criteria for a good testing procedure and families' emotional reactions. A good quality testing procedure involves the parents and child consulting with a geneticist and psychiatrist during the process of deciding whether to pursue genetic testing for the child. Results indicated no association between the nature of the result, age or sex of the child and families' emotional reactions, however, the quality of the testing procedure differentiated between families reactions to receipt of a child's results, with adherence to good testing procedures associated with calm rather than tense reactions.

Key Points
- There is a need for research exploring the experiences of genetic testing for children and adolescents with an FECS. In the absence of FECS specific data, young people at-risk of LFS believe at-risk children should be offered genetic testing and where possible involved in the process of decision making around whether to pursue it.
- Parents of children at risk for MEN2 reported seeking certainty with genetic testing, with feelings of relief and resignation occurring after receiving results.
- Parents of children at risk for VHL were motivated to obtain genetic testing for their children as soon as possible.
- A study of genetic testing for individuals with pathogenic variants in SDH-related genes found highest distress in those who developed tumors and had children.

- In families undergoing genetic testing for children at risk of hereditary paraganglioma and pheochromocytoma, adherence to good testing procedure was associated with "calm" rather than "tense" reactions to test results.

Experiences of Surveillance

If genetic testing identifies that a child or adolescent has a FECS, the young person and their parents/caregivers are recommended to engage in clinical surveillance for their condition. Surveillance protocols are designed to detect disease at an early stage and typically include a combination of physical examinations, imaging (e.g., MRI), and laboratory investigations. Recommended surveillance protocols vary by condition and country with specific age-related interventions advised. Very few studies have explored the attitudes towards, and psychosocial impact of undergoing medical surveillance in patients with a FECS. We identified one study of adolescents' experiences, which describes the experiences of a mixed sample of young people with a cancer predisposition syndrome including four patients with FECS, and a small number of studies which explored families' experiences of surveillance for FECS via studies of adults, including parents. Table 1.1 provides an overview of the studies described below.

Van Engelen et al. [8] interviewed adolescents ($n = 9$) undergoing surveillance for a cancer predisposition syndrome and parents ($n = 11$) whose children were undergoing surveillance for a cancer predisposition syndrome. Study participants included four adolescents with a FECS ($n = 1$ MEN2A, $n = 1$ VHL, $n = 2$ SDH) and three parents of a child undergoing surveillance for a FECS ($n = 1$ MEN2A, $n = 2$ SDH). Other genetic conditions affecting children and parents included in the study included LFS, PTEN hamartoma syndrome, DICER1 syndrome, and rhabdoid tumor predisposition syndrome. Both adolescents and parents reported experiencing worry associated with surveillance, as well as practical and logistical challenges with attending regular appointments. Worries were related to procedure-related risks, and the risk of developing cancer, which surveillance was a reminder of. Worries tended to be cyclical, peaking around surveillance appointments, and decreasing over time as surveillance appointments became part of their routine. Alongside these challenges, adolescents and parents described feeling reassured by the proactive approach, giving some parents a sense of control. Several factors were identified as important in helping adolescents and parents manage the worry associated with surveillance, including positive family connections, shared surveillance experiences, open and honest communication with health care providers, and approaching surveillance with the attitude of not worrying until there is something to worry about.

The findings of van Engelen et al.'s study echoed those of Kasparian et al.'s qualitative study of the experiences of VHL affected adult patients' and caregivers. Participants perceived screening for tumors as a necessary but anxiety provoking process. While screening was perceived as important and effective it was an unavoidable reminder of VHL, with the potential to provoke anxiety. While screening tests were described as a burden by some, most participants reported never having missed a screening appointment. Caregivers typically accompany patients to medical appointments, to help with understanding new information, provide support and to ease their own worries. Participants also talked about surveillance appointments as being a family affair, organizing screening appointments for the same day.

Rasmussen et al.'s [35] study of VHL affected families described earlier also looked at adherence to surveillance among individuals identified as pathogenic variant carriers following genetic testing ($n = 36$, including $n = 10$ children). All were offered screening and annual surveillance for VHL related tumors All undertook the initial screening, however, after 5 years only 14 individuals (38.9%; from $n = 8$ families) continued with surveillance (with $n = 3$ participants having died). Having been symptomatic before undergoing genetic testing was associated with continuing surveillance and having significant pre-test anxiety was associated with prematurely dropping out of surveillance. There was no association between adherence to surveillance and having children, pre-test depression, gender, education, income, marital status or religiosity. The authors noted that in families with multiple gene carriers, family members tended to take the same stance towards long-term surveillance. They also observed that families led by a matriarch tended to have higher levels of engagement in follow-up than those led by a patriarch, although their study lacked the statistical power to confirm this observation.

Key Points
- There is limited research examining the experiences of and attitudes towards surveillance for young people with FECS and their families.
- Data from a study of adolescents and their parents affected by a mix of cancer predisposition syndromes, including FECS, reported worry surrounding cancer surveillance appointments, as well as feeling reassured by continued surveillance. This is consistent with qualitative data from adults with VHL and their caregivers.
- A study of VHL affected families found that despite high uptake of initial screening, less than half of families adhered to surveillance recommendations in the years following.

Reproductive Considerations

The possibility of passing an inherited cancer syndrome down to biological children can have implications for a carrier's reproductive decision making. Advances in reproductive technology mean that in some countries patients now have the option of Pre-implantation Genetic Diagnosis (PGD) in addition to prenatal testing. Giving affected individuals access to these reproductive options is a consideration in decision making around the timing of genetic testing of young people in affected families.

No studies have explored the impacts of having a cancer predisposition syndrome on reproductive considerations among young people with a FECS. The previously described qualitative study of young people at-risk of LFS, while not specific to FECS, confirms the impact of genetic testing on reproductive considerations for young people at-risk of an inherited cancer syndrome [34]. Of the seven young people who were aware of having undergone genetic testing for LFS in this study, four commented on the impact of genetic testing on future plans for having children. There is a need for studies examining the impact of having a FECS on reproductive considerations among affected young people. Below we describe studies of adults with a FECS exploring the impact of carrier status on reproductive considerations, and awareness and acceptability of reproductive technologies.

Impact of Carrier Status on Reproductive Considerations

In Kasparian et al.'s [14] qualitative study of adults living with VHL 4 patients (from a sample of $n = 15$) reported that the diagnosis had made them less willing to have children. One parent in this study, who had been severely affected by tumors himself and had a young child who was symptomatic, said he would not have had children if he had been aware of his carrier status at the time. These findings are consistent with an earlier report of 24 adult men and women living with VHL which suggested carrier status impacted some patients' reproductive intentions [36]. Ten of these patients, including six without children, reported having decided not to have children in the future because of the potential risk to their offspring.

Awareness and Acceptability of Reproductive Options

Decision making about the use of reproductive technology for families affected by a cancer predisposition syndrome is contingent on patient awareness and perceptions of what is available. We currently have very limited data on awareness of reproductive technology among families affected by FECS. A small number of studies have explored the acceptability of reproductive technologies, including prenatal testing and PGD, among families affected by VHL and MEN1 and 2.

A 2014 study looking at attitudes towards PGD among adults with a cancer predisposition syndrome recruited from a Clinical Cancer Genetics Program in the U.S. included patients with MEN1 and MEN2 along with other predisposition syndromes [38]. Ten out of 33 (30.3%) patients with MEN1 and 21/36 (58.3%) patients with MEN2 reported being aware of PGD. This study also compared attitudes towards PGD between patients with different hereditary cancer syndromes including MEN1 and 2. Among patients with MEN1, 27/33 (81.8%) believed that PGD should be offered to individuals with their hereditary cancer syndrome, no patient believed that it should not be offered, and 6/33 (18.2%) were unsure. Among patients with MEN2 34/56 (60.7%) thought PGD should be offered, 8/56 (14.29%) thought it should not and 14/56 (25%) were unsure. Comparing across syndromes, acceptability of PGD was highest among patients with MEN1 (and familial adenomatous polyposis) and lowest among patients with MEN2. In terms of personally considering using PGD, 19/31 (61.3%) of the MEN1 patients reported they would consider using PGD, 4/31 (12.9%) reported they would not, and 8/31 (25.8%) were unsure. Among MEN2 carriers, 23/54 (42.6%) said they would, 21/54 (38.9%) said they would not, and 10/54 (18.5%) were unsure. PGD acceptance was associated with syndrome, age of symptom onset, and perceived disease burden, suggesting acceptability of PGD may be associated with unique aspects of each syndrome.

An early study of attitudes towards prenatal testing among adult VHL patients found 22/31 (71%) of those who wished to have children reported intending to use prenatal diagnosis in pregnancy [36]. Of these, half considered termination of a VHL affected pregnancy acceptable while the other half were either undecided or disapproved of this. The authors note that the decisions of VHL affected patients appear to be individual and difficult to predict but that hope for improved treatment and management of the condition seemed to influence reproductive decisions. In Kasparian et al.'s more recent qualitative study of adults living with VHL, patients expressed a mix of perspectives towards prenatal testing to inform possible pregnancy terminations. Parents expressed more favorable attitudes towards PGD, with the majority of patients (10/15) viewing it as a good option to avoid bearing a child with the syndrome.

Lammens et al. [39] looked at attitudes towards PGD in families affected by VHL or LFS. This study included 95 carriers, 34 family members at 50% risk, and 50 partners in the Netherlands. Two-thirds of respondents were from VHL affected families and one-third LFS affected. None of the participants in the study had used PGD but 35% said they would consider doing so, 27% were uncertain, and 38% would not use PGD. A current desire to have children was associated with a positive attitude towards PGD, but no medical or psychosocial variables were. Attitudes towards PGD among partners were similar to those of affected individuals. Most participants did not endorse any particular advantages or disadvantages of PGD, which the authors suggested may have been due to limited knowledge of the technology.

A study by Dommering et al. [40] compared the uptake of prenatal diagnostic testing in the Netherlands for families affected by retinoblastoma with four other autosomal dominantly inherited cancer syndromes, including VHL. During the period covered by the study (1990-May 2013) 92 families were diagnosed with VHL through genetic testing, of whom 6 couples (6.5%) underwent prenatal diagnostic testing (representing 7 prenatal diagnostic tests). There was no difference between the percentage of VHL, retinoblastoma or LFS affected families seeking prenatal diagnostic testing, but families affected by these syndromes opted for prenatal diagnostic testing more frequently than familial adenomatous polyposis and hereditary breast and ovarian cancer affected families. The authors suggest that differences in uptake of prenatal diagnostic testing in couples affected by different syndromes may be explained by differences in age of symptom onset, disease penetrance, availability of risk-reducing options and perceived disease burden.

Key Points

- PGD and other reproductive technologies may be a consideration for adults with FECS facing reproductive decisions, particularly when weighing risks for potential future children.
- The available evidence on adults with FECs indicates limited awareness of PGD.
- A study of MEN carriers indicated the majority thought PGD should be offered to individuals with a cancer predisposition syndrome, and a smaller proportion would personally consider using it. A study of VHL and LFS affected families found more than a quarter would consider using PGD.
- The available evidence suggests syndrome specific factors such as perceived disease burden and age of onset may impact patients' attitudes towards reproductive technologies.

Ethical Issues That Arise in Genetic Counseling of Familial Endocrine Cancer Syndromes in Pediatrics and Adolescents

This section will focus on the ethical dilemmas that are likely to be encountered by genetic counselors and other clinicians working with pediatric and adolescent patients affected by FECSs and their families.

Review of Guidelines and Framework

In 1995, the American Society of Human Genetics (ASHG) and the American College of Medical Genetics/Genomics (ACMG) published their first joint statement addressing the ethical concerns that genetic counselors faced when working with children and adolescents [41]. The recommendations were geared towards preparing healthcare providers to acknowledge and discuss the ethical issues surrounding the wellbeing of children when a genetic test was requested by the parents [41]. In 2015, 20 years later, an updated statement was published that incorporated the new massive advances in genomic testing [42]. Table 1.2 includes excerpts from this statement summarizing the general recommendations for clinicians involved in offering genetic testing to children and adolescents.

American Society of Human Genetics (ASHG)/American College of Medical Genetics/Genomics (ACMG) guidelines (see Table 1.2) suggest genetic testing in children is justified when a medical intervention is available or when substantial psychosocial distress can be alleviated by the results of the tests. As many

Table 1.2 Excerpts from the American Society of Human Genetics (ASHG)/ American College of Medical Genetics/Genomics (ACMG) statement on ethical concerns that genetic counselors faced when working with children and adolescents

1	Unless there is a clinical intervention appropriate in childhood, parents should be encouraged to defer predictive or pre-dispositional testing for adult-onset conditions until adulthood or at least until the child is an older adolescent who can participate in decision making in a relatively mature manner.
2	Adolescents should be encouraged to defer predictive or pre-dispositional testing for adult-onset conditions until adulthood because of the complexity of the potential impact of the information at formative life stages.
3	Providers should offer to explore the reasons why parents or adolescents are interested in predictive or pre-dispositional testing for adult-onset conditions.
4	Providers can acknowledge that, in some cases, testing might be a reasonable decision, but decisions should follow thorough deliberation.
5	Adolescents should be provided the opportunity to discuss these issues without the presence of their parents, although parents should be involved in, and supportive of, any final decisions for testing. A referral to genetic counselors and mental-health professionals is appropriate if the clinician and family need additional support for decision making or in assessing the psychosocial dynamics.
6	Facilitating predictive or pre-dispositional testing of children for adult-onset conditions can be justified in certain circumstances. For example, after careful deliberations with the family and older child, testing can be justified to alleviate substantial psychosocial distress or to facilitate specific life-planning decisions.
7	The impact of predictive testing on children and families remains uncertain and therefore can be justified in specific cases when it is requested by families after informed deliberations and when the testing is not clearly inconsistent with the welfare of the child.
8	Empirical research on the psychosocial impact of predictive or pre-dispositional testing in children is necessary for future policy recommendations.
9	Genetic testing of children for adult-onset conditions in the research context can be ethically justified because of its social importance and when risks are minimized by appropriate counseling and support and when appropriate parental permission and child assent are obtained.

interventions for FECS commence in childhood, predictive testing in children is endorsed for these syndromes. But the question then remains, who can accurately assess the impact of the test on the psychosocial wellbeing of the child when he/she is an adult? As with many ethical principles, the answer to this question is, at times, unclear. Research exploring the impact of FECS across the lifespan may prove helpful for families and clinicians weighing these complex decisions.

As advances in science and technology continue, genetic testing in children remains a primary subject of ethical and, at times, legal debate. At the core of this debate is the need to balance respect for a child's autonomy with parental rights and responsibilities. In order for a child to be considered able to make decisions about their medical care, they must have sufficiently developed abilities in four capacities: (1) the ability to communicate a choice; (2) understanding of information provided about medical treatment or research; (3) reason and evaluate risks, benefits, and possible consequences, and (4) an appreciation of the relevance of their medical situation and the options provided to them [43]. Provided that development proceeds at an appropriate trajectory, children may begin and are encouraged to have an increasingly active voice in their healthcare decisions. Several organizations including American Society of Human Genetics (ASHG)/ACMG/American College of Medical Genetics/Genomics (ACMG) have released position statements that provide some guidance on the appropriateness of predictive testing for individual family circumstances [3]. Generally, the final decision is made by the parent or legal guardian with advisement and education by medical providers, genetic counselors and mental health professionals.

At times, a parent may make a decision that is not agreed upon by the provider or other members of the multidisciplinary team. The case of Jane Smith, below, illustrates some of the ethical issues that may arise in caring for a patient affected by a FECS:

The Case of Jane Smith

Jane was a G4P3AB1 45 year-old female who presented to the genetic counseling clinic with a previously diagnosed wild-type gastrointestinal stromal tumor (GIST)-epithelioid and spindle type. At the time of her initial evaluation, she was status post-gastrectomy, hepatic and partial hepatectomy with metastases to the liver. She was referred for genetic counseling because the type of GIST she had is often part of a hereditary condition known as Hereditary Paraganglioma-Pheochromocytoma Syndrome (see Chap. 6 for detailed description of these conditions). The pre-test counseling session focused mainly on discussing her risks of having a hereditary cancer predisposing syndrome, the risks and benefits of genetic testing, and the implications of the possible outcomes. Most of her concerns and questions were about the risks to her 3 children who, at the time, were ranging in ages from 5 to 11 years of age. The family history was significant on the paternal side for her uncle who had a paraganglioma and her paternal grandmother who died of "stomach cancer" of unknown type; consanguinity was denied.

After reviewing the pros and cons of genetic testing, Jane consented to having a germline panel of cancer genes that included all currently known pathogenic variants associated with GIST, and a somatic panel of her tumor. The results revealed that her tumor was SDHB-deficient and that she had a pathogenic germline variant in the *SDHA* gene. She was called for an in-person post-test genetic counseling session to discuss the implications of this result for her prognosis/treatment, and the risks to her relatives. She came to the post-test counseling session with her husband; they were both devastated to learn that Jane had a pathogenic variant that could be passed onto her children. Each child had a 50% chance of inheriting this variant and if positive they would be predisposed to developing GIST, paragangliomas, and other tumors.

Testing of asymptomatic relatives of carriers of pathogenic variants in the succinate dehydrogenase sub-unit genes (SDHA/B/C/D) is performed so that preventive and screening guidelines can be implemented before the person develops tumors. The clinical and practice guidelines for the management of patients who are positive for pathogenic variants in the SDHA/B/C/D are evidence-based and have been reviewed by several expert panels [44–46]. In general, the recommendation is to refer the family to a specialized multidisciplinary team that will establish a personalized management plan in order to optimize a favorable outcome.

Jane and her husband were informed of the benefits of these recommendations; she was given examples of the type of medical management that her children (if positive) would undergo (e.g., annual MRIs, biochemical testing). In addition, the recommended age at which these screening guidelines should begin, 8 years of age, were discussed at length [47]. After a long discussion, the couple decided not to test any of their children due to the extreme additional distress a positive finding would bring to the family at a time when they were dealing with treatment decisions and multiple medical visits for Jane. Given that two of their children were within the range of recommended surveillance and one was closely approaching, the genetic counselor was concerned about letting the couple leave the consultation without further discussion. However, genetic counselors are trained to be non-directive and accept the patient's decision as long as this was an informed/educated decision. The issue of nondirectiveness in genetic counseling has been discussed and reviewed extensively [48–50] although recent approaches allow the practitioner to be more "directive" based on clinical circumstances and medical expertise [51]. In the case of Jane's children, there were significant medical consequences of not screening her positive offspring (e.g., undetected tumors may become too large to resect). However, her state of mind at the time led her to avoid the introduction of additional stressors in her life. Hence, she decided not to test the children.

A subsequent visit was scheduled after Jane's upcoming surgery. The couple informed the team that they had decided to have their two older children tested because they wanted to "spare their children all the suffering Jane had been through."

Although difficult at times, healthcare providers are not responsible for determining whether a parent's decision is morally right or wrong. The primary responsibility of the healthcare team is to ensure that a parent's decision is an informed one and that they have adequate support that allows them to consider the risks and benefits to the child both currently and in the future, and to make the best decision for the child's wellbeing. In the case described, the genetic counselor provided the patient and her family with significant education and opportunities to discuss and ask questions. Despite this, the counselor noted that Jane and her family were significantly distressed and as a result, declined further testing. This presents an opportunity for further patient education and support. At the time, Jane and her family expressed their concern that a positive result would lead to increased stress and adverse effects within the family. It would be appropriate to share with the family additional family and individual therapy resources as well as further patient education on the psychological and social impact of genetic testing on children (described elsewhere in this chapter).

General Discussion

Familial endocrine cancer syndromes encompass a number of conditions with varying risks of cancer. Families affected by these conditions must make decisions about whether to pursue genetic testing, and if a family member is found to be a carrier, whether to engage with lifelong management and surveillance. Many of these syndromes have a childhood onset, meaning parents may have to consider these decisions for their at-risk children. Despite recent advances in the diagnosis and management of FECS, and the benefits that come with knowing one's carrier status, available data suggests a FECS diagnosis can have a range of negative psychosocial impacts on patients and introduce challenges for caregivers.

In the absence of studies examining the impact of FECS on children and adolescents we reviewed research exploring the impacts of a FECS on adults in order to understand the psychosocial impact of these conditions. Studies of adults living with a MEN1, MEN2, VHL, and SDH-related syndromes indicate they have a significant psychosocial burden, although the impact varies between syndromes. Adults with a FECS report higher levels of depression, anxiety, fatigue, and pain compared with population norms [10–12, 16]. They describe challenges associated with the uncertainty of their condition and frustration and anxiety accompanying lifelong medical screening [14, 27]. Caregivers, including partners and parents, report anxiety and distress over their loved one's condition, as well as caregiving responsibilities and relationship challenges [14, 17]. Some caregivers who transmit a FECS to their child report experiencing associated guilt and anxiety [13, 14, 26]. Alongside these challenges, adult studies indicate FECS can have some positive impacts on relationships between patients and caregivers, bringing family members closer together [14, 17].

While we found no studies exploring children's and adolescent's experiences of genetic testing for a FECS, research involving adolescents from LFS affected families suggests that young people believe at-risk children should be offered genetic testing, and where possible, be involved in decision making about whether to pursue it [34]. Parents in VHL affected families appear motivated to have their children undergo genetic testing as soon as possible and parents pursuing testing for MEN2 reported doing so in search of certainty, experiencing feelings of relief and resignation after receiving results [14, 36]. The limited data available on the experiences of adolescents engaged in surveillance for a FECS, and their parents, suggests that it is both a trigger for worry as well as a source of reassurance [8].

The available data suggests that living with a FECS has consequences for reproductive planning. While there is limited data from FECS affected families, available evidence indicates limited awareness of available reproductive technologies but a belief that individuals should be given the option to access PGD. Data on acceptability suggests use of these reproductive technologies may be appealing to some individuals living with a FECS but not others, with some data to suggest that the acceptability of PGD may be associated with unique aspects of each syndrome.

The available literature provides some indication of how best to support FECS affected families pursuing genetic testing and living with a positive result. Studies of both patients and caregivers highlighted a desire for specialized psychosocial support, and identified benefits associated with families being able to access information, genetic counseling, and psychological services. Studies highlighted the value of routinely offering FECS affected patients and their caregivers access to such support, especially around the time of genetic testing. As caregivers are an essential source of support for patients [14], and social support can be a buffer between stressful events and psychological distress [17], providing caregivers with ongoing psychosocial support along with those affected, is clearly warranted. Available data suggests families living with a cancer predisposition syndrome and their caregivers can benefit from a highly skilled, interdisciplinary medical team that provides high quality psychosocial support and evidence-based psychosocial interventions along with excellent medical care.

This chapter highlights the need for future research focused on understanding the psychosocial impact of FECS on children and adolescents and their parents/caregivers. The lack of research exploring young peoples' perspectives meant this chapter had to rely on data from FECS affected adults and insights from young people with other cancer predisposition syndromes. The majority of studies involving adults with FECS have been limited by cross-sectional designs. These studies provide valuable insights into patients' experiences at a single point in time but provide no information about how individuals' psychosocial strengths and vulnerabilities may change over time. There is a need for prospective studies, tracking the experiences of at-risk young people from FECS affected families. Where possible, future studies should include quantitative and qualitative measures and biological markers to determine whether symptoms, such as heightened anxiety, could be part of symptoms seen in primary hyperparathyroidism. Given the familial nature of these syndromes, and the indications from adult data of their impacts on family relationships, future studies should include child and adolescent patients as well as their parents and siblings. Many unanswered questions remain regarding the impact of FECS on young people's wellbeing, experiences of genetic testing, and surveillance, and reproductive considerations, and the impacts of caring for a FECS affected young person on parents/caregivers. The lack of data regarding the psychosocial impact of FECS on children and adolescents in part reflects the complexity and challenges associated with researching the impacts of these syndromes. Small absolute numbers and lack of consensus regarding which impacts to measure are two such challenges. We suggest that collaboration across treatment centers, and harmonization of measures used to assess syndrome impacts help to overcome some of these challenges.

Funding

KH is supported by a Cancer Institute Translational Program Grant (2021/TPG2112) as well as the Zero Childhood Cancer National Personalised Medicine Program for children with high-risk cancer, a joint initiative of Children's Cancer Institute and Kids Cancer Centre, Sydney Children's Hospital.

KH and JH are supported by Luminesce Alliance—Innovation for Children's Health. Luminesce Alliance—Innovation for Children's Health, is a not-for-profit cooperative joint venture between the Sydney Children's Hospitals Network, the Children's Medical Research Institute, and the Children's Cancer Institute. It has been established with the support of the NSW Government to coordinate and integrate paediatric research. Luminesce Alliance is also affiliated with the University of Sydney and the University of New South Wales Sydney. CW is supported by the NHMRC of Australia (APP2008300).

LW and MR: This project has been funded in whole or in part with federal funds from the Intramural Program of the National Cancer Institute, National Institutes of Health, under Contract No. [75N91019D00024]. MR: funding provided by the NCI Cancer Moonshot^{SM} for the My Pediatric and Adult Rare Tumor (MyPART) network and by the NCI Intramural Research Program. RL: This project has been funded in whole or in part with federal funds from the Intramural Program of the National Cancer Institute, National Institutes of Health, under Contract No. [75N91019D00024]. LW, MR, RL: The content of this publication does not necessarily reflect the views or policies of the Department of Health and Human Services, nor does mention of trade names, commercial products, or organizations imply endorsement by the U.S. Government.

References

1. Vears DF, Ayres S, Boyle J, Mansour J, Newson AJ. Human Genetics Society of Australasia Position Statement: predictive and presymptomatic genetic testing in adults and children. Twin Res Hum Genet. 2020;23(3):184–9. https://doi.org/10.1017/thg.2020.51.
2. Petr EJ, Else T. Genetic predisposition to endocrine tumors: diagnosis, surveillance and challenges in care. Semin Oncol. 2016;43(5):582–90. https://doi.org/10.1053/j.seminoncol.2016.08.007.
3. Johnson LM, Hamilton KV, Valdez JM, Knapp E, Baker JN, Nichols KE. Ethical considerations surrounding germline next-generation sequencing of children with cancer. Expert Rev Mol Diagn. 2017;17(5):523–34. https://doi.org/10.1080/14737159.2017.1316665.
4. ACMG. Ethical and policy issues in genetic testing and screening of children. Pediatrics. 2013;131(3):620–2. https://doi.org/10.1542/peds.2012-3680.
5. Druker H, Zelley K, McGee RB, Scollon SR, Kohlmann WK, Schneider KA, et al. Genetic counselor recommendations for cancer predisposition evaluation and surveillance in the pediatric oncology patient. Clin Cancer Res. 2017;23(13):e91–7. https://doi.org/10.1158/1078-0432.ccr-17-0834.
6. Newey PJ. Clinical genetic testing in endocrinology: current concepts and contemporary challenges. Clin Endocrinol. 2019;91(5):587–607. https://doi.org/10.1111/cen.14053.
7. Lockridge R, Bedoya S, Allen T, Widemann BC, Akshintal S, Glod J, Wiener L. Psychosocial characteristics and experiences in patients with multiple endocrine neoplasia type 2 (MEN2) and medullary thyroid carcinoma (MTC). Children. 2022;9:774–86.
8. van Engelen K, Barrera M, Wasserman JD, Armel SR, Chitayat D, Druker H, et al. Tumor surveillance for children and adolescents with cancer predisposition syndromes: the psychosocial impact reported by adolescents and caregivers. Pediatr Blood Cancer. 2021;68(8):e29021. https://doi.org/10.1002/pbc.29021.

9. Martins RG, Carvalho IP. Pheochromocytoma and paraganglioma genetic testing: psychological impact. Health Psychol. 2020;39(10):934–43. https://doi.org/10.1037/hea0000993.
10. Mongelli MN, Peipert BJ, Goswami S, Helenowski I, Yount SE, Sturgeon C. Quality of life in multiple endocrine neoplasia type 2A compared with normative and disease populations. Surgery. 2018;164(3):546–52. https://doi.org/10.1016/j.surg.2018.04.036.
11. Peipert BJ, Goswami S, Yount SE, Sturgeon C. Health-related quality of life in MEN1 patients compared with other chronic conditions and the United States general population. Surgery. 2018;163(1):205–11. https://doi.org/10.1016/j.surg.2017.04.030.
12. Goswami S, Peipert BJ, Helenowski I, Yount SE, Sturgeon C. Disease and treatment factors associated with lower quality of life scores in adults with multiple endocrine neoplasia type I. Surgery. 2017;162(6):1270–7. https://doi.org/10.1016/j.surg.2017.07.023.
13. Rodrigues KC, Toledo RA, Coutinho FL, Nunes AB, Maciel RMB, Hoff AO, et al. Assessment of depression, anxiety, quality of life, and coping in long-standing multiple endocrine neoplasia type 2 patients. Thyroid. 2017;27(5):693–706. https://doi.org/10.1089/thy.2016.0148.
14. Kasparian NA, Rutstein A, Sansom-Daly UM, Mireskandari S, Tyler J, Duffy J, et al. Through the looking glass: an exploratory study of the lived experiences and unmet needs of families affected by Von Hippel-Lindau disease. Eur J Hum Genet. 2015;23(1):34–40. https://doi.org/10.1038/ejhg.2014.44.
15. van Hulsteijn LT, Kaptein AA, Louisse A, Smit JWA, Corssmit EPM. Avoiding and non-expressing: coping styles of patients with paragangliomas. J Clin Endocrinol Metab. 2013;98(9):3608–14. https://doi.org/10.1210/jc.2013-1340.
16. van Hulsteijn LT, Louisse A, Havekes B, Kaptein AA, Jansen JC, Hes FJ, et al. Quality of life is decreased in patients with paragangliomas. Eur J Endocrinol. 2013;168(5):689–97. https://doi.org/10.1530/eje-12-0968.
17. Lammens CR, Bleiker EM, Verhoef S, Ausems MG, Majoor-Krakauer D, Sijmons RH, et al. Distress in partners of individuals diagnosed with or at high risk of developing tumors due to rare hereditary cancer syndromes. Psychooncology. 2011;20(6):631–8. https://doi.org/10.1002/pon.1951.
18. Lammens CR, Bleiker EM, Verhoef S, Hes FJ, Ausems MG, Majoor-Krakauer D, et al. Psychosocial impact of Von Hippel-Lindau disease: levels and sources of distress. Clin Genet. 2010;77(5):483–91. https://doi.org/10.1111/j.1399-0004.2010.01333.x.
19. Havekes B, van der Klaauw AA, Hoftijzer HC, Jansen JC, van der Mey AGL, Vriends AHJT, et al. Reduced quality of life in patients with head-and-neck paragangliomas. Eur J Endocrinol. 2008;158(2):247. https://doi.org/10.1530/eje-07-0464.
20. Grosfeld FJ, Beemer FA, Lips CJ, Hendriks KS, ten Kroode HF. Parents' responses to disclosure of genetic test results of their children. Am J Med Genet. 2000;94(4):316–23. https://doi.org/10.1002/1096-8628(20001002)94:4<316::aid-ajmg10>3.0.co;2-n.
21. Grosfeld FJ, Lips CJ, Beemer FA, Blijham GH, Quirijnen JM, Mastenbroek MP, et al. Distress in MEN 2 family members and partners prior to DNA test disclosure. Multiple endocrine neoplasia type 2. Am J Med Genet. 2000;91(1):1–7. https://doi.org/10.1002/(sici)1096-8628(20000306)91:1<1::aid-ajmg1>3.0.co;2-9.
22. Concolino P, Costella A, Capoluongo E. Multiple endocrine neoplasia type 1 (MEN1): an update of 208 new germline variants reported in the last nine years. Cancer Genet. 2016;209(1–2):36–41. https://doi.org/10.1016/j.cancergen.2015.12.002.
23. Giusti F, Marini F, Brandi ML. Multiple endocrine neoplasia type 1. In: Adam MP, Ardinger HH, Pagon RA, Wallace SE, Bean LJH, Mirzaa G, et al., editors. GeneReviews(®). Seattle, WA: University of Washington, Seattle; 2017. Copyright © 1993–2021, University of Washington, Seattle. GeneReviews is a registered trademark of the University of Washington, Seattle. All rights reserved.
24. Berglund G, Lidén A, Hansson MG, Öberg K, Sjöden PO, Nordin K. Quality of life in patients with multiple endocrine neoplasia type 1 (MEN 1). Familial Cancer. 2003;2(1):27–33. https://doi.org/10.1023/a:1023252107120.

25. Eng C. Multiple endocrine neoplasia type 2. In: Adam MP, Ardinger HH, Pagon RA, Wallace SE, Bean LJH, Mirzaa G, et al., editors. GeneReviews(®). Seattle, WA: University of Washington, Seattle; 2019. Copyright © 1993–2021, University of Washington, Seattle. GeneReviews is a registered trademark of the University of Washington, Seattle. All rights reserved.
26. Grey J, Winter K. Patient quality of life and prognosis in multiple endocrine neoplasia type 2. Endocr Relat Cancer. 2018;25(2):T69–77. https://doi.org/10.1530/erc-17-0335.
27. Allen T, Bedoya SZ, Glod J, Widemann B, Wiener L. Baseline characteristics of adolescents and young adults with medullary thyroid cancer and MEN-2B: data from the rare tumor initiative at the National Cancer Institute. Paper presented at the International Psycho-Oncology Society's 21st world congress, Banff, Canada; 2019.
28. van Leeuwaarde RS, Ahmad S, Links TP, Giles RH. Von Hippel-Lindau syndrome. In: Adam MP, Ardinger HH, Pagon RA, Wallace SE, Bean LJH, Mirzaa G, et al., editors. GeneReviews(®). Seattle, WA: University of Washington, Seattle; 2018. Copyright © 1993–2021, University of Washington, Seattle. GeneReviews is a registered trademark of the University of Washington, Seattle. All rights reserved.
29. Schneider K, Zelley K, Nichols KE, Garber J. Li-Fraumeni syndrome. In: Adam MP, Ardinger HH, Pagon RA, Wallace SE, Bean LJH, Mirzaa G, et al., editors. GeneReviews(®). Seattle, WA: University of Washington, Seattle; 2019. Copyright © 1993–2021, University of Washington, Seattle. GeneReviews is a registered trademark of the University of Washington, Seattle. All rights reserved.
30. Else T, Greenberg S, Fishbein L. Hereditary paraganglioma-pheochromocytoma syndromes. In: Adam MP, Ardinger HH, Pagon RA, Wallace SE, Bean LJH, Stephens K, et al., editors. GeneReviews(®). Seattle, WA: University of Washington, Seattle; 2018. Copyright © 1993–2020, University of Washington, Seattle. GeneReviews is a registered trademark of the University of Washington, Seattle. All rights reserved.
31. McGill BC, Wakefield CE, Vetsch J, Barlow-Stewart K, Kasparian NA, Patenaude AF, et al. Children and young people's understanding of inherited conditions and their attitudes towards genetic testing: a systematic review. Clin Genet. 2019;95(1):10–22. https://doi.org/10.1111/cge.13253.
32. Nelson HD, Pappas M, Cantor A, Haney E, Holmes R. Risk assessment, genetic counseling, and genetic testing for BRCA-related cancer in women: updated evidence report and systematic review for the US Preventive Services Task Force. JAMA. 2019;322(7):666–85. https://doi.org/10.1001/jama.2019.8430.
33. Wakefield CE, Hanlon LV, Tucker KM, Patenaude AF, Signorelli C, McLoone JK, et al. The psychological impact of genetic information on children: a systematic review. Genet Med. 2016;18(8):755–62. https://doi.org/10.1038/gim.2015.181.
34. Alderfer MA, Lindell RB, Viadro CI, Zelley K, Valdez J, Mandrell B, et al. Should genetic testing be offered for children? The perspectives of adolescents and emerging adults in families with Li-Fraumeni syndrome. J Genet Couns. 2017;26(5):1106–15. https://doi.org/10.1007/s10897-017-0091-x.
35. Rasmussen A, Alonso E, Ochoa A, De Biase I, Familiar I, Yescas P, et al. Uptake of genetic testing and long-term tumor surveillance in von Hippel-Lindau disease. BMC Med Genet. 2010;11:4. https://doi.org/10.1186/1471-2350-11-4.
36. Levy M, Richard S. Attitudes of von Hippel-Lindau disease patients towards presymptomatic genetic diagnosis in children and prenatal diagnosis. J Med Genet. 2000;37(6):476–8. https://doi.org/10.1136/jmg.37.6.476.
37. Lahlou-Laforêt K, Consoli SM, Jeunemaitre X, Gimenez-Roqueplo AP. Presymptomatic genetic testing in minors at risk of paraganglioma and pheochromocytoma: our experience of oncogenetic multidisciplinary consultation. Horm Metab Res. 2012;44(5):354–8. https://doi.org/10.1055/s-0032-1311568.

38. Rich TA, Liu M, Etzel CJ, Bannon SA, Mork ME, Ready K, et al. Comparison of attitudes regarding preimplantation genetic diagnosis among patients with hereditary cancer syndromes. Familial Cancer. 2014;13(2):291–9. https://doi.org/10.1007/s10689-013-9685-0.
39. Lammens C, Bleiker E, Aaronson N, Vriends A, Ausems M, Jansweijer M, et al. Attitude towards pre-implantation genetic diagnosis for hereditary cancer. Familial Cancer. 2009;8(4):457–64. https://doi.org/10.1007/s10689-009-9265-5.
40. Dommering CJ, Henneman L, van der Hout AH, Jonker MA, Tops CM, van den Ouweland AM, et al. Uptake of prenatal diagnostic testing for retinoblastoma compared to other hereditary cancer syndromes in The Netherlands. Familial Cancer. 2017;16(2):271–7. https://doi.org/10.1007/s10689-016-9943-z.
41. ACMG, ASHG. Points to consider: ethical, legal, and psychosocial implications of genetic testing in children and adolescents. American Society of Human Genetics Board of Directors, American College of Medical Genetics Board of Directors. Am J Hum Genet. 1995;57(5):1233–41.
42. Botkin JR, Belmont JW, Berg JS, Berkman BE, Bombard Y, Holm IA, et al. Points to consider: ethical, legal, and psychosocial implications of genetic testing in children and adolescents. Am J Hum Genet. 2015;97(1):6–21. https://doi.org/10.1016/j.ajhg.2015.05.022.
43. Grootens-Wiegers P, Hein IM, van den Broek JM, de Vries MC. Medical decision-making in children and adolescents: developmental and neuroscientific aspects. BMC Pediatr. 2017;17(1):120. https://doi.org/10.1186/s12887-017-0869-x.
44. Lenders JW, Duh QY, Eisenhofer G, Gimenez-Roqueplo AP, Grebe SK, Murad MH, et al. Pheochromocytoma and paraganglioma: an endocrine society clinical practice guideline. J Clin Endocrinol Metab. 2014;99(6):1915–42. https://doi.org/10.1210/jc.2014-1498.
45. Muth A, Crona J, Gimm O, Elmgren A, Filipsson K, Stenmark Askmalm M, et al. Genetic testing and surveillance guidelines in hereditary pheochromocytoma and paraganglioma. J Intern Med. 2019;285(2):187–204. https://doi.org/10.1111/joim.12869.
46. Raygada M, King KS, Adams KT, Stratakis CA, Pacak K. Counseling patients with succinate dehydrogenase subunit defects: genetics, preventive guidelines, and dealing with uncertainty. J Pediatr Endocrinol Metab. 2014;27(9–10):837–44. https://doi.org/10.1515/jpem-2013-0369.
47. Rednam SP, Erez A, Druker H, Janeway KA, Kamihara J, Kohlmann WK, et al. Von Hippel-Lindau and hereditary pheochromocytoma/paraganglioma syndromes: clinical features, genetics, and surveillance recommendations in childhood. Clin Cancer Res. 2017;23(12):e68–75. https://doi.org/10.1158/1078-0432.ccr-17-0547.
48. Clarke AJ, Wallgren-Pettersson C. Ethics in genetic counselling. J Community Genet. 2019;10(1):3–33. https://doi.org/10.1007/s12687-018-0371-7.
49. Elwyn G, Gray J, Clarke A. Shared decision making and non-directiveness in genetic counselling. J Med Genet. 2000;37(2):135–8. https://doi.org/10.1136/jmg.37.2.135.
50. Oduncu FS. The role of non-directiveness in genetic counseling. Med Health Care Philos. 2002;5(1):53–63. https://doi.org/10.1023/a:1014289418443.
51. Weil J, Ormond K, Peters J, Peters K, Biesecker BB, LeRoy B. The relationship of nondirectiveness to genetic counseling: report of a workshop at the 2003 NSGC annual education conference. J Genet Couns. 2006;15(2):85–93. https://doi.org/10.1007/s10897-005-9008-1.

Chapter 2
Transitions of Care Models

Stéphanie Larose

Introduction

Transition of care is defined as a planned, deliberate process of identifying and meeting the medical and psycho-social needs of adolescents and young adults (AYA) as they move from pediatric to adult care [1]. Transition of care programs, interventions, and clinics can be categorized into transition of care models, each of which has its own common design features [2]. Developing evidence-based transition of care models will become increasingly important in the coming years. The cure rate of endocrine pediatric cancers is increasing, leading to more young adult survivors [3, 4] in need of transition of care planning. These patients can have a variety of late complications, including psychological disorders, secondary malignancies, and end-organ damage. Beyond the scope of endo-oncology, we are also facing increasing numbers of adolescents and young adults surviving a variety of complex diseases, such as hematological cancers, cystic fibrosis, and congenital heart disease [5–8], just to name a few. The literature review of transition of care models presented in this chapter is inclusive, going beyond the frontiers of endo-oncology.

Current State of Transition of Care

Lack of transition of care planification (and thus of models) has negative outcomes on AYA patients. The National Survey of Children's Health found in 2016 that about 64% of American adolescents report not having discussed with their current

S. Larose (✉)
Division of Endocrinology, McGill University Health Center, Montreal, QC, Canada
e-mail: stephanie.larose2@mail.mcgill.ca

© The Author(s), under exclusive license to Springer Nature Switzerland AG 2023
F. Hannah-Shmouni (ed.), *Familial Endocrine Cancer Syndromes*,
https://doi.org/10.1007/978-3-031-37275-9_2

pediatric health care provider (HCP) about transition of care to an adult HCP [9], and only about 17% of those with special health care needs had transition of care discussions and planning with their HCP [10]. This lack of planning diminishes the adolescents' own perceptions of transition readiness and future transition success compared to those who do discuss transition of care [9]. When transition is not properly planned, potential negative outcomes for AYA patients include being lost to follow-up or experiencing lapses in care [11, 12], decreased adherence to treatment [13], increased emergency department visits and hospitalizations [14, 15], use of pediatric center for inpatient admission needs instead of adult centers [16, 17], and increased morbidity, complications [5] (including graft loss [18, 19]), and mortality [5]. Transition of care planning (or lack thereof) can impact psychosocial outcomes as well: young adults with chronic illnesses, disabilities or a history of cancer tend to have poorer social development, with decreased autonomy and employment compared to their peers [5, 20]. On the other hand, having a structured transition of care model has been shown to improve attendance to adult care visits, adherence to therapy, self-care skills and decrease hospitalizations, although results vary by type of intervention and disease studied [21–24], as we will see below.

Transition of Care Models

Various models of transition of pediatric-centered to adult-centered care exist, and there are various ways of naming and classifying these models. It is important to note that outside of oncology survivorship literature, model conceptualization to help direct transition of care studies is often lacking [25] and no formal consensus exists on a taxonomy of models in transition of care literature [26]. Evaluation of the performance outcomes of the various models with the evaluation checklists available [27, 28] is also limited. For example, transition programs' outcomes are inconsistently evaluated by the "Triple Aim" framework, a checklist used to evaluate the programs' experience of care for the patients, impact on population health and care cost [28]. Despite these limitations, we present below one taxonomy and classification of transition of care models that emerge from a broad literature review of transition of care in various chronic disease settings (Table 2.1). One large group, the HCP-based models (PCP-led model, shared-care model and specialized care-led model) are derived in large part from the oncology survivorship literature, which classifies models according to the setting (academic vs. community) and to the type of HCP (generalist vs. specialist) who provides care [29, 30]. The navigator-led model and the intervention-based model are ubiquitous in a variety of settings and diseases. Due to the lack of formal, agreed-upon taxonomy, it is possible that some models do not fit in any one of these descriptions or fit in more than one (e.g., one theoretical model found is a shared-care model with a strong navigator component and even a coaching intervention [31]). Thus, models are not mutually exclusive, but this classification will be useful to compare the advantages, disadvantages, and performance outcomes of each.

Table 2.1 Transition of care models

Transition of care models		Advantages	Disadvantages
HCP-based models	PCP-led model	Wellness-oriented care	PCP less skilled to treat rare, pediatric onset chronic diseases
		Access to routine care and preventive medicine	PCP discomfort in treating AYA patients with special health care needs
		Convenient to the patient	Burden of advocacy for specialized care on patient's shoulders
		Potentially lower health care costs	Potential lack of access to specialized or multidisciplinary resources
		Advantageous for the low-risk AYA patient	
	Specialized care-led model	Disease-oriented care	May discourage AYA patient from finding/ maintaining follow up with PCP
		Access to subspecialized, highly skilled HCPs	Lack of access to routine care and preventive medicine
		Potentially more access to a multidisciplinary team	Potentially higher health care costs
		Disease-specific multidisciplinary resources	
		More advantageous to the high-risk AYA patient	
	Shared-care model	Access to both wellness-oriented and disease-oriented care	Difficulty in implementing and maintaining the model
		Access to routine care and preventive medicine	Burden of constant communication between physicians
			Potential for PCP to be relegated to secondary role in transition planning
Navigator-based model		Burden of transition of care management on navigator rather than HCP	Human resource-intensive
		Potential of systematizing transition planning	Variable costs
		May or may not be a disease-specific navigator	

(continued)

Table 2.1 (continued)

Transition of care models	Advantages	Disadvantages
Intervention-based model	Can be adapted to both a community and specialized center setting	Initial difficulty of intervention implementation
	High engagement from AYA patients with technology-based interventions	High initial costs of more complex interventions
	Potential for cost-effectiveness	

AYA adolescents and young adults, *HCP* health care provider, *PCP* primary care provider
Partially adapted from Shannon [29] and Kinahan et al [32]

Health Care Provider (HCP)-Based Models

HCP-based models can and have been applied to a variety of pediatric onset chronic diseases, but their conceptualization and subclassification is mostly derived from the pediatric oncology literature. The latter tends to subgroup models in either of the following three categories: PCP-led (sometimes called community-based) model, specialized care-led model or shared care (between the PCP and a specialized medical team) [29, 32, 33]. The consultative model is sometimes distinguished from the more general shared-care model [34].

Primary Care Provider (PCP)-Led Model

In this model, a PCP such as a family physician, registered nurse practitioner or general internist in the community leads and assures the long-term follow-up of the patient, in a clinic that may or may not be dedicated specifically to young adults [29, 32, 35, 36]. Often, the AYA patient is simply incorporated into the general mix of the PCP clinic or center [35]. Having at least one communication with the past pediatric team (e.g., to get a medical summary and recommendations) is helpful to better incorporate these patients in a general practice [35].

Advantages of this model include the reintegration into primary care, which tend to be more wellness-centered rather than disease-centered [29, 34, 37]. This wellness focus is important to assure that patients get routine care such as preventive medicine measures [37], which they may not get in a highly specialized center (e.g., pap tests, tobacco smoking cessation, sexually transmitted diseases prevention and screening, etc.) This model of transition of care is also convenient for the AYA patients, easy to access and optimal for those who are at low risk of having late complications of their pediatric disease [32]. Health system costs are potentially lower as well [38, 39].

A disadvantage of this model is that PCPs are often less knowledgeable of the late complications of complex, chronic diseases (such as pediatric cancers) and are also less comfortable treating such patients [32]. They may not be up to date with recent, highly specialized literature on these complications and this may put the burden on AYA patients to advocate for specialized care [34]. Cancer survivor AYA patients in particular are noted to have low confidence in PCPs' abilities to deliver optimal care for them [40]. Depending on the location of the PCP, the latter may also lack easy liaison with subspecialists to support them, and they may lack time (and resources, such as psychologists, social workers, etc.) to devote to their AYA patients' complex medical or psychosocial issues [34, 38], unless they have access to a well implemented multidisciplinary team with them [41]. Finally, the PCP's capacity to do research might be more limited [29, 38].

In a 2016 systematic review of PCP-led transition of care model programs, none of the studies included examined transition of care in all three of the Triple Aim Framework domains (i.e., some programs examined outcomes in only one or two of the domains), giving us limited evidence to support the PCP-led model or guide improvement of the programs formed on this model [42]. However, the PCP-led model has been shown to be effective at implementing evidence-based core elements of a successful transition model in a pilot study [43]. The Comprehensive Care Clinic, implemented by the Geisinger Health System in Pennsylvania was successful in decreasing acute care utilization in AYA patients with special health care needs of all kinds [39].

Specialized Care-Led Model

The specialized care-led model encompasses all transition programs and clinics that are led by an adult specialist, often in the setting of a specialized center. It has many names in the literature and varies according to the disease-specific literature: cancer center care model [32], adult health care program model [44], and the joint adult and pediatric clinics model [45] are just a few of the names found in oncology, endocrinology, and neurology transition of care literature. The model is often embedded in a disease-specific transition clinic centered around the pediatric and the adult specialists; sometimes a multidisciplinary team is present to help manage the transition and take care of the AYA patient's psychosocial needs. The specialized care-led model has been applied, among many other diseases, to epilepsy [46], type 1 diabetes [47, 48], cystic fibrosis [49], HIV [50], liver transplant [51], inflammatory bowel disease clinic [52], and hemophilia [53].

Major advantages of the specialized care-led model are the access to knowledgeable specialists, to disease-focused care (which is especially useful for patients with a high risk of long-term complications or an active disease) and to a multidisciplinary team, if there is one [29]. Indeed, this model may be more likely than the PCP-led model to benefit from a multidisciplinary team (especially in large centers). Those multidisciplinary resources might be more tailored to the needs of certain AYA populations as well (e.g., presence of diabetes educators and dieticians for diabetes patients or support of onco-psychologists for AYA cancer survivors, instead of "generalist" dieticians and psychologists.) This model can also confer a certain familiarity, if the pediatric and adult care specialists work in the same center.

Disadvantages include the risk of discouraging AYA patients from forming or maintaining a relationship with a generalist PCP, and thus missing the wellness-focused, routine care of primary care medicine [29, 32]. Increased use of specialist services contributes to make health care costs higher in young patients with special health care needs [54]. Overall, this type of model is more suited to AYA patients with rare diseases, complex chronic diseases that are still active or patients with a high risk of relapse or late complications.

As noted above, there are multiple examples of implemented programs following this transition of care model and the variability between them makes it difficult to evaluate performance outcomes. A systematic review of various transition of care approaches, including programs fitting the specialized care-led model, found mixed results in terms of health outcomes (e.g., improvements in A1c lowering), development of acute or chronic complications, development of self-management skills and rate of either loss to follow up or clinic attendance for this model [55]. In a more recent systematic review, two of the five programs included followed the specialized care-led model; both focused on diabetes and they had divergent results in terms of success of transfer itself and in glycated hemoglobin measurements [23].

Shared-Care Model

In the shared-care model, both a specialist and a PCP are co-leading transition of care for the AYA patient and are collaborating closely [32, 38]. A broader definition of this model is widely used worldwide with success not just in AYA patients but in patients of all ages living with chronic diseases [30]. The degree of involvement of the specialist depends on how active the chronic condition is; the shared-care model can thus be modulated according to a risk based approach [30], as is the case in the risk-stratified shared-care model developed for AYA cancer survivors: in this variant of the shared-care model, the intensity of follow-up with the PCP and the oncologist is modulated according to the patient's risk of late complications and recurrence [32]. Other oncology authors call it the need-based care model [29]. Follow-up is at least initially with both the specialist and a PCP. Collaboration between the two physicians can take the form of the specialist providing screening recommendations to the PCP, and the PCP in turn reporting to the specialist the evolution of the AYA patient [31, 38]. Part of the process (e.g., sharing recommendations, support) can be done virtually [56, 57].

Advantages include having access to both the generalist's knowledge on routine preventive medicine in adolescents and the specialist's knowledge, and a strong focus on communication and collaboration [29, 32]. There may be less risk to follow up loss as well, as two physicians are following the patient at least initially.

The disadvantages include some of those of the PCP-led model, but also include the fact that many resources are needed, contributing to the difficulty of implementing and maintaining the model [29, 32]. The constant communication can be a burden for both physicians involved, who may be geographically distant. Finally, in one study involving AYA patients with disabilities, it has been found that the PCP may be faced with barriers to participation in the planning of transition of care [58].

Although the shared-care model applied to AYA patients' transition exists outside of the cancer survivor literature [59], it is more explicitly mentioned and evaluated in the latter. In an intervention study comparing the efficacy of a program based on the shared-care model for AYA cancer survivors ($n = 271$), the program improved follow up with the general practitioner in the intervention cohort compared to the control cohort [60]. Finally, in a pilot study of a shared-care program of AYA cancer survivors in the Netherlands, the vast majority of both cancer survivors selected ($n = 123$) and family physicians ($n = 115$) were satisfied with the share-care model [61].

Navigator-Based Model

The transition navigator (also sometimes called case manager [62], transition coordinator or facilitator [63]) can be one person (e.g., a specialized registered nurse, a social worker, a psychologist or an administrative coordinator [2, 64]), a multidisciplinary team that is dedicated to transition planning and visit organization [65, 66], a virtual system or application [67] or even a combination of human and virtual resources [62]. This model creates a triad around the patient: the navigator, the pediatric HCP, and the adult HCP.

A first advantage of this model is that the navigator's presence lifts the burden of transition management on someone else than the treating physicians. Transition planification is less likely to be forgotten, as this is the navigator's primordial task. Furthermore, transition planification has the potential to be systematized if the navigator is virtual, making the process more passive. Finally, navigators are transition of care specialists that do not need to be disease-specific, and thus have the potential to be used in parallel for a wide variety of pediatric subspecialties.

A disadvantage of this model, however, is that a human navigator or a multidisciplinary navigator team are human resources that may not be available in certain settings, especially outside of large academic centers. Costs of such a model vary depending on who (or what) is the navigator and their degree of implication.

In a systematic review evaluating the capacity of various transition programs to assure a successful transfer, three of the five programs fitted the navigator-based model; two of those three had higher rates of successful transfer or clinic attendance among patients in the programs than those in the comparison groups [23]. One example of a successful implementation of the navigator-based model is the Maestro Project, a multi-modal navigator system that was shown to help improve medical surveillance for 2 cohorts of 18–25 year olds with type 1 diabetes in Manitoba, Canada [62].

Intervention-Based Model

The intervention-based model includes programs that are centered around an intervention or a group of interventions that aim to improve transition of care. There are multiple types of interventions. Incentive-based interventions, for example, incentivize the AYA patient to engage more often with the new treating team. A controversial example of an incentive-based intervention is to use a financial incentive to promote autonomy and self-management [68, 69]. Education-based interventions, on the other hand, are often geared towards the development of disease-specific self-care skills (e.g., learning to self-inject a medication) or general self-care skills (teaching the AYA patient how to make an appointment, how to deal with insurance issues, etc.) Transition education programs have been used for AYA patients with esophageal atresia [70], inflammatory bowel disease [71], and heart transplant [72]. Finally, e-coaching on web platforms and via text messages also fit the intervention-based model [73–75]. Intervention programs can include both incentive and educational measures.

The first advantage of the intervention-based model is its flexibility: it can be used in various settings, from a community PCP to the specialist in a large academic center. The intervention-based model is also easy to hybridize with other models, and can be relatively simple in terms of logistics (e.g., automated text messages). AYA patients show high engagement with digital- or technology-based interventions, when they are presented to them [76]. Simple, technology-based interventions have the potential to be cost-effective [74].

A disadvantage may be the initial difficulty in developing and implementing the intervention program. Indeed, this may necessitate the help of both medical and non-medical specialists such as nurses, social workers, software designers, informatic technicians, psychologists, and educators [72, 77]. This, in turn, might make the cost of developing a new intervention program prohibitive.

As the intervention-based model encompasses a wide variety of programs, outcomes of such interventions are mixed, with low certainty evidence that they can slightly improve transition readiness and disease self-management [22]. A systematic review of incentive interventions found that they were often used to promote cessation of adverse behaviors rather than to promote healthy behaviors in transitioning AYAs, and that little follow up had been provided for the intervention itself [78]. In turn, a systematic review of mobile- and web-based applications to promote transition was also unable to provide evidence for their effectiveness overall [79]. However, some incentive-based interventions included were successful at increasing knowledge and therapy adherence (including to medication) [79].

Got Transition

Got transition is a federally funded program from the National Alliance to Advance Adolescent Health that was designed to help health care professionals, health care programs, AYA patients, parents, and caregivers improve transition of care from pediatric centered to adult centered care [80]. It is a resource center entirely dedicated to transition of care that developed and improved over the years the Six Core Elements (Table 2.2), which are not a model in itself but rather an evidence-based approach that can be used to develop transition of care models and implement transition programs [80]. They are, in other words, the "core elements" that should be embedded in all transition of care models.

The Six Core Elements are already being used by treating teams to implement programs and interventions fitting the various transitions of care models, and their use leads to significant improvement in the transition of care process [81]. As an

Table 2.2 Six core elements of got transition

Six core elements	Age group
1. Policy/Guide	12–14 years old
(a) Development a transition and care policy or guide	
(b) Education of treating team members on transition of care approach adopted and on the roles of all stakeholders (AYA patient, caregivers, HCPs on pediatric and adult side)	
(c) Display the policy or guide	
(d) Discuss and share with the AYA patient and their caregiver	
2. Tracking and monitoring	14–18 years old
(a) Development of standardized process to identify AYA patients in need of transition	
(b) Integration of monitoring of the Six Core Elements	
3. Readiness	14–18 years old
(a) Regular assessments of readiness to transition	
(b) Ongoing education of self-care skills	
(c) Identification of adult HCPs	
(d) Orientation of AYA patients to identified adult HCPs	
4. Planning	14–18 years old
(a) Transition of care planification: medical summary preparation and transfer, optimal timing for transfer discussion, young adult plan of care with recommendations, etc.	
5. Transfer of care	18–21 years old
(a) Sharing of key health information	
(b) Communication between the pediatric and adult clinicians	
(c) Confirmation of transfer date to adult care team	
6. Transition completion	18–23 years old
(a) Confirmation of transfer of care completion	
(b) Ongoing communication and collaboration with adult care team	
(c) Solicit feedback on transfer of care experience	

The Six Core Elements of Health Care Transition™ are the copyright of Got Transition®. This version of the Six Core Elements has been modified and is with permission [80]. *AYA* adolescents and young adults, *HCP* health care provider example, the implementation feasibility and customization of the Six Core Elements were examined in a pilot study of AYA patients transitioning from two school-based health centers in Washington D.C. to adult PCPs [82]. The Six Core Elements were also used by a Texas team to successfully implement and then evaluate a transition program for liver transplant AYA patients (specialized care-led model) [51]. Another team from the University of Vermont used the Six Core Elements to implement a text-messaging-based coaching system (intervention-based model) [73]. Finally, the Six Core Elements were also successfully used to develop and implement the Transition Intervention Program at the Virginia Commonwealth University; designed for AYA patients with sickle cell disease, this program is following both the specialized care model and the intervention model (with educators and educational material) [83].

Towards a New Transition of Care Model

Integrating aspects of the existing models and the framework of the Six Core Elements, we now present a new transition of care model that can be adapted to AYA patients with various special health care needs (including endocrine cancer syndromes.) It is called the integrative model, as it integrates features of the risk-based, shared-care model, the navigator-based model, and the Six Core Elements (Fig. 2.1).

In the integrative model, the HCPs (pediatric specialist, adult specialist, and PCP) are assisted by a transition navigator (ideally associated with the pediatric clinic, as this is the starting point of the patient's transition process.) The tasks associated with each Core Element are shared between the navigator, the HCPs and the multidisciplinary team (where available.) The navigator holds the responsibility of assuring both the implementation of the Six Core Elements into the local program and the collaboration and communication between all stakeholders (patient, parents, physicians, multidisciplinary team members). Thus, the navigator will coordinate the HCPs in the creation of a local transition of care policy and plan, and assure the development of a tracking and monitoring system (e.g., the tracking system could be embedded in the electronic medical record, with an automatic pop-up at a patient's 14th birthday to remind the team to start the transition process). Finally, the navigator will also assure transition is complete and transmit constructive feedback between HCPs. As for the HCPs (and their multidisciplinary team), their Six Core Elements tasks will include: readiness assessment of the patients at each visit in the pediatric and primary care offices; education of the patient on disease-specific self-care skills; preparation of care recommendations and of a medical summary to the intention of the PCP and/or adult specialist; and collaboration with the other HCP.

There should be shared care between the pediatric team and at least one adult care provider, ideally one of which is a PCP, to assure that the patient receives routine preventive care and not just disease-oriented care. This feature of the integrative model fits into the broader definition of the shared-care model, making the new

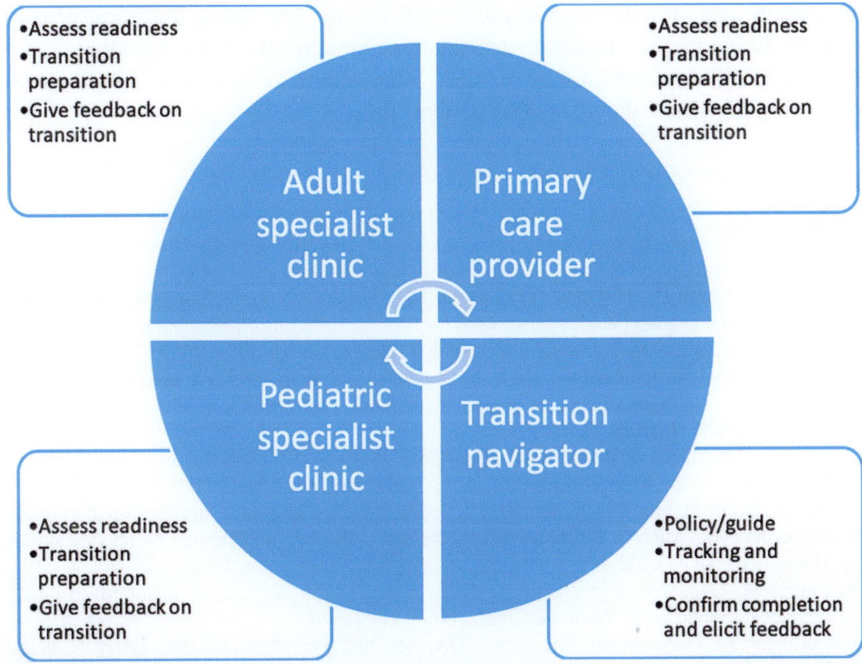

Fig. 2.1 The integrative transition of care model

model adaptable to various realities. Indeed, while shared care may only be applicable with a PCP in specialist-poor, rural regions, it may also be limited to shared care with an adult specialist (not necessarily part of a joint transition clinic) for some patients who do not have yet access to primary care. While some settings face more difficulty accessing specialized care [84], others show limited regular access to a family physician [85]. The shared care is risk-based: collaboration will be more frequent between the pediatric and adult specialists for an active disease, while both specialists may adopt a more distant, consultative role for the PCP in the case of quiet, low-risk disease.

Conclusion

In this chapter, we have presented the existing transition of care models that emerge from the large literature on transition interventions, programs and models themselves. We then presented the new integrative model, which incorporates evidence-based best practices for transition. To help current and future generations of AYA patients with special health care needs, future research on transition of care models should be directed by theory and by a consensus taxonomy [25, 26]. It should examine not only health outcomes but also AYA patients' experience, adherence to visits and health care system use, and costs [86]. Finally, increasing transition of care training during medical residency and adapting systems of care to make them more supportive of transition of care models' implementation will also contribute to improving transition of care of AYA patients [86].

References

1. Blum RW, Garell D, Hodgman CH, Jorissen TW, Okinow NA, Orr DP, et al. Transition from child-centered to adult health-care systems for adolescents with chronic conditions. A position paper of the Society for Adolescent Medicine. J Adolesc Health. 1993;14(7):570–6.
2. Marani H, Fujioka J, Tabatabavakili S, Bollegala N. Systematic narrative review of pediatric-to-adult care transition models for youth with pediatric-onset chronic conditions. Child Youth Serv Rev. 2020;118:105415.
3. Binderup MLM, Jensen AM, Budtz-Jørgensen E, Bisgaard ML. Survival and causes of death in patients with von Hippel-Lindau disease. J Med Genet. 2017;54(1):11–8.
4. Raue F, Dralle H, Machens A, Bruckner T, Frank-Raue K. Long-term survivorship in multiple endocrine neoplasia type 2B diagnosed before and in the new millennium. J Clin Endocrinol Metab. 2018;103(1):235–43.
5. Viner RM. Transition of care from paediatric to adult services: one part of improved health services for adolescents. Arch Dis Child. 2008;93(2):160–3.
6. Oeffinger KC, Argenbright KE, Levitt GA, McCabe MS, Anderson PR, Berry E, et al. Models of cancer survivorship health care: moving forward. Am Soc Clin Oncol Educ Book. 2014;34:205–13.
7. Mackie AS, Fournier A, Swan L, Marelli AJ, Kovacs AH. Transition and transfer from pediatric to adult congenital heart disease care in Canada: call for strategic implementation. Can J Cardiol. 2019;35(12):1640–51.
8. Coyne I, Sheehan AM, Heery E, While AE. Improving transition to adult healthcare for young people with cystic fibrosis: a systematic review. J Child Health Care. 2017;21(3):312–30.
9. Syverson EP, McCarter R, He J, D'Angelo L, Tuchman LK. Adolescents' perceptions of transition importance, readiness, and likelihood of future success: the role of anticipatory guidance. Clin Pediatr (Phila). 2016;55(11):1020–5.
10. Lebrun-Harris LA, McManus MA, Ilango SM, Cyr M, McLellan SB, Mann MY, et al. Transition planning among US youth with and without special health care needs. Pediatrics. 2018;142(4):e20180194.
11. Heery E, Sheehan AM, While AE, Coyne I. Experiences and outcomes of transition from pediatric to adult health care services for young people with congenital heart disease: a systematic review. Congenit Heart Dis. 2015;10(5):413–27.
12. Sheehan AM, While AE, Coyne I. The experiences and impact of transition from child to adult healthcare services for young people with type 1 diabetes: a systematic review. Diabet Med. 2015;32(4):440–58.
13. Fredericks EM. Nonadherence and the transition to adulthood. Liver Transpl. 2009;15(Suppl 2):S63–9.
14. Nakhla M, Daneman D, To T, Paradis G, Guttmann A. Transition to adult care for youths with diabetes mellitus: findings from a Universal Health Care System. Pediatrics. 2009;124(6):e1134-41.
15. Pyatak EA, Sequeira PA, Vigen CL, Weigensberg MJ, Wood JR, Montoya L, et al. Clinical and psychosocial outcomes of a structured transition program among young adults with type 1 diabetes. J Adolesc Health. 2017;60(2):212–8.
16. Edwards JD, Houtrow AJ, Vasilevskis EE, Dudley RA, Okumura MJ. Multi-institutional profile of adults admitted to pediatric intensive care units. JAMA Pediatr. 2013;167(5):436–43.

17. Goodman DM, Mendez E, Throop C, Ogata ES. Adult survivors of pediatric illness: the impact on pediatric hospitals. Pediatrics. 2002;110(3):583–9.
18. Watson AR. Non-compliance and transfer from paediatric to adult transplant unit. Pediatr Nephrol. 2000;14(6):469–72.
19. Foster BJ. Heightened graft failure risk during emerging adulthood and transition to adult care. Pediatr Nephrol. 2015;30(4):567–76.
20. Colver A, Rapley T, Parr JR, McConachie H, Dovey-Pearce G, Le Couteur A, et al. Programme Grants for Applied Research. Facilitating the transition of young people with long-term conditions through health services from childhood to adulthood: the transition research programme. Southampton: NIHR Journals Library. Copyright © Queen's Printer and Controller of HMSO 2019. This work was produced by Colver et al. under the terms of a commissioning contract issued by the Secretary of State for Health and Social Care. This issue may be freely reproduced for the purposes of private research and study and extracts (or indeed, the full report) may be included in professional journals provided that suitable acknowledgement is made and the reproduction is not associated with any form of advertising. Applications for commercial reproduction should be addressed to: NIHR Journals Library, National Institute for Health Research, Evaluation, Trials and Studies Coordinating Centre, Alpha House, University of Southampton Science Park, Southampton SO16 7NS, UK; 2019.
21. Gabriel P, McManus M, Rogers K, White P. Outcome evidence for structured pediatric to adult health care transition interventions: a systematic review. J Pediatr. 2017;188:263–9.e15.
22. Campbell F, Biggs K, Aldiss SK, O'Neill PM, Clowes M, McDonagh J, et al. Transition of care for adolescents from paediatric services to adult health services. Cochrane Database Syst Rev. 2016;4:CD009794.
23. Chu PY, Maslow GR, von Isenburg M, Chung RJ. Systematic review of the impact of transition interventions for adolescents with chronic illness on transfer from pediatric to adult healthcare. J Pediatr Nurs. 2015;30(5):e19–27.
24. Schmidt A, Ilango SM, McManus MA, Rogers KK, White PH. Outcomes of pediatric to adult health care transition interventions: an updated systematic review. J Pediatr Nurs. 2020;51:92–107.
25. Betz CL, Ferris ME, Woodward JF, Okumura MJ, Jan S, Wood DL. The health care transition research consortium health care transition model: a framework for research and practice. J Pediatr Rehabil Med. 2014;7(1):3–15.
26. Ryan D, Moorehead PC, Chafe R. Standardizing the categorizations of models of aftercare for survivors of childhood cancer. BMC Health Serv Res. 2019;19(1):850.
27. Campagna V, Nelson SA, Krsnak J. Improving care transitions to drive patient outcomes: the triple aim meets the four pillars. Prof Case Manag. 2019;24(6):297–305.
28. Prior M, McManus M, White P, Davidson L. Measuring the "triple aim" in transition care: a systematic review. Pediatrics. 2014;134(6):e1648–61.
29. Shannon S. Foundations for long-term follow-up. In: Landier W, editor. Establishing and enhancing services for childhood cancer survivors: long-term follow-up program resource guide. Arcadia: Children's Oncology Group; 2007. p. 1–16.
30. Oeffinger KC, McCabe MS. Models for delivering survivorship care. J Clin Oncol. 2006;24(32):5117–24.
31. Vaks Y, Bensen R, Steidtmann D, Wang TD, Platchek TS, Zulman DM, et al. Better health, less spending: redesigning the transition from pediatric to adult healthcare for youth with chronic illness. Healthc (Amst). 2016;4(1):57–68.
32. Kinahan KE, Sanford S, Sadak KT, Salsman JM, Danner-Koptik K, Didwania A. Models of cancer survivorship care for adolescents and young adults. Semin Oncol Nurs. 2015;31(3):251–9.
33. Heirs M, Suekarran S, Slack R, Light K, Gibson F, Glaser A, et al. A systematic review of models of care for the follow-up of childhood cancer survivors. Pediatr Blood Cancer. 2013;60(3):351–6.
34. Oncology ASoC. Models of long-term follow-up care. https://www.asco.org/practice-policy/cancer-care-initiatives/prevention-survivorship/survivorship/survivorship-3.

35. Hart LC, Mouw MS, Teal R, Jonas DE. What care models have generalists implemented to address transition from pediatric to adult care?: a qualitative study. J Gen Intern Med. 2019;34(10):2083–90.
36. Wright C, Steinway C, Jan S. The genesis of systems of care for transition to adulthood services: emerging models in primary and subspecialty care. Curr Opin Pediatr. 2018;30(2):303–10.
37. Graves L, Leung S, Raghavendran P, Mennito S. Transitions of care for healthy young adults: promoting primary care and preventive health. South Med J. 2019;112(9):497–9.
38. Singer S, Gianinazzi ME, Hohn A, Kuehni CE, Michel G. General practitioner involvement in follow-up of childhood cancer survivors: a systematic review. Pediatr Blood Cancer. 2013;60(10):1565–73.
39. Maeng DD, Snyder SR, Davis TW, Tomcavage JF. Impact of a complex care management model on cost and utilization among adolescents and young adults with special care and health needs. Popul Health Manag. 2017;20(6):435–41.
40. Signorelli C, Wakefield CE, Fardell JE, Foreman T, Johnston KA, Emery J, et al. The role of primary care physicians in childhood cancer survivorship care: multiperspective interviews. Oncologist. 2019;24(5):710–9.
41. Ciccarelli MR, Gladstone EB, Armstrong Richardson EA. Implementation of a transdisciplinary team for the transition support of medically and socially complex youth. J Pediatr Nurs. 2015;30(5):661–7.
42. Bhawra J, Toulany A, Cohen E, Moore Hepburn C, Guttmann A. Primary care interventions to improve transition of youth with chronic health conditions from paediatric to adult healthcare: a systematic review. BMJ Open. 2016;6(5):e011871.
43. McManus M, White P, Pirtle R, Hancock C, Ablan M, Corona-Parra R. Incorporating the Six Core Elements of health care transition into a Medicaid managed care plan: lessons learned from a pilot project. J Pediatr Nurs. 2015;30(5):700–13.
44. Agarwal S, Raymond JK, Schutta MH, Cardillo S, Miller VA, Long JA. An adult health care-based pediatric to adult transition program for emerging adults with type 1 diabetes. Diabetes Educ. 2017;43(1):87–96.
45. Carrizosa J, An I, Appleton R, Camfield P, Von Moers A. Models for transition clinics. Epilepsia. 2014;55(Suppl 3):46–51.
46. Geerlings RP, Aldenkamp AP, Gottmer-Welschen LM, de With PH, Zinger S, van Staa AL, et al. Evaluation of a multidisciplinary epilepsy transition clinic for adolescents. Eur J Paediatr Neurol. 2016;20(3):385–92.
47. Cadario F, Prodam F, Bellone S, Trada M, Binotti M, Trada M, et al. Transition process of patients with type 1 diabetes (T1DM) from paediatric to the adult health care service: a hospital-based approach. Clin Endocrinol. 2009;71(3):346–50.
48. Lane JT, Ferguson A, Hall J, McElligott M, Miller M, Lane PH, et al. Glycemic control over 3 years in a young adult clinic for patients with type 1 diabetes. Diabetes Res Clin Pract. 2007;78(3):385–91.
49. Gravelle AM, Paone M, Davidson AG, Chilvers MA. Evaluation of a multidimensional cystic fibrosis transition program: a quality improvement initiative. J Pediatr Nurs. 2015;30(1):236–43.
50. Griffith D, Jin L, Childs J, Posada R, Jao J, Agwu A. Outcomes of a comprehensive retention strategy for youth with HIV after transfer to adult care in the United States. Pediatr Infect Dis J. 2019;38(7):722–6.
51. Shapiro JM, Himes R, Khaderi S, Economides J, El-Serag HB. A multidisciplinary approach to improving transition readiness in pediatric liver transplant recipients. Pediatr Transplant. 2020;25:e13839.
52. Erős A, Soós A, Hegyi P, Szakács Z, Eröss B, Párniczky A, et al. Spotlight on transition in patients with inflammatory bowel disease: a systematic review. Inflamm Bowel Dis. 2020;26(3):331–46.
53. Breakey VR, Blanchette VS, Bolton-Maggs PH. Towards comprehensive care in transition for young people with haemophilia. Haemophilia. 2010;16(6):848–57.

54. Marshall DA, Benchimol EI, MacKenzie A, Duque DR, MacDonald KV, Hartley T, et al. Direct health-care costs for children diagnosed with genetic diseases are significantly higher than for children with other chronic diseases. Genet Med. 2019;21(5):1049–57.
55. Crowley R, Wolfe I, Lock K, McKee M. Improving the transition between paediatric and adult healthcare: a systematic review. Arch Dis Child. 2011;96(6):548–53.
56. Blaauwbroek R, Barf HA, Groenier KH, Kremer LC, van der Meer K, Tissing WJ, et al. Family doctor-driven follow-up for adult childhood cancer survivors supported by a web-based survivor care plan. J Cancer Surviv. 2012;6(2):163–71.
57. Costello AG, Nugent BD, Conover N, Moore A, Dempsey K, Tersak JM. Shared care of childhood cancer survivors: a telemedicine feasibility study. J Adolesc Young Adult Oncol. 2017;6(4):535–41.
58. Dressler PB, Nguyen TK, Moody EJ, Friedman SL, Pickler L. Use of transition resources by primary care providers for youth with intellectual and developmental disabilities. Intellect Dev Disabil. 2018;56(1):56–68.
59. Culnane E, Loftus H, Efron D, Williams K, Di Iorio N, Shepherd R, et al. Development of the fearless, tearless transition model of care for adolescents with an intellectual disability and/or autism spectrum disorder with mental health comorbidities. Dev Med Child Neurol. 2020;63:560.
60. Ducassou S, Chipi M, Pouyade A, Afonso M, Demeaux JL, Ducos G, et al. Impact of shared care program in follow-up of childhood cancer survivors: an intervention study. Pediatr Blood Cancer. 2017;64(11).
61. Blaauwbroek R, Tuinier W, Meyboom-de Jong B, Kamps WA, Postma A. Shared care by paediatric oncologists and family doctors for long-term follow-up of adult childhood cancer survivors: a pilot study. Lancet Oncol. 2008;9(3):232–8.
62. Van Walleghem N, Macdonald CA, Dean HJ. Evaluation of a systems navigator model for transition from pediatric to adult care for young adults with type 1 diabetes. Diabetes Care. 2008;31(8):1529–30.
63. Nguyen T, Embrett MG, Barr NG, Mulvale GM, Vania DK, Randall GE, et al. Preventing youth from falling through the cracks between child/adolescent and adult mental health services: a systematic review of models of care. Community Ment Health J. 2017;53(4):375–82.
64. Betz CL, O'Kane LS, Nehring WM, Lobo ML. Systematic review: health care transition practice service models. Nurs Outlook. 2016;64(3):229–43.
65. Razon AN, Greenberg A, Trachtenberg S, Stollon N, Wu K, Ford L, et al. A multidisciplinary transition consult service: patient referral characteristics. J Pediatr Nurs. 2019;47:136–41.
66. Szalda D, Steinway C, Greenberg A, Quinn S, Stollon N, Wu K, et al. Developing a hospital-wide transition program for young adults with medical complexity. J Adolesc Health. 2019;65(4):476–82.
67. Kreuzer M, Prüfe J, Bethe D, Vogel C, Großhennig A, Koch A, et al. The TRANSNephro-study examining a new transition model for post-kidney transplant adolescents and an analysis of the present health care: study protocol for a randomized controlled trial. Trials. 2014;15:505.
68. Malik FS, Senturia KD, Lind CD, Chalmers KD, Yi-Frazier JP, Shah SK, et al. Adolescent and parent perspectives on the acceptability of financial incentives to promote self-care in adolescents with type 1 diabetes. Pediatr Diabetes. 2020;21(3):533–51.
69. Shah S, Malik F, Senturia KD, Lind C, Chalmers K, Yi-Frazier J, et al. Ethically incentivising healthy behaviours: views of parents and adolescents with type 1 diabetes. J Med Ethics. 2020;47:e55.
70. Dingemann J, Szczepanski R, Ernst G, Thyen U, Ure B, Goll M, et al. Transition of patients with esophageal atresia to adult care: results of a transition-specific education program. Eur J Pediatr Surg. 2017;27(1):61–7.
71. Schmidt S, Markwart H, Bomba F, Muehlan H, Findeisen A, Kohl M, et al. Differential effect of a patient-education transition intervention in adolescents with IBD vs. diabetes. Eur J Pediatr. 2018;177(4):497–505.

72. Anton CM, Anton K, Butts RJ. Preparing for transition: the effects of a structured transition program on adolescent heart transplant patients' adherence and transplant knowledge. Pediatr Transplant. 2019;23(7):e13544.
73. Beaudry J, Consigli A, Clark C, Robinson KJ. Getting ready for adult healthcare: designing a chatbot to coach adolescents with special health needs through the transitions of care. J Pediatr Nurs. 2019;49:85–91.
74. Huang JS, Terrones L, Tompane T, Dillon L, Pian M, Gottschalk M, et al. Preparing adolescents with chronic disease for transition to adult care: a technology program. Pediatrics. 2014;133(6):e1639–46.
75. Tornivuori A, Tuominen O, Salanterä S, Kosola S. A systematic review on randomized controlled trials: coaching elements of digital services to support chronically ill adolescents during transition of care. J Adv Nurs. 2020;76(6):1293–306.
76. Radovic A, McCarty CA, Katzman K, Richardson LP. Adolescents' perspectives on using technology for health: qualitative study. JMIR Pediatr Parent. 2018;1(1):e2.
77. Le Marne FA, Butler S, Beavis E, Gill D, Bye AME. EpApp: development and evaluation of a smartphone/tablet app for adolescents with epilepsy. J Clin Neurosci. 2018;50:214–20.
78. Yu CH, Guarna G, Tsao P, Jesuthasan JR, Lau AN, Siddiqi FS, et al. Incentivizing health care behaviors in emerging adults: a systematic review. Patient Prefer Adherence. 2016;10:371–81.
79. Virella Pérez YI, Medlow S, Ho J, Steinbeck K. Mobile and web-based apps that support self-management and transition in young people with chronic illness: systematic review. J Med Internet Res. 2019;21(11):e13579.
80. Got Transition. http://www.gottransition.org/.
81. Jones MR, Hooper TJ, Cuomo C, Crouch G, Hickam T, Lestishock L, et al. Evaluation of a health care transition improvement process in seven large health care systems. J Pediatr Nurs. 2019;47:44–50.
82. White PH, Ilango SM, Caskin AM, la Guardia MGA, McManus MA. Health care transition in school-based health centers: a pilot study. J Sch Nurs. 2020;38:1059840520975745.
83. Smith WR, Sisler IY, Johnson S, Lipato TJ, Newlin JS, Owens ZS, et al. Lessons learned from building a pediatric-to-adult sickle cell transition program. South Med J. 2019;112(3):190–7.
84. Timbie JW, Kranz AM, Mahmud A, Damberg CL. Specialty care access for Medicaid enrollees in expansion states. Am J Manag Care. 2019;25(3):e83–7.
85. Smithman MA, Brousselle A, Touati N, Boivin A, Nour K, Dubois CA, et al. Area deprivation and attachment to a general practitioner through centralized waiting lists: a cross-sectional study in Quebec, Canada. Int J Equity Health. 2018;17(1):176.
86. White PH, Cooley WC. Supporting the health care transition from adolescence to adulthood in the medical home. Pediatrics. 2018;142(5):e20182587.

Chapter 3
Genomic Endocrinology, Genome Sequencing, and Applications in Genetic Testing

Fady Hannah-Shmouni and Constantine A. Stratakis

Introduction

Medicine is an ever-changing art, continuously adjusting to the shifting principles of ethics and society and adapting the constant discoveries of science; this was beautifully said by Hippocrates: "…η δε ιητρικη νυν τε και αυτικα ου το αυτο ποιεει…" ("…*medicine does not do the same thing at this moment and the next…*") [1]. In the mid-1980s, two advances revolutionized medicine in a way that is comparable only to some of the most important events in the approximately 3000 years of its history. The first was theoretical; it was the introduction of the concept of "positional cloning," the idea that one can identify genes for human disease without knowing anything, or with knowing very little, about their function. The second was technical; the method of polymerase chain reaction (PCR) made DNA (the genome in essence) available to biomedical researchers and, more importantly, clinicians. Cancer medicine and traditional human genetics were the fields that benefited most from the first applications of the new genomic concepts and technologies. The human genome project (HGP) was then completed in 2003 using mostly PCR-based Sanger sequencing. The latter was expensive, laborious, and impractical for studying whole genomes; thus, HGP technologies that were grown out of necessity led to

F. Hannah-Shmouni
Division of Endocrinology, University of British Columbia, Vancouver, BC, Canada

C. A. Stratakis (✉)
Hormones, Athens, Greece

Human Genetics & Precision Medicine, IMBB, FORTH, Heraklion, Greece

Medical Genetics, H. Dunant Hospital, Athens, Greece

ELPEN Research Institute, Athens, Greece

NIH Clinical Center, SEGEN, NICHD, NIH, Bethesda, MD, USA

F. Hannah-Shmouni (ed.), *Familial Endocrine Cancer Syndromes*,
https://doi.org/10.1007/978-3-031-37275-9_3

the development of next-generation sequencing methods that are now widely available [2]. The HGP also determined that the human genome is composed of 3.3 billion pairs of nucleotide bases and that all human beings share 99.9% similarity at the DNA level with only 0.1% of genetic variation, the latter mostly due to single-nucleotide polymorphisms (SNPs). Thus, there are about ten million SNPs in the human genome. On the average, these SNPs occur once in every 300 nucleotides mostly in non-coding DNA that is located between approximately 20,000 and 25,000 coding genes. Decades after the first successful disease-causing gene identifications in endocrinology, the gene mutations in congenital adrenal hyperplasia (CAH), the insulin and steroid hormone receptors, and *RET, GNAS, MEN1, PTE,N* and *PRKAR1A* in the various forms of multiple endocrine tumor syndromes, a number of other genetic causes have been identified in diseases affecting the pituitary, thyroid, parathyroid, pancreas, adrenal, the gonads, and so on [3]. In fact, progress is so fast that we are already talking about post-genomic medicine in endocrinology [4]. However important these discoveries were in helping us understand cellular processes, glandular development, disease pathophysiology, even leading in some cases to new, molecularly designed treatments, it is only now that genomic medicine is in fact altering clinical practice. The changes are fast and far-reaching, from defining the genotypes of each one of us, to linking electronic medical records to genomic data, to direct-to-consumer genetic testing and its implications for patient-doctor interactions, disease surveillance, ethics and beyond. Hippocrates, again, noted that *"Medicine cannot be learned quickly because it is impossible to create any established principle in it, the way that a person who learns writing according to one system that people teach understands everything; for all who understand writing in the same way, do so because the same symbol does not sometimes become opposite, but is always steadfastly the same and not subject to chance. Medicine, on the other hand, does not do the same thing at this moment and the next, and it does opposite things to the same person, and at those things that are self-contradictory"* [1]. The continuous shifting of ideas and practices is indeed very real in modern medicine and endocrinology and is due to the advances of genetics.

Genetics in Pediatric and Adolescent Clinical Practice and Next-Generation Sequencing Applications

The vast majority of our pediatric and adolescent patients with genetic conditions including familial endocrine cancer syndromes were not, up until recently, candidates for genetic testing. For most practicing endocrinologists, encountering a patient with familial glucocorticoid resistance (FGR), for example, would be almost unheard of. In these rare cases, a referral to a research academic center would be the solution; there the patient of our example, with FGR, would undergo genetic testing that could lead to the identification of the causative mutation in the glucocorticoid receptor gene [5]. The discovery would lead to a publication but would remain relatively obscure for the average clinician. This was the case for most of medicine.

However, today, there are more than 10,000 rare diseases and even though each is extraordinarily rare (like FGR), collectively, these diseases affect large numbers of patients and represent an exceedingly disproportionate share of health care costs [6]. The International Rare Disease Research Consortium (IRDRC; Paris, France) estimates that a significant number of patients with rare diseases are seen and remain undiagnosed at clinical practices [6]. Several of our patients with complex symptoms and signs are now offered genetic testing in routine clinical settings.

In addition, the chances are that most clinicians in developed countries will encounter patients that have already been the recipients of direct-to-consumer genetic testing [7]. In February 2019, it was estimated that over 26 million people had taken home DNA tests. In 2015, a company known as "23andMe" was granted approval by the federal drug administration (FDA; MD, USA) to include health risk assessments in genetic reports. There are several such companies today from those providing direct-to-consumer genetic testing for ancestry and various traits for a relatively inexpensive fee, to others that provide full genome sequence analysis data and discuss health risks for a higher price.

Genetic testing is a powerful tool in clinical practice for patients and their families. The identification of the underlying genetic etiology will allow estimations of recurrence risk, which will inform family planning decisions, facilitate preimplantation genetic testing, and allow accurate prenatal screening. Additionally, genetic information will allow for the monitoring of disease progression and the introduction of timely treatment regimens to minimize complications and also provides important knowledge of the underlying disease mechanism or mechanisms. The complexity of these decisions, with their significant medical and psychosocial implications, is an important aspect of managing patients and their families.

The identification of the genes responsible for the various pediatric or adolescent familial endocrine cancer syndromes has enabled the genetic diagnosis and early identification of patients and their at-risk family members. Genetic testing in clinical practice for familial syndrome has become widely spread and considered routine in tertiary medical centers. Most pediatric syndromes are familial and rarely sporadic. When faced with a rare endocrinopathy in pediatrics, such as pheochromocytoma, Cushing disease or thyroid cancer, clinicians are encouraged to obtain a detailed family history and pedigree to deduce dominance and distinguish autosomal from X-linked inheritance. Pattern recognition, age of onset, radiological and histopathological features are key in distinguishing between the various CPSs. Thus, when a clinician encounters a pediatric patient with any of the syndromic features, genetic testing and counseling regardless of family history should be considered as many of these conditions may have decreased penetrance and first-degree relatives that are carriers may not be affected. A low threshold for exploring genetic testing is important particularly if the clinical phenotype warrants it. Genetic counseling and testing strategies in the pediatric population are not without complexities and ethical challenges which need to be considered. Screening should also be offered to a first-degree relative when a germline pathogenic variant in a disease-causing gene has been identified. Additionally, the identification of a germ-line pathogenic variant should prompt periodic clinical, biochemical, and radiological screening for the syndrome in question. Periodic reassessment of the medical literature and raw genetic data is encouraged to identify new genes or syndromes in individuals with a suspected syndrome and an unidentified genetic mutation.

Genetic screening may begin as early as infancy in at-risk individuals, especially with conditions that can manifest with early mortality, such as Carney complex, an autosomal dominant condition manifesting with multiple endocrine neoplasia. Given the complexity of choosing between the multiple candidate genes with overlapping clinical phenotypes, testing genes either singly or in a panel, particularly in patients without known syndromic features, should be considered. Several sequencing technologies exist. The growing availability and use of whole genome sequencing (WGS), whole exome sequencing (WES), whole genome arrays, and multigene panels increase the likelihood of detecting unintentionally or unexpectedly pathogenic mutations or variances of undetermined significance (e.g., detection of *TP53* mutations that predispose to adrenocortical cancers). After identifying a pathogenic mutation, pro-band's parents, siblings, and offsprings should be tested. If the mutation is transmitted in an autosomal dominant fashion, then each sibling has a 50% risk of having the mutation. In the case of *TP53* and other genes, if neither parent carries the mutation, the risk to siblings is low, but the possibility of germline mosaicism exists.

On another front, it is not unusual for the average clinical practitioner to encounter pharmacogenomics (PGx) [8]. For example, in testing for abnormal cortisol levels in response to the 1 mg overnight dexamethasone test, it is essential to know whether the patient is a rapid or slow dexamethasone metabolizer. There are several testing sites that now test for cytochrome P450, the liver enzymes responsible for dexamethasone metabolism. In areas of medicine other than endocrinology, PGx is already in daily practice from infectious diseases and the right choice of an antibiotic for a rapid or slow metabolizer, respectively, to how certain ethnic groups respond to a drug, based on gene-specific and ethnicity-related genetic variants. There are now more than 200 drugs that have PGx information included in their FDA-approved labels and new clinical practice guidelines based on PGx are now published frequently [9].

Finally, there is increasing use of genetic screening for preventive health and for prenatal diagnostic testing. There are several efforts across USA and other countries and in several health systems, private or government-run, to link cancer, cardiovascular, and other risk factors to medical records (electronic medical records and other types of records) with the intent to lead to behavior, diet and other modifications, diagnostic and even invasive procedures that prevent disease [8].

Non-invasive prenatal testing relies on the detection of cell-free DNA (cfDNA) on parental samples for the detection of trisomies and increasingly other genetic defects [10]. Non-invasive prenatal testing represents one of the fastest adopted tests by everyday clinical practice in the history of medicine and has revolutionized the detection of fetal aneuploidies and other disorders, obviating the need for amniocentesis and several other procedures [2, 10].

What made all the above possible were advances emanating from the HGP, mostly massively parallel DNA sequencing technologies, which were first introduced in 2005 and keep improving and becoming cheaper every day [2]. Collectively, these new DNA sequencing technologies are known as next-generation sequencing (NGS) and they can generate billions of short sequencing reads within hours; the current cost for a near-comprehensive determination of one's genome by NGS for both frequent and rare variants is approximately $1000, whereas the cost is significantly less for exome-only versions and even less if specific regions or a collection of genes are targeted [11, 12].

In addition to NGS, a product of HGP was high density DNA microarrays based on SNPs. They were first introduced in the late 1990s; however, at the beginning, these microarrays were mostly used in population- or other large cohort-based research studies to genotype human genomes for genetic variation and other association studies. Now, high density DNA microarrays are also used in clinical practice for the identification of structural variants of the human genome but also for the rapid identification of any sequence variation: in fact, the most popular genetic tests today are not sequencing-based tests, but genotyping tests utilizing technology derived from the DNA microarrays that were first developed by HGP researchers [11, 12].

It is hard to predict the future in which NGS is heading [2]. It is safe to say, however, that it will expand in ways and applications that will intrude in every aspect of medicine and indeed life. It is therefore essential for endocrinologists to understand the basics of NGS, how it is applied today, and its impact on how we practice medicine.

Genome Versus Exome Sequencing, Variant Interpretation, Other Challenges

The goal of NGS is to provide a high-quality map of genome variation for each sample. Whole genome sequencing (WGS) provides exactly that, with short-read NGS technology that is widely available today [12]. Yet, it remains prohibitively expensive for clinical use and cumbersome in data management. Since nearly 99% of the ~3.3 billion nucleotides that constitute the human genome do not code for proteins, and most human diseases are caused by variations of or defects of coding genes (the exome), the alternative approach is whole exome sequencing (WES), which currently costs less than $1000 and is widely available in developed countries.

Single-nucleotide variants and small insertion or deletion variants (indels) that are less than 50 base pairs (bp)-long represent most variants in the human genome: there are 3–4 million single-nucleotide variants and 0.4–0.5 million indels in every human sample when compared with the reference genome [12]. However, only approximately a few more than 100 lead to a premature stop codon for a coding gene and only about 20 or so are potentially deleterious in everyone. Nevertheless, practically every variant can cause a phenotype: the variants that change the sequence of molecules may affect the protein by an amino acid substitution—a deletion or an insertion—whereas the variants that do not change the sequence may affect binding of transcription factors, interactions with other molecules, RNA stability, and so on. Sequence variants that are identified by WGS or WES are reported, therefore, as variants of unknown significance because unless there is previously existing data documenting their function, they may not be called mutations and cannot be linked to disease or even a risk factor [11, 12].

Structural variation (SV) is another form of genome variation, by definition larger than 50 bp that includes copy number variants, which represent amplifications or deletions of variable size DNA segments, chromosomal rearrangements, and mobile element insertions [12]. SVs account for approximately 0.2% of total variants but they have much more of an effect on phenotype, representing, for example, as many as 4–12% of high-impact coding alleles. Their phenotypic effect typically is proportionate to their size, although exceptions to this rule exist. SVs are not easily detectable by short-read WGS and even less so by WES. Their architectural diversity also poses additional challenges in their detection. For one to see the impact of methodology, a typical human genome contains as many as 10,000 SVs detectable by the commonly used short-read WGS but more than 20,000 SVs identified by long-read WGS. The complexity of variant interpretation increases when one considers repetitive elements, such as short or variable number tandem repeats and mobile element insertions.

Functional annotation for each one of the variants, whether they are variants of unknown significance, SV (copy number variants or otherwise) or a repeat variant, is constantly updated based on information in publicly available databases to which genotypic and phenotypic data are added daily [8]. It is estimated that up to 25% of patients with a rare disease may be found to have a causative defect upon first application and reading of a WES test in specific cohorts studied by experienced clinical centers [6]. Due to continuously available new information, reanalysis of previously "negative" WES data may increase yield by more than 10% and even higher when family and other data are added to the analysis [6, 12].

Variants may be classified as pathogenic or likely pathogenic variants, and benign or likely benign, based on the structural effect on DNA and/or the coding gene or protein, functional studies, in silico data, variant frequency in control populations, family studies (segregation analysis), and other factors [13]. There are stringent and explicit guidelines followed now by all genetic testing laboratories and endorsed by professional societies. Variant assessment also includes carefully searching the available literature, but one must be careful with older nomenclature, different gene symbols, sequence numbering, and phenotypic interpretations.

During NGS, one may also identify what have been called "secondary" findings, which is understandable given the number of variations in the human genome, as stated above. Currently, the American College of Medical Genetics and Genomics (ACMGG; MD, USA) and other organizations have identified 59 medically actionable genes in which if variants are identified, they need to be reported as secondary findings, which may lead to additional testing and even invasive procedures [11,

13]. Examples include the *BRCA1* and *BRCA2* genes, associated with early breast, ovarian, and other cancers; *BMPR1A* and *SMAD4* associated with increased risk for colorectal and other cancers, and other genes [11].

NGS and Cell-Free (cf)DNA in Cancer Medicine and Prenatal Testing

Plasma-borne DNA was first described in 1948 but for years its origin and significance were unknown [11]. In the 1980s, it was realized that tissues such as tumors, the placenta, and the human fetus, shed DNA. In cancer medicine, cfDNA can lead to early detection, identification of the mutational profile of a given tumor, and provide means for follow-up as a tumor marker and in response to therapy. The notion of "liquid biopsy" is now well accepted in many oncological settings, despite the challenges that remain: the relatively low proportion of tumor-derived cfDNA in the circulation, the difficulty in assessing such abnormalities early during malignancy and the high rates of false positives [11].

On the other hand, sequence analysis of cfDNA fragments that circulate in the blood of pregnant women, along with the translation of this method into screening for fetal chromosome abnormalities, is clearly a great success story of modern genetics [2, 10]: as of late 2017, a total of 4–6 million pregnant women had had DNA from their plasma analyzed to screen for fetal aneuploidy [10]. During pregnancy, DNA fragments are released from the placenta into the maternal circulation; plasma contains both maternal and placental DNA and one calculates the ratio of placental to total cfDNA, which is known as the "fetal fraction," and increases as pregnancy advances. Testing is performed from the tenth week of gestation onward. The testing has revolutionized aneuploidy detection and obviated the need for more invasive procedures (for example, amniocentesis). However, there are issues with the relatively high rate of false positives, and the identification of secondary findings governed by the same ACMGG-sponsored guidelines referred to in the previous section [13].

NGS, Mosaicism and Its Applications in Detecting Somatic Genetic Defects

A "negative" WGS or WES in a tissue sample may be not only due to some of the issues discussed above but also due to the increasingly recognized as frequent issue of mosaicism: most commercially available NGS technologies may not detect mosaicism for a pathogenic variant because the latter may not be present in the tissue tested (for example, in peripheral blood in most cases), picking a variant at low levels from the "noise" of a sequence is often impossible (unless one increases the "depth" of the sequence), and mosaicism levels for a variant change with aging at various tissues (sequence variants detectable in blood in infancy may not be there in adolescence) [11]. There are new diagnostic tools under development to detect mosaicism but for most cases it remains a difficult issue to solve.

On the other hand, NGS is used frequently for the detection of the mutational spectrum in cancers [11]. Tumors have a hugely variable genome that offers diagnostic and treatment opportunities if identified by NGS. Just like what was mentioned above in cfDNA analysis, challenges include the relatively high heterogeneity of tumor samples, low frequency of single clonal DNA changes, and the high rate of false positivity.

In endocrine diseases, McCune-Albright syndrome is a classic disorder due to postzygotic mosaicism for an activating mutation of the *GNAS* gene [14]. NGS may be used for the detection of mosaicism in peripheral tissues since frequently the mutation is not detectable in peripheral blood. It is expected that the wider application of NGS will lead to the identification of many more instances of mosaicism in endocrine diseases, just like it did in other areas of medicine.

Disclosures Dr. Stratakis holds patents on technologies involving *GPR101*, *PRKAR1A, PDE11A*, and related genes causing adrenal, pituitary and other tumors. In addition, his laboratory has received research funding support by Pfizer Inc. for investigations on growth-hormone producing pituitary adenomas. Dr. Stratakis has consulting relationships with ELPEN, Sterotherapeutics, Human Longevity, Lundbeck pharmaceuticals, and sits in the Editorial Boards of several journals.

Funding This study was supported in part by the Intramural Research Program of the *Eunice Kennedy Shriver* National Institute of Child Health & Human Development, National Institutes of Health (project number Z1A HD008920), and now by intramural funding of the Foundation for Research & Technology Hellas, Heraklion, Greece.

Author Contribution Statement All authors have contributed to the conception, design and execution of the study, and the writing of the manuscript.

References

1. Potter P, editor. Hippocrates "places in man". Cambridge, MA: Harvard University Press; 1995. p. 81.
2. Green ED, Rubin EM, Olson MV. The future of DNA sequencing. Nature. 2017;550:179–81.
3. Stratakis CA. Clinical genetics of multiple endocrine neoplasias, Carney complex and related syndromes. J Endocr Invest. 2001;24(5):370–83.
4. Stratakis CA. Genetics and the new (precision) medicine and endocrinology: in medias res or ab initio? Endocrinol Metab Clin North Am. 2017;46(2):xv–xvi.

5. Stratakis CA, Karl M, Schulte HM, Chrousos GP. Glucocorticoid resistance in humans: elucidation of the molecular mechanisms and implications for pathophysiology. Ann N Y Acad Sci. 1994;746:362–76.
6. Boycott KM, Hartley T, Biesecker LG, et al. A diagnosis for all rare genetic diseases; the horizon and the next frontiers. Cell. 2018;177:32–7.
7. Crow D. A new wave of genomics for all. Cell. 2018;177:5–7.
8. Abul-Husn NS, Kenny EE. Personalized medicine and the power of electronic health records. Cell. 2018;177:58–69.
9. Sirugo G, Williams SW, Tishkoff SA. The missing diversity in human genetic studies. Cell. 2018;177:26–31.
10. Bianchi DW, Chiu RWK. Sequencing of circulating cell-free DNA during pregnancy. N Engl J Med. 2018;379:464–73.
11. Shendure J, Findlay GM, Snyder MW. Genomic medicine—progress, pitfalls, and promise. Cell. 2018;177:45–57.
12. Lappalainen T, Scott AJ, Brandt M, Hal IM. Genomic analysis in the age of human genome sequencing. Cell. 2018;177:70–84.
13. Richards S, Aziz N, Bale S, et al. Standards and guidelines for the interpretation of sequence variants: a joint consensus recommendation of the American College of Medical Genetics and Genomics and the Association for Molecular Pathology. Genet Med. 2015;17(5):405–24.
14. Salpea P, Stratakis CA. Carney complex and McCune Albright syndrome: an overview of clinical manifestations and human molecular genetics. Mol Cell Endocrinol. 2014;386(1–2):85–91.

Chapter 4
Familial Endocrine Cancer Syndromes with Pediatric and Adolescent Presentation

Joselyne Tessa Tonleu, Rachel Wurth, and Skand Shekhar

Introduction

Benign and malignant endocrine neoplasms in childhood and adolescence form a widely heterogeneous group of disorders often presenting with subtle clinical or biochemical features that are often missed or misdiagnosed during a clinical encounter [1]. Endocrine neoplasia developing in young patients are quite characteristic for certain familial endocrine cancer syndromes that are usually inherited. A wide spectrum of non-malignant and malignant tumors within each syndrome exists, with poor genotype-to-phenotype correlation [1]. Thus, experienced clinicians working in established centers of excellence are best suited to care for at-risk or affected individuals with these syndromes.

The identification of the genes responsible for various pediatric-onset familial endocrinopathies has enabled the genetic diagnosis and early identification of patients and their at-risk family members [1]. Most pediatric endocrine syndromes are familial and rarely sporadic (Table 4.1). When faced with a rare endocrine neoplasm in pediatric patients, such as pheochromocytoma, Cushing disease and thyroid cancer, pattern recognition, age of onset, radiological and histopathological features are key in distinguishing various subtypes (Table 4.1). Genetic testing in

J. T. Tonleu
Clinical Research Branch, National Institute of Environmental Health Sciences, National Institutes of Health (NIH), Research Triangle Park, NC, USA

R. Wurth
Mayo Clinic Graduate School of Biomedical Sciences, Mayo Clinic, Rochester, MN, USA

S. Shekhar (✉)
Clinical Research Branch, National Institute of Environmental Health Sciences, National Institutes of Health (NIH), Research Triangle Park, NC, USA
e-mail: skand.shekhar@nih.gov

F. Hannah-Shmouni (ed.), *Familial Endocrine Cancer Syndromes*,
https://doi.org/10.1007/978-3-031-37275-9_4

Table 4.1 Genetics and pathogenesis of familial endocrine cancer syndromes

Familial Endocrine Cancer Syndrome	Genetics and Pathogensis
Multiple endocrine neoplasia type 1 [1]	• *MEN1*, autosomal dominant
	• Gastro-entero-pancreatic neuroendocrine tumors (typically pancreatic), primary hyperparathyroidism adrenocortical tumors, pituitary tumors
	• Multiple facial angiofibromas, collagenomas, lipomas
Multiple endocrine neoplasia type 2a/familial medullary thyroid carcinoma [2, 3]	• *RET*, autosomal dominant
	• Medullary thyroid cancer, primary hyperparathyroidism, pheochromocytoma, and paragangliomas, pituitary adenoma
	• Cutaneous lichen amyloidosis
Multiple endocrine neoplasia type 2b (also referred to as MEN-3) [4, 5]	• *RET*, autosomal dominant
	• Medullary thyroid cancer, C-cell hyperplasia, pituitary adenoma (seen in MEN2A)
	• Lip/tongue/eyelid mucosal neuromas, medullated corneal nerve fibers, marfanoid habitus, ganglioneuromatosis of the GI tract
Multiple endocrine neoplasia type 4 [1, 6]	• *CDKN1B*, other
	• Primary hyperparathyroidism, adrenocortical tumors, neuroendocrine tumors, pituitary adenoma, differentiated thyroid carcinoma
	• Tumors of the kidney, ovary, meninges
von Hippel-Lindau [7, 8]	• *VHL*, autosomal dominant
	• Pancreatic neuroendocrine tumors, pheochromocytoma and paragangliomas
	• Renal cysts, renal cell carcinoma (clear cell), hemangioblastoma (retina/CNS) endolymphatic sac tumors, pancreatic cysts, cystadenomas of the epididymis and broad ligament
Neurofibromatosis type 1 [9, 10]	• *NF1*, autosomal dominant
	• Pheochromocytoma and paragangliomas, growth hormone excess, precocious puberty, pituitary adenomas, neuroendocrine tumors
	• Gastrointestinal stromal tumors, axillary/inguinal freckling, neurofibroma, malignant peripheral nerve sheath tumor, lisch nodules, optic pathway glioma, learning disabilities, café-au-lait spots
X-linked acrogigantism [11, 12]	• *GPR101*, sporadic > AD
	• Pituitary adenoma, somatotropinoma or somatomammotropinoma
PTEN hamartoma tumor syndrome [13–15]	• *PTEN*, autosomal dominant
	• Nodular thyroid hyperplasia
	• Thyroid carcinoma, macrocephaly, autism/developmental delay, skin features (oral papillomas, trichilemmomas, lipomas, penile freckling), gastrointestinal polyps, arteriovenous malformations, hemangioma

(continued)

Table 4.1 (continued)

Familial Endocrine Cancer Syndrome	Genetics and Pathogensis
Beckwith-Wiedemann syndrome [16, 17]	• *CDKN1C*, other; variable inheritance
	• Adrenocortical cancer, hyperinsulinism, cytomegaly of the fetal adrenal cortex
	• Wilms tumor, hepatoblastoma, lateralized overgrowth, macrosomia, macroglossia, omphalocele/umbilical hernia, neonatal hypoglycemia
Carney complex [18, 19]	• *PRKAR1A*, other; autosomal dominant
	• Primary pigmented nodular adrenocortical disease, thyroid cancer, pituitary adenoma
	• Skin pigmentary anomalies (lentigines), myxoma of the heart, breast and skin, large calcifying Sertoli cell tumors of the testis, psammomatous melanotic schwannomas
Carney-Stratakis syndrome [20]	• *SDHA*, *SDHB*, *SDHC*, *SDHD*; autosomal dominant
	• Pheochromocytoma and paragangliomas, adrenocortical tumors
	• Gastrointestinal stromal tumors
Carney triad [21, 22]	• *SDHC* promoter methylation
	• Pheochromocytoma and paragangliomas, adrenocortical tumors, primary pigmented nodular adrenocortical disease (PPNAD)
	• Gastrointestinal stromal tumors, pulmonary chondroma, esophageal leiomyoma, sarcoma
DICER1 syndrome [23–25]	• *DICER1*, autosomal dominant
	• Multinodular goiter, pituitary blastoma, differentiated thyroid carcinoma
	• Pleuropulmonary blastoma, ovarian Sertoli-Leydig cell tumor, cystic nephroma, embryonal rhabdomyosarcoma of the cervix, ciliary body medulloepithelioma, pineoblastoma
Familial adenomatous polyposis [26, 27]	• *APC*, autosomal dominant
	• Non-medullary thyroid carcinoma
	• Gastrointestinal adenomas, colorectal cancer, desmoid tumors, Gardner fibroma, hepatoblastoma, medulloblastoma, odontomas, osteomas
Familial isolated pituitary adenoma [28]	• *AIP*, autosomal dominant
	• Pituitary adenoma, including somatotropinoma, somatomammotropinoma, corticotropinoma, prolactinoma, and non-functional adenoma
Familial pheochromocytoma and paraganglioma [29]	• *SDHA*, *SDHB*, *SDHC*, *SDHD*, *SDHAF2*; autosomal dominant
	• Pheochromocytoma and paraganglioma
	• Renal cell carcinoma

(continued)

Table 4.1 (continued)

Familial Endocrine Cancer Syndrome	Genetics and Pathogensis
Hereditary leiomyomatosis renal cell carcinoma [30–32]	• *FH*, autosomal dominant
	• Renal cell carcinoma (papillary type II), cutaneous and uterine leiomyomatosis
	• Pheochromocytoma and paragangliomas, adrenocortical tumors, primary bilateral macronodular adrenocortical hyperplasia
Hyperparathyroidism-jaw tumor syndrome/familial isolated hyperparathyroidism [33]	• *CDC73*, autosomal dominant
	• Primary hyperparathyroidism, parathyroid carcinoma
	• Ossifying fibroma of the jaw, renal cysts, and tumors
Li-Fraumeni syndrome [34]	• *TP53*, autosomal dominant
	• Adrenocortical cancer
	• Hypodiploid acute lymphoblastic leukemia, pre-menopausal breast cancer, choroid plexus carcinoma, brain tumors, bone and soft-tissue sarcomas
Werner syndrome [35]	• *WRN*, autosomal recessive
	• Premature features of normal aging starting in the second decade and the development of multiple cancer types including non-medullary thyroid cancer

clinical practice for familial syndrome has become widely spread and considered routine in tertiary medical centers [36]. Most pediatric and adolescent cancer-predisposing syndromes are familial and rarely sporadic. Thus, when a clinician encounters a pediatric patient with any of the syndromic features, genetic testing, and counseling, regardless of family history should be considered as many of these conditions may have decreased penetrance and first-degree relatives that are carriers may not be affected. This review outlines several familial multiple neoplasia syndromes with prominent endocrine presentations, summarized in Table 4.1.

Syndromes with Prominent Endocrine Presentations

Multiple Endocrine Neoplasia, Type 1

Background and Prevalence

Multiple endocrine neoplasia type 1 (MEN-1, OMIM #131100) is an autosomal dominant disorder caused by heterozygous germline pathogenic variants in the *MEN1* gene [36] (Table 4.1). The clinical manifestations of MEN-1 can vary substantially, with over 20 reported endocrine and non-endocrine tumors [36]. However, three endocrine tumors are common features of the disease, including parathyroid hyperplasia with hyperparathyroidism, anterior pituitary adenomas, and entero-pancreatic tumors [1, 37]. The presence of two of the three main endocrine tumors, along with family history of one case of MEN-1 and one first-degree relative with at least one of the three main endocrine tumors, and genetic screening strongly supports a diagnosis of MEN-1 [36]. Age of affected individuals can range from 5 to 82 years, but 83% of MEN-1 patients present after the age of 21 [38] and 12% of MEN-1 patients will receive a diagnosis in the first two decades of life [1, 39]. A study of 734 MEN-1 patients indicated a 57.8% female predominance, indicating the disease may have a slight female predilection, and a delayed diagnosis in women [39]. The prevalence of MEN-1 in the general population is estimated at 1:30,000 [1].

Clinical Characteristics

Parathyroid hyperplasia with hyperparathyroidism is present in 90% of MEN-1 patients with nearly 100% penetrance by age 50 [1, 36, 37]. Typical age of onset is between 20 and 25 but presentation as early as 4 has been reported [1, 37]. Hyperparathyroidism is typically mild, and the recommended treatment is a subtotal parathyroidectomy, a 3 and ½ gland resection, and associated removal of the cervical thymus [38]. Rarely, parathyroid carcinoma may occur, and indicates a poor prognosis [39].

Anterior pituitary adenomas previously associated with MEN-1 include: prolactinomas, growth hormone (GH)-secreting, TSH-secreting, ACTH-secreting, and non-functioning adenomas, with prolactinomas occurring most frequently [36]. While the prevalence of pituitary adenomas is 45%, less than 10% of MEN-1 cases will present with a pituitary adenoma initially [1, 37]. A prolactinoma variant of MEN-1 with an unusually high penetrance of prolactinomas and low penetrance of gastrinomas has been reported [37, 40, 41].

Gastro-entero-pancreatic neuroendocrine tumors are found in 30–75% of MEN-1 patients [1, 37]. They can present as Zollinger-Ellison syndrome (ZES), which has a prevalence of 20–25% of MEN-1 and an earlier age of onset [42]. The development of medical therapies, such as proton pump inhibitors and Histamine H2-receptor antagonists, have reduced the mortality in MEN-1 due to uncontrolled gastric acid secretion associated with ZES [38].

Pancreatic adenomas or carcinomas in MEN-1 remain life-threatening due to limitations in detection until they gain biochemical activity and become invasive [37, 40]. While glucagonomas and VIPomas occur occasionally, insulinomas, which typically manifest as a single benign nodule with multiple islet macroadenomas, are the second most common functioning pancreatic tumors in MEN-1 [38, 39].

Adrenocortical tumors, which are typically non-functioning bilateral hyperplasia or adenomas, occur in 36–41% of MEN-1 patients [1, 37]. Additional adrenal manifestations include adrenocortical carcinoma in 1.4– 6% of cases, and pheochromocytomas [36, 37, 39].

Additionally, tumors previously reported in MEN-1 include cutaneous and visceral lipomas, facial angiofibromas, collagenomas, as well as thymic, gastric, and bronchopulmonary carcinoid tumors [36, 37]. Approximately 33% of patients have lipomas, which are typically non-recurrent after surgical resection. Multiple facial angiofibromas occur in 40–80% of MEN-1 cases [37]. Ultimately, carcinoid tumors in MEN-1 are rare, however, type II gastric enterochromaffin-like cell carcinoid tumors occur more frequently. Thymic carcinoid tumors have also been reported, more frequently in men compared to women and are often treated with a thymectomy [37, 38].

Multiple Endocrine Neoplasia, Type 2

Background and Prevalence

Multiple endocrine neoplasia type 2 (MEN-2) is an autosomal dominant disorder caused by activating pathogenic variants in the rearranged during transfection (*RET*) proto-oncogene (Table 4.1). The syndrome primarily affects three endocrine glands: the thyroid, adrenal, and parathyroid glands. MEN-2 can be subclassified into three phenotypic presentations: MEN-2A (OMIM #171400), MEN-2B (OMIM #162300, also referred to as MEN-3), and familial medullary thyroid carcinoma (FMTC, OMIM #155240) although FMTC is thought to be a variant of MEN-2A [2, 37, 43, 44]. MEN-2A makes up the majority (70–80%) of all MEN-2 cases whereas MEN-2B is the least frequent but most aggressive phenotype [37, 45]. Biochemical screening for tumors associated with the MEN-2 syndrome will be positive in 93% of disease carriers by 31 years of age [46]. The prevalence of MEN-2 in the general population is estimated at 1:35,000 [2].

Clinical Characteristics

While each subclassification of MEN-2 has discrete phenotypic characteristics, all have a high penetrance for medullary thyroid cancer (MTC), with approximately 90% of patients showing some evidence of MTC [37, 47]. MEN-2A is characterized by MTC, pheochromocytoma, and multi-gland parathyroid tumors [2, 37]. MTC often acts as the first sign of MEN-2A, typically around the ages of 20–30, with C-cell hyperplasia and multifocal carcinomas affecting the thyroid bilaterally [38, 45, 48]. In both MEN-2A and MEN-2B, bilateral MTC occurs in 100% of patients and bilateral (sometimes unilateral) pheochromocytomas affect approximately 50% of patients. Of the classifications of MEN-2, only MEN-2A presents with primary hyperparathyroidism in 20–30% of cases [37, 38, 45]. Unlike other subgroups, 20–30% of MEN-2A patients also develop parathyroid hyperplasia and adenomas [37]. Non-endocrine presentations which may occur in MEN-2A include Hirschsprung's disease [2, 37, 45].

The MEN-2B phenotype includes characteristic facial features such as enlarged lips and eyelids, marfanoid habitus, and mucosal neuromas of the lips and tongue in addition to MTC and pheochromocytomas [2, 37]. MTC presents in the first year of life, is more aggressive, has greater metastatic potential and occurs universally in

MEN-2B patients [37, 45]. If left untreated, MTC may lead to mortality by age 30 [38]. Other MEN-2B manifestations include gastrointestinal symptoms, and gastrointestinal ganglioneuromatosis occurs in approximately 40% of MEN-2B patients [4, 49, 50].

Patients with a family history of MEN-2 and a *RET* mutation should be screened at 5 years of age (or earlier). Surgical removal of the thyroid gland is recommended if found to be affected during screening and if the thyroid gland is affected, it should be surgically removed. Given the lethality of MTC in MEN-2B, thyroidectomy and central lymph node dissection should be performed early. Management of a confirmed pheochromocytoma takes precedence over MTC and usually includes a unilateral or bilateral adrenalectomy [38].

FMTC presents with isolated MTC and a very low likelihood of developing endocrine or non-endocrine manifestations of the MEN-2 syndrome. FMTC accounts for 10–20% of all MEN-2 cases, however, the prevalence may be underestimated due to the absence of other signs and symptoms outside of MTC, which complicates the diagnosis [2, 45, 47].

Multiple Endocrine Neoplasia, Type 4

Background and Prevalence

Multiple endocrine neoplasia, type 4 (OMIM #610755) is the most recently recognized MEN phenotype [1, 51, 52] (Table 4.1). In 2006, MEN-4 was recognized in rat models who developed pituitary adenomas, thyroid C-cell hyperplasia, parathyroid hyperplasia, as well as intra- and extra-adrenal pheochromocytomas due to a pathogenic variant in the cyclin-dependent kinase inhibitor 1B (*CDKN1B*) gene [1]. This finding led to the MEN-4 subclassification, which has been reported less than 30 times to date. Therefore, accurate assessments of prevalence, penetrance, and genotype-to-phenotype correlations have not been performed [6, 51].

Clinical Characteristics

A formal clinical guideline for the diagnosis of MEN-4 has not been established, however, the diagnosis is typically ascertained by age 40. The most frequently reported manifestations of MEN-4 are parathyroid hyperplasia or adenomas, pituitary adenoma, and entero-pancreatic neuroendocrine tumors [1, 6, 51].

There is considerable overlap between the clinical manifestations in MEN-1 and MEN-4, with some differences [51]. Hyperparathyroidism has an incidence rate of 81% and is most frequently due to a parathyroid tumor. Compared to MEN-1, hyperparathyroidism has a later age of onset in MEN-4, ranging from ages 46 to 74 [1, 51]. Pituitary adenomas occur in 41% of MEN-4 patients. The absence of prolactinomas in MEN-4 distinguishes it from MEN-1, however, gastrinomas and non-functioning pancreatic tumors occur in approximately 25% of MEN-4 patients [6]. Adrenal masses, neuroendocrine carcinomas of the cervix, as well as bronchial and stomach carcinoid tumors have been reported in MEN-4 [6, 51].

von Hippel-Lindau Syndrome

Background and Prevalence

von Hippel-Lindau syndrome (VHL) is an autosomal dominant multi-tumoral syndrome caused by germline pathogenic variants in the *VHL* gene encoding the VHL protein (pVHL) and has [1] a prevalence of 1:36,000 among live births [53]. VHL is characterized by highly vascularized tumors, including CNS and retinal hemangioblastomas, clear cell renal cell carcinoma (ccRCC), pheochromocytomas and paragangliomas (PHEO/PGL), and pancreatic neuroendocrine tumors (pNET) [1, 54, 55]. Most children (80%) have an affected parent, however, 20% of cases are due to de novo pathogenic variants [1, 55].

Clinical Characteristics

Clinical manifestations of VHL syndrome vary within and between affected families, but most commonly include CNS and retinal hemangioblastomas, ccRCC, PHEO/PGL, and endolymphatic sac tumors (ESTs) [54]. Patients usually develop VHL syndrome between the ages of 18 and 30, with a mean age of onset of 26 [53]. Patients without a family history must present with at least two main tumor presentations and a *VHL* pathogenic variant, whereas only one tumor manifestation is required when a family history is present [54–56]. VHL syndrome has been subclassified into Type 1 and Types 2a, 2b, and 2c, based upon genotype–phenotype characteristics [1, 53, 57] (Table 4.2).

CNS hemangioblastomas are the most frequent tumor presentation in VHL and the leading cause of mortality [1, 56]. Hemangioblastomas occur in 60–80% of patients and are most commonly localized in the cerebellum, spinal cord, and brain stem [58]. Retinal hemangioblastomas have a prevalence of 70% and are often multifocal and bilateral [54, 59]. The second leading cause of mortality in VHL syndrome patients is ccRCC [1, 56] with a mean onset age of 39% and 70% of affected patients developing the tumor by age 60 [54, 59].

PHEO/PGL occur in 10–20% of patients with a mean age of onset of 20–25 years [1, 59]. PGLs are usually non-functional and affect the sympathetic axis of the thorax and abdomen [54]. Approximately 47% of VHL syndrome patients develop pNETs, with a mean age of onset of 33–35 years and the greatest risk of onset by late 30s. pNETs are typically multifocal and non-functional, whereas pancreatic lesions are cystic and uniformly distributed across the pancreas [54, 60].

Table 4.2 Genetic and phenotypic characteristics of von Hippel-Lindau (VHL) syndrome subtypes. **Source:** [54]

von Hippel-Lindau syndrome subtypes			
Type 1	Type 2A	Type 2B	Type 2C
Type 1b with pathogenic truncating and exon deletions (1a), or gene deletions (1b) and a 0.5–10% risk of developing pheochromocytoma and paraganglioma	All Type 2 are characterized by missense pathogenic variants and a >60% chance of developing tumors	Type 2b is associated with a higher risk for renal cell carcinoma	Type 2c patients present with pheochromocytoma
Presents a reduced risk for renal cell carcinoma	Type 2a is associated with a low risk for renal cell carcinoma	Type 2b consists of clear cell renal cell carcinoma, and in some cases, type 2a tumors	
The risk of tumors is non-existent or less than 10%	Presence of retinal and CNS hemangioblastomas and pheochromocytomas		

ESTs occur in 10–16% of patients with VHL; however, bilateral ESTs are pathognomonic and occur in 30% of patients with ESTs [56]. The average age of diagnosis with this tumor is 28 years [56]. Rarely, adenomas are bilateral and may lead to infertility [54]. Interestingly, papillary cystadenomas, the female equivalent, are extremely rare [54, 59].

Conclusion

There are a host of familial endocrine neoplasms that occur in childhood and adolescence. Our improved understanding of these syndromes coupled with advancements in genetics has enabled improved recognition and care of these patients. Due to complexities and nuances in the management of these syndromes, experienced clinicians working in established centers are best suited to care for these patients.

References

1. Goudie C, et al. 65 YEARS OF THE DOUBLE HELIX: endocrine tumour syndromes in children and adolescents. Endocr Relat Cancer. 2018;25(8):T221–44.
2. Charis E. Multiple endocrine neoplasia type 2. In: Adam MP, Mirzaa GM, Pagon RA, et al., editors. GeneReviews®. Seattle, WA: University of Washington, Seattle; 1999.
3. Verga U, et al. Frequent association between MEN 2A and cutaneous lichen amyloidosis. Clin Endocrinol. 2003;59(2):156–61.

4. Cohen MS, et al. Gastrointestinal manifestations of multiple endocrine neoplasia type 2. Ann Surg. 2002;235(5):648–54; discussion 654–5.
5. Moline J, Eng C. Multiple endocrine neoplasia type 2: an overview. Genet Med. 2011;13(9):755–64.
6. Frederiksen A, et al. Clinical features of multiple endocrine neoplasia type 4: novel pathogenic variant and review of published cases. J Clin Endocrinol Metab. 2019;104(9):3637–46.
7. Kim E, Zschiedrich S. Renal cell carcinoma in von Hippel-Lindau disease-from tumor genetics to novel therapeutic strategies. Front Pediatr. 2018;6:16.
8. Castro-Teles J, et al. Pheochromocytomas and paragangliomas in von Hippel-Lindau disease: not a needle in a haystack. Endocr Connect. 2021;10(11):R293–304.
9. Adil A, Koritala T, Munakomi S, et al. Neurofibromatosis type 1. In: StatPearls. Treasure Island, FL: StatPearls Publishing; 2023.
10. Gruber LM, et al. Pheochromocytoma and paraganglioma in patients with neurofibromatosis type 1. Clin Endocrinol. 2017;86(1):141–9.
11. Beckers A, et al. X-linked acrogigantism syndrome: clinical profile and therapeutic responses. Endocr Relat Cancer. 2015;22(3):353–67.
12. Gadelha MR, Kasuki L, Korbonits M. The genetic background of acromegaly. Pituitary. 2017;20(1):10–21.
13. Plamper M, et al. Phenotype-driven diagnostic of PTEN hamartoma tumor syndrome: macrocephaly, but neither height nor weight development, is the important trait in children. Cancers (Basel). 2019;11(7):975.
14. Tan WH, et al. The spectrum of vascular anomalies in patients with PTEN mutations: implications for diagnosis and management. J Med Genet. 2007;44(9):594–602.
15. Smith JR, et al. Thyroid nodules and cancer in children with PTEN hamartoma tumor syndrome. J Clin Endocrinol Metab. 2011;96(1):34–7.
16. Brioude F, et al. Mutations of the imprinted CDKN1C gene as a cause of the overgrowth Beckwith-Wiedemann syndrome: clinical spectrum and functional characterization. Hum Mutat. 2015;36(9):894–902.
17. Borjas Mendoza PA, Mendez MD. Beckwith Wiedemann syndrome. In: StatPearls. Treasure Island, FL: StatPearls Publishing; 2023.
18. Horvath A, Stratakis CA. Carney complex and lentiginosis. Pigment Cell Melanoma Res. 2009;22(5):580–7.
19. Stergiopoulos SG, et al. Pituitary pathology in Carney complex patients. Pituitary. 2004;7(2):73–82.
20. Stratakis CA, Carney JA. The triad of paragangliomas, gastric stromal tumours and pulmonary chondromas (Carney triad), and the dyad of paragangliomas and gastric stromal sarcomas (Carney-Stratakis syndrome): molecular genetics and clinical implications. J Intern Med. 2009;266(1):43–52.
21. Daumova M, et al. SDHC methylation pattern in patients with Carney triad. Appl Immunohistochem Mol Morphol. 2021;29(8):599–605.
22. Boikos SA, et al. Carney triad can be (rarely) associated with germline succinate dehydrogenase defects. Eur J Hum Genet. 2016;24(4):569–73.
23. Khan NE, et al. Quantification of thyroid cancer and multinodular Goiter risk in the DICER1 syndrome: a family-based cohort study. J Clin Endocrinol Metab. 2017;102(5):1614–22.
24. Doros L, et al. DICER1 mutations in embryonal rhabdomyosarcomas from children with and without familial PPB-tumor predisposition syndrome. Pediatr Blood Cancer. 2012;59(3):558–60.
25. Liu APY, et al. Clinical outcomes and complications of pituitary blastoma. J Clin Endocrinol Metab. 2021;106(2):351–63.
26. Carr S, Anup K. Familial adenomatous polyposis. In: StatPearls. Treasure Island, FL: StatPearls Publishing; 2023.
27. Schäfer M, et al. Neonatal Gardner fibroma leads to detection of familial adenomatous polyposis: two case reports. Eur J Pediatr Surg Rep. 2016;4(1):17–21.

28. Beckers A, et al. Familial isolated pituitary adenomas (FIPA) and the pituitary adenoma predisposition due to mutations in the aryl hydrocarbon receptor interacting protein (AIP) gene. Endocr Rev. 2013;34(2):239–77.
29. Else T, Greenberg S, Fishbein L. Hereditary paraganglioma-pheochromocytoma syndromes. In: Adam MP, Mirzaa GM, Pagon RA, et al., editors. GeneReviews®. Seattle, WA: University of Washington, Seattle; 2008.
30. Alam NA, et al. Genetic and functional analyses of FH mutations in multiple cutaneous and uterine leiomyomatosis, hereditary leiomyomatosis and renal cancer, and fumarate hydratase deficiency. Hum Mol Genet. 2003;12(11):1241–52.
31. Menko FH, et al. Hereditary leiomyomatosis and renal cell cancer (HLRCC): renal cancer risk, surveillance and treatment. Familial Cancer. 2014;13(4):637–44.
32. Charchar HLS, Fragoso MCBV. An overview of the heterogeneous causes of cushing syndrome resulting from primary macronodular adrenal hyperplasia (PMAH). J Endocr Soc. 2022;6(5):bvac041.
33. Mehta A, et al. Hyperparathyroidism-jaw tumor syndrome: results of operative management. Surgery. 2014;156(6):1315–24; discussion 1324–5.
34. Swaminathan M, et al. Hematologic malignancies and Li-Fraumeni syndrome. Cold Spring Harb Mol Case Stud. 2019;5(1):a003210.
35. Oshima J, Martin GM, Hisama FM. Werner syndrome. In: Adam MP, Mirzaa GM, Pagon RA, et al., editors. GeneReviews®. Seattle, WA: University of Washington, Seattle; 2002.
36. Giusti F, Marini F, Brandi ML. Multiple endocrine neoplasia type 1. In: GeneReviews®. Seattle, WA: University of Washington, Seattle; 2022.
37. Brandi ML, et al. Guidelines for diagnosis and therapy of MEN type 1 and type 2. J Clin Endocrinol Metab. 2001;86(12):5658–71.
38. Norton JA, Krampitz G, Jensen RT. Multiple endocrine neoplasia: genetics and clinical management. Surg Oncol Clin N Am. 2015;24(4):795–832.
39. Mele C, et al. Phenotypes associated with MEN1 syndrome: a focus on genotype-phenotype correlations. Front Endocrinol (Lausanne). 2020;11:591501.
40. Skogseid B, et al. Multiple endocrine neoplasia type 1: a 10-year prospective screening study in four kindreds. J Clin Endocrinol Metab. 1991;73(2):281–7.
41. Marx S, et al. Multiple endocrine neoplasia type 1: clinical and genetic topics. Ann Intern Med. 1998;129(6):484–94.
42. Roy PK, et al. Zollinger-Ellison syndrome. Clinical presentation in 261 patients. Medicine (Baltimore). 2000;79(6):379–411.
43. Donis-Keller H, et al. Mutations in the RET proto-oncogene are associated with MEN 2A and FMTC. Hum Mol Genet. 1993;2(7):851–6.
44. Mulligan LM, et al. Germ-line mutations of the RET proto-oncogene in multiple endocrine neoplasia type 2A. Nature. 1993;363(6428):458–60.
45. Romei C, et al. Genetic and clinical features of multiple endocrine neoplasia types 1 and 2. J Oncol. 2012;2012:705036.
46. Easton DF, et al. The clinical and screening age-at-onset distribution for the MEN-2 syndrome. Am J Hum Genet. 1989;44(2):208–15.
47. Wells SA Jr, et al. Revised American Thyroid Association guidelines for the management of medullary thyroid carcinoma. Thyroid. 2015;25(6):567–610.
48. Machens A, et al. Early malignant progression of hereditary medullary thyroid cancer. N Engl J Med. 2003;349(16):1517–25.
49. Barwick KW. Gastrointestinal manifestations of multiple endocrine neoplasia, type IIB. J Clin Gastroenterol. 1983;5(1):83–7.
50. Wray CJ, et al. Failure to recognize multiple endocrine neoplasia 2B: more common than we think? Ann Surg Oncol. 2008;15(1):293–301.
51. Lee M, Pellegata NS. Multiple endocrine neoplasia type 4. Front Horm Res. 2013;41:63–78.
52. Pellegata NS, et al. Germ-line mutations in p27Kip1 cause a multiple endocrine neoplasia syndrome in rats and humans. Proc Natl Acad Sci U S A. 2006;103(42):15558–63.

53. Ben-Skowronek I, Kozaczuk S. Von Hippel-Lindau syndrome. Horm Res Paediatr. 2015;84(3):145–52.
54. van Leeuwaarde RS, Ahmad S, Links TP, et al. Von Hippel-Lindau syndrome. In: Adam MP, Mirzaa GM, Pagon RA, et al., editors. GeneReviews®. Seattle, WA: University of Washington, Seattle; 2000.
55. Nielsen SM, et al. Von Hippel-Lindau disease: genetics and role of genetic counseling in a multiple neoplasia syndrome. J Clin Oncol. 2016;34(18):2172–81.
56. Dornbos D III, et al. Review of the neurological implications of von Hippel-Lindau disease. JAMA Neurol. 2018;75(5):620–7.
57. Kim WY, Kaelin WG. Role of VHL gene mutation in human cancer. J Clin Oncol. 2004;22(24):4991–5004.
58. Maher ER, Neumann HP, Richard S. von Hippel-Lindau disease: a clinical and scientific review. Eur J Hum Genet. 2011;19(6):617–23.
59. Lonser RR, et al. von Hippel-Lindau disease. Lancet. 2003;361(9374):2059–67.
60. Keutgen XM, et al. Evaluation and management of pancreatic lesions in patients with von Hippel-Lindau disease. Nat Rev Clin Oncol. 2016;13(9):537–49.

Chapter 5
Familial Thyroid Cancer Syndromes in Children and Adolescents

Ghadah Al-Naqeeb, Neelam Baral, James Welch, and Joanna Klubo-Gwiezdzinska

Abbreviations

AFP	Alpha-fetoprotein
ATA	American Thyroid Association
ATM	Ataxia telangiectasia mutated
CS	Cowden syndrome
CT	Computed tomography
DNA	Deoxyribonucleic acid
EBRT	External beam radiotherapy
FMTC	Familial medullary thyroid cancer
FNAB	Fine needle aspiration biopsy
FNMTC	Familial non-medullary thyroid cancer
FOXE1	Fork-head box E1
FTC	Follicular thyroid cancer
HABP2	Hyaluronan binding protein 2
MAP2K5	Mitogen-activated protein kinase 5
MEN2A	Multiple endocrine neoplasia 2A
MEN2B	Multiple endocrine neoplasia 2B

Ghadah Al-Naqeeb and Neelam Baral contributed equally with all other contributors.

G. Al-Naqeeb · J. Klubo-Gwiezdzinska (✉)
Metabolic Diseases Branch, National Institutes of Diabetes, Digestive and Kidney Diseases, National Institutes of Health, Bethesda, MD, USA
e-mail: joanna.klubo-gwiezdzinska@nih.gov

N. Baral
Department of Endocrinology, Medstar Georgetown University Hospital, Washington, DC, USA

J. Welch
Metabolic Diseases Branch, Office of the Clinical Director, National Institutes of Diabetes, Digestive and Kidney Diseases, National Institutes of Health, Bethesda, MD, USA
e-mail: James.Welch@nih.gov

F. Hannah-Shmouni (ed.), *Familial Endocrine Cancer Syndromes*, https://doi.org/10.1007/978-3-031-37275-9_5

MNG	Multinodular goiter
MRI	Magnetic resonance imaging
MTC	Medullary thyroid cancer
NGS	Next generation sequencing
PHTS	PTEN hamartoma syndrome
PKA	Protein kinase A
PPNAD	Primary pigmented nodular adrenocortical disease
PRKAR1A	Protein kinase A regulatory subunit type 1-alpha
PRN	Papillary renal neoplasia
PTC	Papillary thyroid cancer
PTEN	Phosphatase and tensin homolog
RET	Rearranged during transfection
SEC23B	SEC23 homolog B COPII coat complex component
SEER	Surveillance epidemiology and end results
SRGAP	Slit-Robo rho GTPase activating protein
TCO	Thyroid carcinoma with oxyphilia locus
TITF-1	Thyroid transcription factor-1
TREC	T-cell receptor excision circle
VEGFR	Vascular endothelial growth factor receptor

Introduction

Familial thyroid cancer syndromes are classified into familial medullary thyroid carcinoma (FMTC) and familial non-medullary thyroid cancer (FNMTC). FMTC syndromes are associated with the development of thyroid cancer derived from neuroendocrine C cells, either as the sole presentation (FMTC) or as a part of multiple endocrine neoplasia type II (MEN2A or B) [1] (Fig. 5.1). Approximately 25% of patients with medullary thyroid cancer (MTC) have one of these familial forms, which are typically caused by specific germline pathogenic variants in the *RET* proto-oncogene.

FNMTC is associated with the development of thyroid malignancy of epithelial origin—either papillary (PTC) or follicular thyroid cancer (FTC)—and again could present as an isolated cancer or in a syndromic form associated with other manifestations [2] (Fig. 5.1). Most cases of PTCs and FTCs are sporadic, but approximately 3–9% may have familial disease [1, 3].

Given the inherited component of FMTC and FNMTC oncogenesis, it is expected that thyroid malignancies may develop in childhood and adolescence, dependent on the penetrance of certain germline molecular drivers and their modulation by environmental factors. According to the Surveillance, Epidemiology and End Results

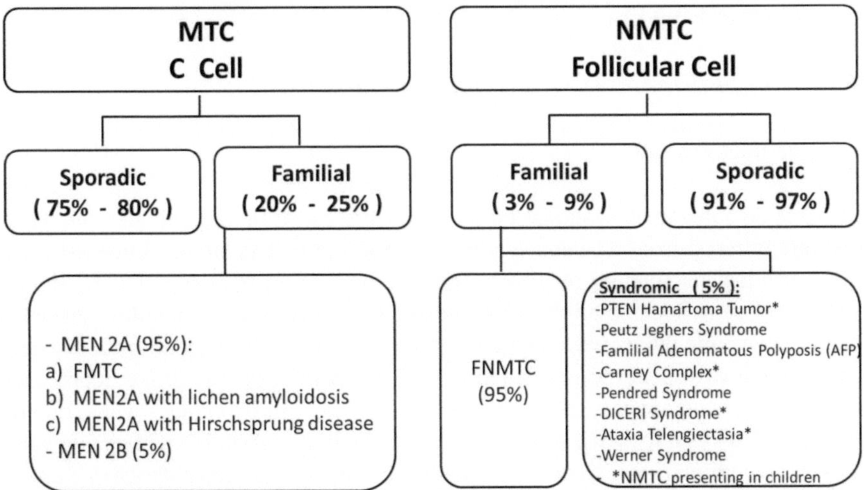

Fig. 5.1 Overview of sporadic and familial thyroid cancer presentations. *MTC* medullary thyroid cancer, *NMTC* non-medullary thyroid cancer, *FMTC* familial medullary thyroid cancer, *FNMTC* familial non-medullary thyroid cancer, *MEN* multiple endocrine neoplasia

(SEER) program, new cases of thyroid cancer in children and adolescents younger than 20 years old represent 1.8% of all thyroid malignancies diagnosed in the USA. The incidence appears to be increasing among 15–19-year-old adolescents, and thyroid cancer is the eighth most diagnosed cancer in this age group. Adolescents have a ten times higher likelihood of developing thyroid cancer than younger children, with a significantly higher incidence in females compared with males, resulting in a ratio of 5:1 [2]. In fact, thyroid cancer is the second most common malignancy in female adolescents [4, 5]. Such gender disbalance is not observed in younger children [2].

The most common presentation of thyroid cancer in children is a thyroid nodule, but more aggressive cancer forms may present as either local or distant metastases [2]. The diagnostic work-up usually includes fine needle aspiration biopsy (FNAB) of the thyroid nodule and/or metastatic lesion with the appropriate malignancy risk stratification based on the Bethesda system of cytologic classification of thyroid nodules [3, 6]. The subsequent surgical and adjuvant therapy is guided by the histological type of the tumor, disease stage, likelihood of recurrence, and risks to benefit estimates [6].

The goal of this chapter is to review the genetics, epidemiology, presentation, and management of syndromic and non-syndromic forms of thyroid cancer that can affect children and adolescents.

Syndromic FNMTC

PTEN Hamartoma Tumor Syndrome (PHTS)

Genetic Background

PHTS is an autosomal dominant inherited disease spectrum that includes the more commonly recognized Cowden syndrome (CS). The molecular signature of PHTS is a germline inactivation of the phosphatase and tensin homolog (*PTEN*) tumor suppressor gene, located on chromosome 10q23.3. It is believed that this gene produces an enzyme that is responsible for removing a phosphate group from proteins and lipids involved in the regulation of cell division. A classic tumor suppressor gene, *PTEN* gene appears to follow the Knudson two-hit hypothesis where one of the two alleles is knocked out in every cell of the body (germline pathogenic variant) and then tumorigenesis occurs following a somatic acquired pathogenic variant (or epigenetic downregulation) knocking out the working wild-type allele in one of the cell types that relies on this gene to prevent aberrant cell division (second hit) [7]. While a tumor or cancer of one of the PTHS-associated tissues can occur in someone from the general population as the result of both *PTEN* alleles being knocked out in the same cell through somatic acquired pathogenic variants, the germline inactivation of one of the two *PTEN* alleles in every cell of the body in someone with PTHS greatly increases the likelihood of developing one of more of the tumors associated with this disorder and also makes it more likely to occur early in life, such as in childhood or adolescence [7].

Epidemiology

The disease spectrum involves a group of disorders that include CS, Cowden-like syndrome, Bannayan-Riley-Ruvalcaba syndrome, PTEN-related Proteus syndrome, and Proteus-like syndrome. It has been reported that these disorders are likely underdiagnosed as they may be hard to recognize; therefore, the determination of their exact incidence and prevalence is difficult to assess. It has been reported that CS is estimated to affect 1 in 200,000 individuals in the general population [8]. Proteus syndrome and Proteus-like syndrome are rare complex syndromes with an estimated prevalence of less than 1:1,000,000 live births [9] (Table 5.1).

Clinical Presentation in Children and Adolescents

CS is the best-known of the PHTS group of disorders. It is named after the first family that was diagnosed with this condition, which was identified by Lloyd and Dennis in 1963. While most of the data on the increased cancer risks associated with PTHS come from studies of CS, it is believed that all individuals with a germline pathogenic variant in *PTEN* carry the same increased risks for certain cancers, including a one in three chance of developing thyroid cancer during their life [10].

CS can involve several organs and various systems. One way to diagnose CS is based on pathognomonic criteria, either with central nervous system involvement and/or skin pathology including dysplastic cerebellar gangliocytoma, facial trichilemmomas, acral keratosis or papillomatous lesions. The diagnosis could be established also based on any two major criteria with or without minor criteria; or one

Table 5.1 Summary of genetics, epidemiology, and screening strategies in FNMTC and FMTC

Syndrome	Genetics	Prevalence	Clinical manifestations	Screening for thyroid cancer
Syndromic FNMTC				
PTEN Hamartoma	Inheritance: autosomal dominant	Cowden Syndrome	Thyroid pathology: Adenoma, MNG, Hashimoto thyroiditis, FTC	Screening for germline *PTEN* in children with thyroid cancer, and macrocephaly
	PTEN gene following the Knudson two-hit hypothesis	~1:200,000 in the general population	Non-thyroid pathology: macrocephaly, dysplastic cerebellar gangliocytoma, facial trichilemmomas, acral keratosis or papillomatous lesions, hamartomas, epidermal nevi, hamartomas, fibrocystic breast disease, breast cancer uterine fibroid/cancer, renal cell carcinoma	Germline *PTEN* present: baseline and annual thyroid US before the age of 18 or 5–10 years before the earliest cancer diagnosis, whichever occurs first
		Proteus syndrome and Proteus like syndrome 1:1,000,000		

(continued)

Table 5.1 (continued)

Syndrome	Genetics	Prevalence	Clinical manifestations	Screening for thyroid cancer
DICER 1	Inheritance: autosomal dominant	Ranging between 1:10,500 and 1:2500	Thyroid pathology: multinodular goiter, NMTC	Genetic counseling and testing are recommended for individuals who have clinical features of DICER1 and for those with a family history of DICER1
	DICER 1 (14q32.13) including missense variants in the RNaseIIIb domain responsible for the processing of microRNAs		Non-thyroid pathology: cystic nephromas, ovarian sec cord-stromal tumors, Sertoli, Leydig cell tumor, nasal, eye, pituitary blastoma, pinealoblastoma, Wilms tumors, and pleuro-pulmonary blastomas	Annual thyroid ultrasound during childhood/ adulthood recommended
	DICER1 operates under the two-hit tumor suppressor gene model			
Carney Complex	Inheritance: autosomal dominant	>750 cases since 1985	Thyroid pathology: multinodular goiter, follicular adenoma	Screening for thyroid nodules with ultrasound after the second decade of life
	PRKAR1A (17q24.2)		PTC, FTC	
	PRKACA and *PRKACB*		Non-thyroid pathology: spotty skin pigmentation or blue nevi, muco-cutaneous, breast or cardiac myxomas, primary pigmented adrenal hyperplasia, growth hormone producing adenomas, Sertoli cell tumors, schwannomas, osteochondromyxomas	

Table 5.1 (continued)

Syndrome	Genetics	Prevalence	Clinical manifestations	Screening for thyroid cancer
Ataxia Telangiectasia	Inheritance: autosomal recessive	1:40,000 to 1:300,000 in general population	Thyroid pathology: PTC—2 case reports reported in children	Lack of data regarding screening results given the rare occurrence of thyroid cancer
	ATM gene		Non-thyroid pathology: leukemias, lymphomas. cerebellar ataxia, oculomotor apraxia, choreoathetosis, oculocutaneous telangiectasia, immunological deficiency, premature aging, insulin-resistant diabetes mellitus and premature ovarian failure	

Non-syndromic FNMTC

Syndrome	Genetics	Prevalence	Clinical manifestations	Screening for thyroid cancer
FNMTC	Inheritance: autosomal dominant with incomplete penetrance	3–9% of all NMTC	Thyroid pathology: PTC, HTC, FTC	There is no specific recommendation by the American Thyroid Association for or against screening, but screening with thyroid ultrasound every 2–3 years should be considered in families with 3 or more first-degree relatives affected by FNMTC starting at teenage years
	The genetic susceptibility is not well-defined		Non-thyroid pathology: not applicable	

(continued)

Table 5.1 (continued)

Syndrome	Genetics	Prevalence	Clinical manifestations	Screening for thyroid cancer
MEN2A	Inheritance: autosomal dominant	1:35,000 in general population	Thyroid pathology: MTC	Annual assessments that include physical examination, cervical ultrasound, and serum calcitonin measurement in all children with MEN-2A beginning at 3–5 years of age. Prophylactic thyroidectomy at or before the age of 5 for high-risk *RET* mutation. For moderate-risk *RET* mutation thyroidectomy when calcitonin level becomes elevated.
	Activating mutations in *RET* gene:		Non-thyroid pathology: primary hyperparathyroidism, pheochromocytoma, cutaneous lichen amyloidosis, Hirschsprung's disease	
	High-risk *RET* mutation codon 634. Moderate risk RET mutations: codon 321; 531, 515, 533; 600, 603 606; 649 666; 768, 777, 790 791; 804, 819, 833 844; 866, 891, 912, 609, 611, 618, 620; 630, 631 and 633,			

Table 5.1   (continued)

Syndrome	Genetics	Prevalence	Clinical manifestations	Screening for thyroid cancer
MEN2B	Inheritance: autosomal dominant	0.9–1.6:1,000,000 general population	Thyroid pathology: MTC	ATA guidelines recommend early thyroidectomy before the age of 1 year in children carrying the M918T mutation and by the age of 5 for affected with germline p.Ala883Phe *RET* mutation
	Activating mutations in *RET* gene:		Non-thyroid pathology: pheochromocytoma, mucosal neuromas, intestinal ganglioneuromas, skeletal abnormalities, ophthalmologic abnormalities	
	Highest risk: p.Met918Thr *RET*			
	High risk: p.Ala883Phe *RET* mutation			

major and two minor criteria; or three minor criteria. Among major diagnostic criteria are macrocephaly, as well as different types of malignancies, including breast cancer, NMTC, and endometrial cancer. The minor criteria are less specific and consist of hamartomas, multinodular goiter, intellectual disability, fibrocystic breast disease, fibromas, uterine fibroids, and renal cell carcinoma.

Thyroid diseases like adenomatoid nodules, lymphocytic thyroiditis, follicular adenomas or carcinomas are the most common presentations observed in about 50–68% of patients with CS [11, 12]. After breast cancer, NMTC is the second most common malignancy in patients with CS, as it has been reported in about 3–14% of patients. CS is associated with a high lifetime risk of thyroid cancer of about 35% [13, 14]. FTC is more common than PTC in patients with PHTS. This is opposite to non-syndromic forms of thyroid cancers, as PTC is the most common non-syndromic thyroid cancer. NMTC in patients with CS has been reported as early as at 6–7 years of age. Classic papillary and Hürthle cell cancers have also been described in children with PTIIS [15, 16].

Bannayan-Riley-Ruvalcaba syndrome is associated with a wide spectrum of phenotypic presentations [12]. It can manifest as angiomatosis, lipomatosis, and macrocephaly [15]. Several types of thyroid tumors may occur in

Bannayan-Riley-Ruvalcaba syndrome including follicular and Hürthle cell adenomas, multinodular goiter, PTC, and FTC. FTC has the highest prevalence in this syndrome [17].

Proteus syndrome and Proteus-like syndrome are characterized by several connective tissue abnormalities such as hamartomas, epidermal nevi, and hyperostosis. These features are present at birth and persist throughout life, with a tendency to progress. The connective tissue nevi are pathognomonic for diagnosis. Patients with Proteus syndrome have a high risk of developing thyroid cancer, breast cancer, and endometrial cancer. The management of Proteus syndrome is usually symptom-based per standard care.

PHTS-Associated Thyroid Cancer Management

Initially, extensive medical and family history investigation is recommended to assess the possible manifestations of PHTS. Genetic testing can be considered if there is any evidence of the typical features in the proband or patients' relatives. Thyroid ultrasound is more accurate than physical examination to diagnose thyroid nodules, and especially helpful in the pediatric population [13]. Baseline thyroid ultrasound is recommended regardless of age. It is recommended to repeat the ultrasound on an annual basis in all patients harboring typical pathogenic variants causing PHTS [16, 18].

Ultrasound-guided fine needle aspiration (FNA) is indicated for any detected thyroid nodule that is 1 cm or larger in a child with a normal TSH [19]. Surgical resection and adjuvant therapy should follow the standard guidelines of the management of thyroid nodules and cancer in children and adolescents [6].

Genetic Counseling

Identifying the causative *PTEN* pathogenic variant in an affected family member allows for genetic counseling and testing of at-risk relatives, which can promote early diagnosis of PHTS in those who carry the predisposition and early identification and management of malignancies associated with PHTS. PHTS can exhibit variable expressivity, meaning that the conditions can affect different people differently, even within the same family and the same mutation. However, PTHS exhibits nearly complete penetrance with almost all individuals with CS developing mucocutaneous lesions by the fourth decade of life and most having macrocephaly [19].

Making a molecular diagnosis in the proband can allow for in-depth genetic counseling about the increased risks for developing certain cancers and the recommended screening and surveillance available to the patient. It is important for both the patients and their physicians to understand these increased risks because, as opposed to a member of the general population who develops cancer, a person with PHTS is seven times more likely to develop a second primary cancer in their lifetime [20]. It also allows for counseling about the risk of passing the disorder on to offspring, which is 50% chance for each child.

Testing for *PTEN* should be considered in children presenting with thyroid cancer, especially where macrocephaly co-exists [5, 6]. In a child found to have PHTS, both parents should have targeted genetic testing for the pathogenic variant in *PTEN* to determine if it was inherited, allowing for appropriate care of that parent and cascade testing of that side of the family, or if it is a de novo pathogenic variant. Approximately half of patients with CS inherited it from a parent, and up to half of patients with PHTS in general have a de novo pathogenic variant in *PTEN,* with almost all of *PTEN*-related Proteus syndrome and Proteus-like syndrome being caused by de novo germline pathogenic variants [18]. If the parents of a child diagnosed with PHTS are found not to carry the pathogenic variant, confirming it as de novo, then the risk for a sibling of the patient is low, probably <1%, although still higher than the general population because of the small possibility of gonadal mosaicism (postfertilization genetic changes that is confined to the gamete precursors and is not detected in somatic tissues) in one of the parents.

DICER1 Syndrome

Genetic Background

DICER1 syndrome is an autosomal dominant disorder caused by germline pathogenic variants in the *DICER1* gene. The gene is located on chromosome 14q32.13 and is responsible for the processing of microRNAs (miRNA). Like *PTEN*, it is believed that *DICER1* operates under the two-hit tumor suppressor gene model whereby tumors and cancer associated with this syndrome, including NMTC, occur after a somatic second hit alters the remaining working copy of the gene in a particular type of cell [21]. However, *DICER1* is different from the classic tumor suppressor genes, which are associated with biallelic loss-of-function pathogenic variants, because one of the hits to the gene must be a missense variant in the RNaseIIIb domain, while the other is usually a truncating loss-of-function variant. It is hypothesized that missense variants in this specific region of the gene lead to aberrant miRNA processing that has downstream oncogenic effects, and this imbalance in processed miRNA is covered up by a working second allele of *DICER1*. This explains why the loss-of-function second hit is needed for tumorigenesis [22]. Moreover, the RNaseIIIb domain missense variant must occur in one of five key amino acids and, for certain tissues, may need to be present at certain points of embryogenesis or development to have an oncogenic effect.

This unique molecular etiology of DICER1 syndrome leads to a highly variable presentation with reduced penetrance. On the other hand, if patients present with the pathogenic RNaseIIIb missense variant, then it is much more likely for them to acquire loss-of-function second hit in one or more cell types, leading to a more severe variant of DICER1 syndrome with greater number of neoplasms and perhaps increased risk for the non-neoplastic manifestations. However, there is evidence that suggests that a *DICER1* pathogenic missense variant in the RNaseIIIb domain cannot be inherited in the germline, suggesting that it would be incompatible with life if present in every cell of the body, so this more severe type of DICER1 is associated with mosaic de novo cases, adding further variability to the phenotype, since the presentation will be affected by which tissues were hit and missed in that individual [22].

Epidemiology

The prevalence of *DICER1* pathogenic variants in the general population has been calculated to be between ~1 in 10,500 people to as common as ~1 in 2500 [23] with a second similar analysis using a different database arriving at a prevalence of ~1 in 4500 [24].

Clinical Presentation in Children and Adolescents

One copy of the altered *DICER1* gene is sufficient to cause an increased risk of developing tumors, but the penetrance and presentation of DICER1 syndrome are highly variable [25]. Typically, a patient starts with a pathogenic germline loss-of-function variant and then, when certain tissues acquire a specific second somatic hit that affects the catalytic activity of the enzyme, it leads to malignant transformation and growth. This can happen at different times and locations of the body during development, growth, and life, leading to different outcomes in the patients.

The disease may present with neoplastic and non-neoplastic manifestations. The neoplastic manifestations include benign and malignant thyroid lesions, cystic nephromas, ovarian sex cord-stromal tumors, nasal, eye, pituitary and pineal tumors, Wilms tumors and renal sarcomas, and pleuropulmonary blastomas. Many of these neoplasms are rare outside of DICER1, so one should consider this syndrome when encountering NMTC or multinodular goiter in a person or family with other DICER1-associated manifestations, especially pleuropulmonary blastoma, pulmonary cysts or pneumothorax in a child, Sertoli-Leydig cell tumor, gynandroblastoma, pituitary blastoma, or pineoblastoma [26]. Non-neoplastic manifestations can include retinal changes, macrocephaly, and kidney and urinary tract anomalies. Thirteen percent of male patients harboring *DICER1* pathogenic variants develop multinodular goiter by the age of 20, while it affects up to 30% of females younger than 20 years. Moreover, thyroid nodules in these patients are characterized by 16–24-fold higher risk of malignant transformation leading to NMTC [27].

Treatment of patients with DICER1 using chemotherapy and/or bone marrow transplantation for pleuropulmonary blastomas can also be a predisposing risk factor for NMTC, as it may lead to second somatic hits in the thyroid tissue. In fact, PTC has been reported to be associated with germline and somatic pathogenic variants of *DICER1* [28]. Moreover, five cases of PTC/FTC associated with a history of high dose chemotherapy have been reported in patients with DICER1 syndrome [21, 29]. Subsequently, Khan et al. reported six additional cases of NMTC developing after chemo-and radiotherapy to the lungs, all in female patients with a median age of 10 years [27]. NMTC usually presents as a thyroid nodule, and follows an indolent course, without an increased risk of invasion or metastasis [16]. Therefore, the outcome is usually favorable.

DICER1-Associated Thyroid Cancer Management

Thyroid carcinoma in DICER1 syndrome is typically well-differentiated with low likelihood for invasion, extrathyroidal extension, or metastasis; poorly differentiated NMTC in DICER1 has been reported very rarely [30]. In 2018, Shultz et al. established DICER1 surveillance guidelines that recommend annual thyroid physical examination for thyroid nodules or asymmetry along with the consideration of thyroid ultrasounds starting at the age of 8 years and repeating every 3–5 years, if normal [30]. If a patient develops MNG or NMTC, then management should follow the standard guidelines as in sporadic cases [20, 29]. Given usually low risk of persistent/recurrent disease at initial NMTC presentation, the surgical intervention with total thyroidectomy is commonly sufficient, without radioactive iodine as adjuvant therapy [3].

Genetic Counseling

DICER1 is an autosomal dominant disorder caused by germline heterozygous pathogenic variants. Up to 10% of pathogenic *DICER1* variants are large deletions of an exon or more that could be missed by gene sequencing (e.g., Sanger single-gene sequencing or Next Generation Sequencing exome sequencing), so deletion/duplication testing must be included in the genetic testing to thoroughly rule out *DICER1* as the cause of the affected patient's manifestations [26].

Genetic counseling and testing are recommended for individuals who have clinical features of DICER1 and for those with a family history of DICER1. For at-risk individuals in affected families, surveillance measures should be discussed as the treatment approach unless or until germline genetic testing rules out the familial *DICER1* pathogenic variant [30, 31]. Due to the reduced penetrance exhibited by DICER1 syndrome, a lack of identified clinical manifestations in a parent or sibling is insufficient to rule them out as carriers. While a significant number of DICER1 cases may be caused by a de novo DICER1 pathogenic variant, with one study of patients with pleuropulmonary blastomas showing 20% of cases being de novo, molecular genetic testing of both parents for the pathogenic variant identified in the patient is necessary to confirm the de novo occurrence and clarify the recurrence risk to siblings, which is 50% if a parent carries the variant and 1% if not [26].

In an apparently-sporadic case of DICER1 syndrome, if no *DICER1* pathogenic variant is identified through germline testing (sequencing and deletion/duplication testing of blood or saliva), there is a possibility of somatic mosaicism; up to 10% of de novo pathogenic variants have been found to exhibit mosaicism wherein germline genetic testing might miss the pathogenic variant but tumor testing will reveal biallelic pathogenic variants in the gene. In these cases, sequencing of buccal tissue or of normal tissue around the tumor tissue, or deep sequencing of blood or saliva DNA, can be helpful to confirm the mosaic diagnosis. Siblings of a patient with mosaic disease are not at increased risk since the de novo pathogenic variant occurred post-zygotically and was not inherited from a parent. If the pathogenic variant that is present in multiple tissues of the patient (mosaic) is the missense RNaseIIIb variant, which would often be the case in severe cases, then any children that the patient might have in the future would be unlikely to inherit this condition since these pathogenic missense variants have never been found in the germline, suggesting they would be incompatible with life and would likely result in a miscarriage [22, 26, 32].

Carney Complex

Genetic Background

Carney complex is an autosomal dominant condition which was first described in 1985 as "myxomas, spotty pigmentation and endocrine overactivity" [33]. Most cases of Carney complex are caused by a germline loss-of-function variant in *PRKAR1A*, which encodes protein kinase A regulatory subunit type 1-alpha on chromosome 17q24.2. This leads to activation of protein kinase A (PKA), as the regulatory subunit normally inhibits PKA activity. Other rare pathogenic variants have been identified in patients who do not have *PRKAR1-a* and have been associated with specific abnormalities. Pathogenic variants in *PRKACA*, the catalytic subunit alpha of PKA located on 1p31.1, has been seen in isolated primary pigmented nodular adrenocortical disease (PPNAD) [34] and variants in *PRKACB*, the catalytic subunit beta of the PKA, located in 19p, have been seen in Carney complex with acromegaly [35].

Epidemiology

Since 1985, over 750 cases of Carney complex have been reported but the exact prevalence is unknown [36]. Carney Complex is slightly more common in females (57%) compared to males (43%). The diagnosis can be made at birth in some cases but median age at diagnosis was found to be 20 years [37]. In a specific study of ten patients with Carney complex and thyroid tumors or thyrotoxicosis, the youngest age at first diagnosis was 13 years and the oldest age was 57 years with median age of 34 years [38].

Clinical Presentations in Children and Adolescents

Carney complex is characterized by multiple neoplasias, including cardiac, skin, and breast myxomas, endocrine tumors, spotty skin pigmentation, and endocrinopathies [39]. Spotty skin pigmentation is the most common clinical manifestation although it is not invariably present.

Major Diagnostic Criteria:

1. Skin: Spotty skin pigmentations or blue nevi.
2. Myxomas: cutaneous or mucosal or cardiac or breast tissue.
3. Adrenal: primary pigmented nodular adrenal hyperplasia.
4. Pituitary: growth hormone producing adenoma causing acromegaly.
5. Gonadal: large cell calcifying Sertoli cell tumors.
6. Thyroid: Thyroid carcinoma or multiple hypoechoic nodules on thyroid ultrasonography.
7. Psammomatous melanotic schwannomas.
8. Breast ductal adenomas.
9. Osteochondromyxomas.

   Supplemental Criteria

(a) Inactivating *PPKAR1A* variants.
(b) Positive family history in first-degree relatives.

Diagnosis is made when any two major diagnostic criteria are found or any one of the major criteria along with one of the supplemental criteria is met [37].

Thyroid gland disease is a late developing feature of Carney complex and can manifest as a spectrum from follicular hyperplasia and nodular disease to carcinoma [40]. Thyroid nodules are detected usually as small hypoechoic lesions on ultrasonography in up to 60% of all patients and two-thirds among children and adolescent [41]. Thyroid nodules often appear during the first 10 years of life [40]. Follicular adenoma is the most common diagnosis, whereas PTC and FTC can be seen in up to 10% of Carney complex patients with thyroid nodules [37, 42].

Carney Complex-Associated Thyroid Cancer Management

Thyroid nodules are rarely detected at an age less than 10 years, therefore screening with physical examination and thyroid ultrasound do not have to be assessed until the second decade of life [43]. Thyroid nodules detected by ultrasound are further assessed based on the American Thyroid Association (ATA) guidelines with biochemical examination and fine needle aspiration biopsy [41]. Follicular thyroid adenomas can be treated conservatively, while PTC and FTC require thyroidectomy with or without lymph node dissection, as appropriate. Patients are selected for radioactive iodine therapy based on post-operative risk stratification per ATA pediatric guidelines. Usually, RAI is indicated for children with tumors exceeding 4 cm, with extrathyroidal extension or extensive regional nodal involvement, as well as iodine-avid pulmonary metastases. Long-term follow-up for a child with differentiated thyroid cancer is essential because disease can recur decades after initial diagnosis and therapy [44]. Prognosis of familial thyroid cancer is similar to sporadic cases after treatment [45].

Genetic Counseling

Any patients who meet diagnostic criteria for Carney complex should have *PRKAR1A* germline analysis, regardless of family history. Carney complex is an autosomal dominant disorder caused by germline heterozygous loss-of-function variants which can include large deletions of an exon or more that would be missed by gene sequencing (e.g., single-gene Sanger or NGS exome sequencing), so deletion/duplication testing must be included in the genetic test to thoroughly rule out *PRKAR1A* variants as the cause of the affected patient's manifestations. If a germline cause is identified, all first-degree relatives of affected patients should be offered targeted genetic analysis for that same pathogenic variant as early as the first 2 years of life [46]. Carriers of the pathogenic variant have a 50% chance of passing on the disorder to each child. Males with Carney complex may have reduced fertility and pregnancies that inherit the *PRKAR1A* pathogenic variant from either parent may be more likely to result in miscarriage, although the finalized data on this are not yet available [47].

Approximately 30% of patients with Carney complex carry a de novo germline pathogenic variant in *PRKAR1A* [47, 48]. If a parent carries the pathogenic variant, then each sibling of the affected patient has a 50% chance of having inherited it as well. If neither parent carries the variant and it is presumed de novo, the recurrence risk for another child is greater than for the general population but still less than 1%. Prenatal genetic counseling is available to discuss prenatal genetic testing options.

Most cases (~60–80%) of Carney complex arise from pathogenic variants in *PRKAR1A*. Meanwhile, approximately 20% of families with Carney complex have been linked to chromosome 2q16, and these have been referred to as having Carney complex 2, although the causative gene in that region has not yet been established [47, 49]. If a causative *PRKAR1A* variant is not found, especially in patients with isolated PPNAD, it may be possible to pursue analysis of additional genes that have been implicated in rare cases of Carney complex, including *PRKACA* and *PRKACB*, the so-called Carney complex 3 [41].

Ataxia Telangiectasia

Genetic Background

Ataxia telangiectasia is an autosomal recessive neurodegenerative disorder characterized by immunodeficiency and an increased risk of developing cancer caused by pathogenic variants in the Ataxia Telangiectasia Mutated (*ATM*) gene located on chromosome 11q22–23 [50]. Most affected individuals in the USA inherit different pathogenic variants from each parent; thus, molecularly, they present as compound heterozygotes. However, there are population-specific pathogenic biallelic homozygotes observed in Amish, North African Jewish, and Sardinian populations [51]. The *ATM* tumor suppressor gene encodes the protein kinase ATM which plays a key role in the cellular response to DNA (Deoxyribonucleic acid) damage and multiple cell cycle checkpoint pathways. The *ATM* pathogenic variants result in the absence of ATM protein expression or a lack of its kinase activity. Therefore, ataxia telangiectasia is characterized by an extreme sensitivity of DNA to radiation-induced damage which is a significant risk factor for oncogenesis [52]. The most common *ATM* pathogenic variants are missense and truncating, detected by a sequence analysis in single-gene testing or multi-gene panels (>90% of cases), while deletion/duplication analysis reveals pathogenic *ATM* variants in 1–2% of patients [53–55] .

Notably, even though the full spectrum of disease manifests in biallelic homozygotes or compound heterozygotes, carriers of a single *ATM* pathogenic variant are also at approximately four times increased risk of developing cancer compared to the general population, attributed mainly to a breast cancer predisposition [51, 56, 57]. Carriers are also at increased risk of developing coronary artery disease [58].

Moreover, there is a genotype-phenotype correlation in ataxia telangiectasia observed for some *ATM* variants. There are variants associated with milder phenotypic presentation of neurogenerative disorder, such as c.5762-1050A > G, c.1A > G, c.7271T > G, c.8147T > C, and c.8494C > T, as well as variants associated with a higher cancer risk such as c.6679C > T [56, 57, 59–63].

Epidemiology

The frequency of heterozygous *ATM* gene carriers varies between 0.1% and 5% in the general population [64] and prevalence of the autosomal recessive disorder is estimated to be 1:40,000 to 1:300,000 in the general population [51, 65]. The incidence has been reported to be significantly higher in consanguineous marriages [66]. Neurodegenerative features can be seen as early as at the age of 1–4 years. Although thyroid carcinoma in adult patients with ataxia telangiectasia has been reported, its occurrence in children is very rare—with only two case reports discussed below [67, 68].

Clinical Features

The classical form of ataxia telangiectasia is a childhood-onset disease characterized by progressive cerebellar ataxia, oculomotor apraxia, choreoathetosis, oculocutaneous telangiectasia, and immunological deficiency associated with frequent infections [68]. Ataxia telangiectasia is also associated with premature aging, insulin-resistant diabetes mellitus, and premature ovarian failure [51]. The clinical diagnosis becomes most apparent after the age of 10 years when ataxia, apraxia, telangiectasia, and dysarthria are fully expressed. MRI shows cerebellar atrophy at this age, unlike in infants where diagnosis can be elusive and confused with mild cerebral palsy, acute infectious or episodic ataxia. The three routine tests to support a diagnosis are: (1) newborn screening for severe combined immunodeficiency revealing reduced T-cell receptor excision circle (TREC) levels and lymphopenia, (2) elevated serum alpha-fetoprotein (AFP) seen in 95% of patients, and (3) translocation of chromosome 7;14 in peripheral blood cells [51, 69]. The diagnosis is confirmed in a proband either by molecular genetic testing documenting the presence of biallelic *ATM* pathogenic variants or by immunoblotting showing absent or significantly reduced ATM protein levels.

The occurrence of malignancies is approximately 100 times greater than in the general population, most commonly consisting of lymphoproliferative disorders such as leukemia or lymphoma. The thyroid malignancies are very rare in childhood consisting of two case reports documented. PTC along with lymph node involvement was seen in a 9-year-old female with ataxia telangiectasia as well as in a 13-year-old girl with follicular variant of PTC confined to the thyroid gland [67, 70].

Ataxia Telangiectasia-Associated Thyroid Cancer Management

There is a lack of data regarding screening results and prognosis of ataxia telangiectasia associated with PTC. When diagnosed, it should be treated according to standard guidelines and treatment recommendations [71]. However, given the predisposition to DNA damage in patients with ataxia telangiectasia, treatment with radioactive iodine should be implemented only in patients with metastatic disease, preferably utilizing dosimetry to quantify the exposure to radiation of normal organs [72].

Genetic Counseling

Notably, ataxia telangiectasia is one of the incidental findings of newborn screening for severe combined immunodeficiency. Based on the study focusing on the parent's perspectives, early ataxia telangiectasia diagnosis in the pre-symptomatic phase of the disorder via newborn screening is a preferred approach [73]. Molecular testing of *ATM* can provide additional information for genetic counseling since certain variants in the gene have a known genotype-phenotype correlation that may allow for a more customized conversation and anticipatory guidance. Genetic counseling can help parents understand the recurrence risk for this autosomal recessive condition, which is a one in four chance to have another affected child. A discussion about the carriers in the family is especially important for this disorder since heterozygous pathogenic variants also predispose to cancer development. This includes the parents, who are both obligate carriers, and any unaffected siblings, who have a 2/3 likelihood of having inherited one of the *ATM* pathogenic variants.

Non-syndromic FNMTC

Non-syndromic FNMTC was first described by Robinson and Orr in 1955 when it was identified in monozygotic twins. Non-syndromic FNMTC is defined by the presence of thyroid cancer of follicular origin in two or more first-degree family members in the absence of hereditary or environmental causes like radiation [74]. However, several studies suggest that the FNMTC diagnosis should be established only if three or more first-degree relatives are affected [2, 75, 76].

Genetic Background

FNMTC is inherited in an autosomal dominant pattern with incomplete penetrance. The genetic susceptibility is not well-defined [4]. Some investigators suggest that FNMTC is a polygenic disorder characterized by a low-to-moderate number of pathogenic alleles with variable penetrance [4, 77, 78] Genome-wide association studies reveal at least 10 loci associated with odds ratio of FNMTC development ranging from 1.2 to 1.8, indicating that low penetrance predisposition may play an important pathogenic role [78]. These loci include but are not limited to, thyroid carcinoma with oxyphilia locus (*TCO*), first described in a French family and subsequently confirmed with other pedigrees [79, 80], and *fPTC/PRN* the first locus discovered in an American family, identified at position 1q21, and associated with FNMTC and papillary renal neoplasia (PRN), hence the locus name [81]. Additional susceptibility loci for "non-medullary thyroid carcinoma-1" NMTC-1 have been identified on chromosome 2q21 [82].

Several additional low penetrance susceptibility risk loci or genes have been identified, although none has been uniformly shown to have a causative role. These include the Slit-Robo Rho GTPase activating protein (*SRGAP*), thyroid-specific-enhancer-binding protein/thyroid transcription factor-1 (*TITF-1/NKX2–1*), Forkhead Box E1 (*FOXE1*), SEC23 Homolog B COPII Coat Complex Component (*SEC23B*), hyaluronan binding protein 2 (*HABP2*), and mitogen-activated protein kinase 5 (MAP2K5) [83–88]. None of the above-mentioned germline variants have been shown to be uniformly associated with FNMTC or to be a common causative factor for several families. There is also no genotype-phenotype correlation identified. Hence, there are no definitively known causative germline drivers of FNMTC to date.

Epidemiology

FNMTC is diagnosed in 3–9% of patients with thyroid cancer [3]. There are limited data on the prevalence of non-syndromic FNMTC in children. However, the disease could present in children as early as the age of 8 years [89].

Clinical Presentation in Children and Adolescents

FNMTC-associated tumors present at an early age are often bilateral and multifocal and have more nodal involvement and higher recurrence rate, although the latter feature has not been uniformly reported [4, 74, 90, 91]. PTC is the most common form of FNMTC. Benign thyroid diseases are also common in FNMTC families and can manifest as follicular adenoma, MNG, and Hashimoto's thyroiditis [74, 92].

There are mixed data about the clinical behavior of FNMTC whether following a more aggressive or less aggressive course compared to sporadic NMTC [4, 78]. These conflicting data are likely due to a bias inherently associated with the low-quality evidence coming from retrospective case-control studies characterized by limited sample sizes. It was also reported that the second generation may develop more aggressive disease, reflecting the clinical anticipation phenomenon, suggestive of genetic background of FNMTC [91].

There are limited data on the presentation of FNMTC in pediatric and adolescent population. However, in a recent study, Capezzone et al. showed that pediatric FNMTC is more prevalent in males and associated with higher rate of bilateral and multifocal tumors as well as lymph node metastases compared to sporadic NMTC in this age group [4].

Management of FNMTC

There are limited data on screening and surveillance as well as clinical course and prognosis of FNMTC compared to sporadic NMTC. However, ultrasound surveillance of family members of affected probands has been shown to detect earlier stages of disease in which tumors are smaller, characterized by a lower incidence of extrathyroidal extension and fewer lymph node metastasis [2]. There is no specific recommendation by the ATA for or against thyroid ultrasound screening, since there is no evidence of decreased morbidity or mortality with screening [3, 6]. However, based on the average age of presentation, screening with thyroid ultrasound occurring in regular intervals (every 2–3 years) is justified to be implemented 10 years before the peak incidence (starting in teenage years) or 10 years before the earliest age of the diagnosis in the family, whichever occurs first [2]. There is no role for prophylactic thyroidectomy in children of the affected parent, due to a very variable disease penetration in individual patients.

The most common and definite treatment of FNMTC is total thyroidectomy in patients with biopsy-proven thyroid cancer. There is also a lower threshold for a surgical intervention in patients with indeterminate thyroid nodules [90]. Lymph node dissection is highly considered, given the likelihood of lymph node involvement, if there is a suspected evidence of nodal involvement on pre-surgical neck ultrasound [91]. Adjuvant therapy with radioactive iodine is considered for children and adolescents with either locally advanced FNMTC or distant metastases.

Genetic Counseling

Increased awareness and screening for familial thyroid cancer can help with earlier detection of the disease and a timely intervention. In clinical genetics, in the absence of a known molecular etiology for which to test, we revert to the pedigree and epidemiological data for risk assessment and genetic counseling. Most patients intuitively know that they are at an increased risk to have or to develop a condition that someone closely related to them has, and this is true for FNMTC. A recently-published large epidemiological study in Korea calculated odds ratios of 4.76 (2.59–8.74), 6.59 (2.05–21.21), and 9.53 (6.92–13.11), respectively, for those with a mother, father, or sibling who had a history of thyroid cancer [93].

Since there are no definitive causative genes to test in those affected with FNMTC at this time, one cannot remove the risk conferred by the family history of FNMTC, but there is still a benefit to discussing the increased risk to family members, facilitating decision making around screening options, and supporting patients psychosocially, including in their communication about these matters to their relatives. Furthermore, it is important for molecularly unsolved patients to know that clinical genetics is a rapidly progressing field and that it is always a good idea to check back in with genetics in the future to get the latest information.

Syndromic Forms of FMTC: Multiple Endocrine Neoplasia Type 2 (MEN2)

MEN-2A

Genetic Background

MEN2A is an autosomal dominant hereditary cancer syndrome that results from pathogenic missense variants in the rearranged during transfection (*RET*) proto-oncogene located on chromosome 10. The *RET* germline pathogenic variants lead to gain-of-function of the tyrosine kinase receptors, promoting uncontrolled cell growth and differentiation in various developing tissues, including those developed from the neural crest. As many as 95% of patients with MEN2A will have germline variants in codon 634 of exon 11 or codons 609, 611, 618, 620 of exon 10 [1, 94]. MEN2A syndrome consists of MTC, pheochromocytoma (often bilateral) and/or tumors of the parathyroid glands that usually manifest as primary hyperparathyroidism (PHPT) within a single patient or family and can sometimes include skin and gastrointestinal manifestations in a form of cutaneous lichen amyloidosis and Hirschsprung disease, respectively. There is a clear association between the genotypes and the phenotype in terms of age of onset, aggressiveness of MTC, and the evidence of other neoplasms. Notably, variants in codon 634 are associated with high risk for aggressive MTC (up to 100% penetrance), while the penetrance for pheochromocytoma is about 50%, primary hyperparathyroidism ~10–30%. There is also an association with cutaneous lichen amyloidosis [1]. Other pathogenic *RET* variants, including exon 5, codon 321; exon 8, codons 531, 515, and 533; exon 10, codons 600, 603, and 606; exon 11, codons 649 and 666; exon 13, codons 768, 777, 790, and 791; exon 14, codons 804, 819, 833, and 844; and exon 15, codons 866, 891, and 912, exon 10, codons 609, 611, 618, and 620; and exon 11, codons 630, 631, and 633, are associated with a moderate risk of aggressive MTC and a later average age of onset as well as a variable presentation of pheochromocytoma, with penetrance ranging from 10 to 30%, and PHPT ranging from 0 to 10%. These genotype–phenotype correlations help with determining the recommendations regarding the age at which to perform prophylactic thyroidectomy and begin biochemical assessments for catecholamine overproduction or hypercalcemia [94, 95].

Epidemiology

MEN-2A is the most common among MEN2 syndromes, representing 95% of cases, and consists of classical MEN2A, MEN2A with cutaneous lichen amyloidosis, MEN2A with Hirschsprung disease, and FMTC diagnosed in families or individuals with RET germline mutations who have MTC but neither pheochromocytoma nor hyperparathyroidism [1, 94].

The prevalence of MEN-2A is about 1/35,000 and depending on the type of genetic background, may lead to MTC in children younger than 5 years old [1, 96].

Clinical Presentation in Children and Adolescents

MTC is generally the first manifestation of MEN-2A, occurring in 95% of patients harboring a pathogenic *RET* variant, and it can develop in early years between 5 and 25 years of age, suggesting that C cells are more prone to oncogenic *RET* gene activation than adrenal medullary or parathyroid cells. Notably, solitary presentation of FMTC has been recently categorized as MEN2A, as there are families diagnosed initially solely with FMTC, for whom development of other endocrine tumors occurred later in life. Hence to avoid any misdiagnosis, particularly of life-threatening conditions, such as pheochromocytoma, FMTC is now a part of MEN2A to assure that the management is similar to all patients with MEN2A [1].

PHPT has been reported in as young as 9 years old and can extend up to 70 years of age. However, the most common age range is between 17 and 49 years [97]. Although PHPT is not common among children, with reported incidence of 2–5/100,000, it is associated with increased morbidity when it affects this age group, as most of the children with PHPT will experience symptomatic hypercalcemia [98]. Pheochromocytoma is very rarely diagnosed during childhood. The average age at diagnosis has been reported in case series as ranging from 23 to 40 year of age. There are few case reports of pheochromocytoma diagnosis at the age of 8 years of age in the setting of underlying MEN2A [99].

MEN2A-Associated Thyroid Cancer Management

Total thyroidectomy before the age of 5 years is recommended for high-risk patients harboring *RET 634* mutation. There are no specific recommendations about the best timing of surgery for patients with moderate risk *RET* variants and prophylactic thyroidectomy is suggested in the teen age years [1]. The timing is guided by the yearly screening with calcitonin measurements and thyroid ultrasound. Annual assessments that include physical examination, cervical ultrasound, and serum calcitonin measurement are recommended in all children harboring germline *RET* proto-oncogene variants and should begin at 3–5 years of age [1]. Children with *RET634* variants should also undergo screening for pheochromocytoma by the measurement of plasma or urine metanephrines and normetanephrines starting at the age of 11-years-old, while those with moderate risk variants listed above, should start screening at the age of 16 years. For practical reasons this screening, occurring every 1–3 years, should be accompanied by testing calcium levels to rule out hyperparathyroidism [1].

If thyroid nodules and/or elevated calcitonin levels are detected in children or adolescents, the extent of surgical treatment depends on the risk of metastatic disease. Although there is a controversy regarding the calcitonin thresholds in decision making process, for calcitonin levels exceeding 20–40 pg/mL, central neck dissection is advocated, as this concentration of calcitonin is associated with increased risk of central neck lymph node metastases. Lateral neck dissection is recommended if there is any evidence of pathologic lymph nodes determined by neck ultrasound. However, when calcitonin levels exceed 200 pg/mL, bilateral lateral neck dissection is proposed to treat likely macro- and micro-metastatic foci in the lateral neck lymph nodes [1]. If serum calcitonin level is greater than 500 pg/mL, suggesting the presence of distant metastases, computed tomography (CT) of the neck and chest as well as imaging evaluation of the liver with three-phase CT or contrast enhanced magnetic resonance imaging (MRI), as well as axial MRI and bone scintigraphy to screen for bone metastases, are recommended. In such patients with distant metastases, less surgical involvement in treating the neck disease can be considered to preserve speech, swallowing, parathyroid function, and shoulder mobility, as priority is given to systemic therapies [1]. Non-surgical treatment can also include external beam radiotherapy (EBRT) to the neck as well as to the bone lesions, and local thermo-or chemo-ablation of the liver metastases.

There are two tyrosine kinase inhibitors approved for the treatment of MTC, vandetanib, and cabozantinib, in children older than 5 years as well as two specific *RET* inhibitors, pralsetinib and selpercatininb, approved for children and adolescents older than 12 years [1, 100]. Interestingly, it appears that vandetanib is more effective in children than in adults, as median progression free survival in children with MEN2 was 6.7 years and 5-year survival rate was 88.2% [101], while in adults median progression free survival was 30.5 months compared with placebo 19.3 months [102]. Less is known about the efficacy of cabozantinib in the pediatric population, while in adults treatment with this tyrosine kinase inhibitor results in the improvement of median progression free survival from 4 months in the placebo group to 11.2 months in cabozantinib-treated patients [103]. However, therapy with tyrosine kinase inhibitors, due to their wide spectrum targets including vascular endothelial growth factor receptor (VEGFR), is associated with significant side effects including, but not limited to hypertension, proteinuria or palmar-plantar erythrodysesthesia [102, 103]. Treatment with specific *RET* inhibitors is associated with a significant reduction of these VEGFR-mediated side effects. Moreover, although the results of head-to-head comparisons between thyroid kinase inhibitors and RET inhibitors from ongoing LIBRETTO-431 and AcceleRET-MTC are not yet available, RET inhibitors have shown very promising efficacy in RET-mutant tumors, with an overall response rate of 60% for those previously treated with tyrosine kinase inhibitors MTC and 71% for treatment-naive MTC [100]. That said, the exact efficacy of RET inhibitors in children is currently unknown.

Genetic Counseling

Given that MEN2A is a monogenic disorder with an autosomal dominant pattern of inheritance, affected individuals have a 50% chance of transmitting the defective gene to each child. Because this disorder is caused by gain-of-function variants, sequencing of *RET* will detect all pathogenic variants that cause MEN2 and deletion/duplication testing is not needed.

Genetic testing of at-risk family members, including parents and siblings of patients diagnosed with MEN2A, promotes early treatment and high likelihood of cure from MTC [31]. The established genotype–phenotype correlations in MEN2 allow for more tailored genetic counseling discussion about the risks associated with the family's pathogenic variant and the corresponding surveillance recommendations.

MEN2B Syndrome

Genetic Background

MEN2B syndrome is a rare autosomal dominant condition caused by specific germline pathogenic variants in *RET*. The most common is p.Met918Thr, accounting for 95% of MEN2B and characterized by the highest risk of aggressive MTC of all known *RET* variants [2]. The next most common cause of MEN2B is *RET* p.Ala883Phe. MTC is seen in 100% of patients with MEN2B. These aforementioned gain-of-function *RET* variants are associated with about 50% chance of developing pheochromocytoma, and approximately half of those will be multiple or bilateral [6]. Unlike MEN2A, parathyroid tumors are uncommon in MEN2B. Approximately 50–75% of patients with MEN2B have de novo germline *RET* variants, while the rest inherit the disease from a parent [1].

Epidemiology

MEN2B accounts for 5–10% of MEN2 cases. The prevalence is about one in a million [104]. MEN2B-associated aggressive MTC affects children as early as in the first year of life.

Clinical Manifestations in Children and Adolescents

MTC due to germline *RET*918 variants develops within the first year of life, even as early as the first few months of life, and lymph node metastases have been identified within the first year as well [105]. The stage of MTC disease at diagnosis is the strongest predictor of survival. MEN2B has a worse prognosis, with a 10-year survival of 75.5% compared with 97.4% in MEN2A. Moreover, patients with MEN2B are also characterized by marfanoid habitus and skeletal deformations including narrow long facies, pes cavus, pectus excavatum, high-arched palate, scoliosis, and slipped capital femoral epiphysis, mucosal neuromas, intestinal ganglioneuromatosis, ophthalmologic abnormalities such as dry eyes, thickened and everted eyelids, ptosis, and prominent corneal nerves as well as presence of pheochromocytomas.

Management of MEN-2B Associated Thyroid Cancer

Surgery is the first line treatment for MTC. The probability of surgical cure is undoubtedly lower in MEN2B than that in MEN2A, likely due to an earlier age of MTC appearance and a delayed diagnosis [106]. To avoid the risk of incurable MTC, ATA guidelines recommend early thyroidectomy before the age of 1 year in children carrying the *RET*918 variant [1, 107]. The surgery should be done in tertiary referral centers by experienced surgeons. Carriers of *RET*883 can undergo prophylactic thyroidectomy by the age of 5 years, as the risk of aggressive MTC is similar to the risk of *RET*634 carriers. Screening for pheochromocytoma should be implemented at the age of 11 years old. Since these patients do not develop hyperparathyroidism, screening for hypercalcemia is not necessary. The management of metastatic MTC in the setting of MEN2B is like that in the setting of MEN2A. Appropriate education of pediatricians and other health care professionals to recognize the early endocrine and nonendocrine manifestations of disease is needed to improve outcomes [108].

Genetic Counseling

Because of the physical manifestations of MEN2B that affect appearance, including mucosal neuromas of the tongue and lips, distinctive facies, and marfanoid habitus, it is much less likely to go undiagnosed than MEN2A or other cancer predisposition syndromes. Nonetheless, it may be appropriate to offer targeted germline genetic testing to the parents of an affected patient either to confirm the diagnosis in an affected parent or to confirm that the child's pathogenic variant occurred de novo. Up to 75% of MEN2B cases occur due to de novo germline mutations [2]. In that case, the recurrence risk for a sibling is greater than for the general population but still less than 1%.

In addition to discussions of the tumor and cancer risks associated with MEN2B, there is also significant psychosocial genetic counseling to be done related to the physical differences caused by this syndrome. Some patients or their parents may find syndrome-specific support groups to be helpful for navigating these psychosocial issues and finding community. For those affected patients who choose to have children, genetic counseling can help them understand their reproductive options, including targeted genetic testing of a baby allowing for prophylactic thyroidectomy before 1 year of age if the child inherits the pathogenic variant (50% chance), targeted genetic testing of a fetus, in vitro fertilization with pre-implantation genetic screening, adoption, or use of a donor egg or sperm.

Conclusion

In summary, several genetic disorders are associated with the presence of thyroid nodules and thyroid cancer in children and adolescents. The diagnostic work-up usually involves thyroid ultrasound and fine needle aspiration biopsy, but the criteria for biopsy in children and adolescents should focus on clinical context and ultrasound features more than on size of the nodules, as thyroid volume continues to change with age.

Unlike FNMTC, the familial forms of MTC are characterized by a well-known genotype-phenotype correlation that can successfully guide the optimal management. The aggressiveness and age of onset of familial MTC differs depending on the specific germline genetic mutation and this should determine the timing and extent of thyroid surgery [109]. Genetic testing helps to detect pre-invasive disease early allowing prophylactic thyroidectomy even in infancy when indicated. Prophylactic thyroidectomy is not routinely practiced in patients with syndromic or non-syndromic FNMTC, as the penetrance of thyroid cancer is highly variable. Children with thyroid cancer should be treated in centers with a multidisciplinary team, including high volume surgeons and expertise in the disease, to minimize the complications.

Areas of Future Research

Management of thyroid cancer is evolving toward a personalized approach based on clinical context, risk stratification, and molecular and anatomical pathology leading to the appropriate staging. More data are required for risk stratification of children and adolescents who would qualify for radioactive iodine therapy and to overcome the challenges of defining the subgroup who will not experience increased morbidity and mortality with deferred treatment. Studies are limited regarding the use of tyrosine kinase inhibitors and systemic treatment for advanced thyroid cancer unresponsive to initial treatment in children.

The genetic background of FNMTC is not elucidated, thus further studies should focus on potential polygenic mode of inheritance or epigenetic modifications as the underlying etiology of this familial disorder. Overcoming the limitations of existing evidence could be achieved by a collaborative international multicenter clinical and molecular data collection.

References

1. Wells SA Jr, Asa SL, Dralle H, Elisei R, Evans DB, Gagel RF, et al. Revised American Thyroid Association guidelines for the management of medullary thyroid carcinoma: the American Thyroid Association Guidelines Task Force on medullary thyroid carcinoma. Thyroid. 2015;25(6):567–610.
2. Klubo-Gwiezdzinska J, Yang L, Merkel R, Patel D, Nilubol N, Merino MJ, et al. Results of screening in familial non-medullary thyroid cancer. Thyroid. 2017;27(8):1017–24.
3. Haugen BR, Alexander EK, Bible KC, Doherty GM, Mandel SJ, Nikiforov YE, et al. 2015 American Thyroid Association management guidelines for adult patients with thyroid nodules and differentiated thyroid cancer: the American Thyroid Association guidelines task force on thyroid nodules and differentiated thyroid cancer. Thyroid. 2016;26(1):1–133.
4. Capezzone M, Maino F, Sagnella A, Campanile M, Dalmiglio C, Pilli T, et al. Clinical features of pediatric familial non-medullary thyroid cancer (FNMTC). J Endocrinol Investig. 2021;44:2319.
5. Hogan AR, Zhuge Y, Perez EA, Koniaris LG, Lew JI, Sola JE. Pediatric thyroid carcinoma: incidence and outcomes in 1753 patients. J Surg Res. 2009;156(1):167–72.
6. Francis GL, Waguespack SG, Bauer AJ, Angelos P, Benvenga S, Cerutti JM, et al. Management guidelines for children with thyroid nodules and differentiated thyroid cancer. Thyroid. 2015;25(7):716–59.
7. Dragoo DD, Taher A, Wong VK, Elsaiey A, Consul N, Mahmoud HS, et al. PTEN hamartoma tumor syndrome/Cowden syndrome: genomics, oncogenesis, and imaging review for associated lesions and malignancy. Cancers. 2021;13(13):3120.
8. Chevalier B, Dupuis H, Jannin A, Lemaitre M, Do Cao C, Cardot-Bauters C, et al. Phakomatoses and endocrine gland tumors: noteworthy and (not so) rare associations. Front Endocrinol. 2021;12:678869.
9. Biesecker LG, Sapp JC. Proteus syndrome. In: Adam MP, Ardinger HH, Pagon RA, Wallace SE, Bean LJH, Mirzaa G, et al., editors. GeneReviews(®). Seattle, WA: University of Washington, Seattle; 1993. Copyright © 1993-2021, University of Washington, Seattle. GeneReviews is a registered trademark of the University of Washington, Seattle. All rights reserved.
10. Tan MH, Mester JL, Ngeow J, Rybicki LA, Orloff MS, Eng C. Lifetime cancer risks in individuals with germline PTEN mutations. Clini Cancer Res. 2012;18(2):400–7.
11. Eng C. Cowden syndrome. J Genet Couns. 1997;6(2):181–92.
12. Marsh DJ, Kum JB, Lunetta KL, Bennett MJ, Gorlin RJ, Ahmed SF, et al. PTEN mutation spectrum and genotype-phenotype correlations in Bannayan-Riley-Ruvalcaba syndrome suggest a single entity with Cowden syndrome. Hum Mol Genet. 1999;8(8):1461–72.

13. Starink TM, van der Veen JP, Arwert F, de Waal LP, de Lange GG, Gille JJ, et al. The Cowden syndrome: a clinical and genetic study in 21 patients. Clin Genet. 1986;29(3):222–33.
14. Hanssen AM, Fryns JP. Cowden syndrome. J Med Genet. 1995;32(2):117–9.
15. Bannayan GA. Lipomatosis, angiomatosis, and macrencephalia. A previously undescribed congenital syndrome. Arch Pathol. 1971;92(1):1–5.
16. Smith JR, Marqusee E, Webb S, Nose V, Fishman SJ, Shamberger RC, et al. Thyroid nodules and cancer in children with PTEN hamartoma tumor syndrome. J Clin Endocrinol Metab. 2011;96(1):34–7.
17. Laury AR, Bongiovanni M, Tille JC, Kozakewich H, Nose V. Thyroid pathology in PTEN-hamartoma tumor syndrome: characteristic findings of a distinct entity. Thyroid. 2011;21(2):135–44.
18. Yehia L, Eng C. PTEN hamartoma tumor syndrome. In: Adam MP, Ardinger HH, Pagon RA, Wallace SE, Bean LJH, Mirzaa G, et al., editors. GeneReviews(R). Seattle, WA: University of Washington, Seattle; 1993.
19. Bennett KL, Mester J, Eng C. Germline epigenetic regulation of KILLIN in Cowden and Cowden-like syndrome. JAMA. 2010;304(24):2724–31.
20. Ngeow J, Stanuch K, Mester JL, Barnholtz-Sloan JS, Eng C. Second malignant neoplasms in patients with Cowden syndrome with underlying germline PTEN mutations. J Clin Oncol. 2014;32(17):1818–24.
21. Rutter MM, Jha P, Schultz KA, Sheil A, Harris AK, Bauer AJ, et al. DICER1 mutations and differentiated thyroid carcinoma: evidence of a direct association. J Clin Endocrinol Metab. 2016;101(1):1–5.
22. Brenneman M, Field A, Yang J, Williams G, Doros L, Rossi C, et al. Temporal order of RNase IIIb and loss-of-function mutations during development determines phenotype in pleuropulmonary blastoma/DICER1 syndrome: a unique variant of the two-hit tumor suppression model. F1000Research. 2015;4:214.
23. Kim J, Field A, Schultz KAP, Hill DA, Stewart DR. The prevalence of DICER1 pathogenic variation in population databases. Int J Cancer. 2017;141(10):2030–6.
24. Kim J, Schultz KAP, Hill DA, Stewart DR. The prevalence of germline DICER1 pathogenic variation in cancer populations. Mol Genet Genomic Med. 2019;7(3):e555.
25. Robertson JC, Jorcyk CL, Oxford JT. DICER1 syndrome: DICER1 mutations in rare cancers. Cancers. 2018;10(5).
26. Schultz KAP, Stewart DR, Kamihara J, Bauer AJ, Merideth MA, Stratton P, et al. DICER1 tumor predisposition. In: Adam MP, Ardinger HH, Pagon RA, Wallace SE, Bean LJH, Mirzaa G, et al., editors. GeneReviews(®). Seattle, WA: University of Washington, Seattle; 1993. Copyright © 1993-2021, University of Washington, Seattle. GeneReviews is a registered trademark of the University of Washington, Seattle. All rights reserved.
27. Khan NE, Bauer AJ, Schultz KAP, Doros L, Decastro RM, Ling A, et al. Quantification of thyroid cancer and multinodular goiter risk in the DICER1 syndrome: a family-based cohort study. J Clin Endocrinol Metab. 2017;102(5):1614–22.
28. Mirshahi UL, Kim J, Best AF, Chen ZE, Hu Y, Haley JS, et al. A genome-first approach to characterize DICER1 pathogenic variant prevalence, penetrance, and phenotype. JAMA Netw Open. 2021;4(2):e210112.
29. de Kock L, Sabbaghian N, Soglio DB, Guillerman RP, Park BK, Chami R, et al. Exploring the association between DICER1 mutations and differentiated thyroid carcinoma. J Clin Endocrinol Metab. 2014;99(6):E1072–7.
30. Schultz KAP, Williams GM, Kamihara J, Stewart DR, Harris AK, Bauer AJ, et al. DICER1 and associated conditions: identification of at-risk individuals and recommended surveillance strategies. Clin Cancer Res. 2018;24(10):2251–61.
31. Wells SA Jr, Asa SL, Dralle H, Elisei R, Evans DB, Gagel RF, et al. Revised American Thyroid Association guidelines for the management of medullary thyroid carcinoma. Thyroid. 2015;25(6):567–610.

32. de Kock L, Wang YC, Revil T, Badescu D, Rivera B, Sabbaghian N, et al. High-sensitivity sequencing reveals multi-organ somatic mosaicism causing DICER1 syndrome. J Med Genet. 2016;53(1):43–52.
33. Son EJ, Nose V. Familial follicular cell-derived thyroid carcinoma. Front Endocrinol (Lausanne). 2012;3:61.
34. Beuschlein F, Fassnacht M, Assie G, Calebiro D, Stratakis CA, Osswald A, et al. Constitutive activation of PKA catalytic subunit in adrenal Cushing's syndrome. N Engl J Med. 2014;370(11):1019–28.
35. Forlino A, Vetro A, Garavelli L, Ciccone R, London E, Stratakis CA, et al. PRKACB and Carney complex. N Engl J Med. 2014;370(11):1065–7.
36. Vindhyal MR, Elshimy G, Elhomsy G. Carney complex. Treasure Island, FL: StatPearls; 2021.
37. Stratakis CA, Kirschner LS, Carney JA. Clinical and molecular features of the Carney complex: diagnostic criteria and recommendations for patient evaluation. J Clin Endocrinol Metab. 2001;86(9):4041–6.
38. Carney JA, Lyssikatos C, Seethala RR, Lakatos P, Perez-Atayde A, Lahner H, et al. The spectrum of thyroid gland pathology in Carney complex: the importance of follicular carcinoma. Am J Surg Pathol. 2018;42(5):587–94.
39. Matyakhina L, Pack S, Kirschner LS, Pak E, Mannan P, Jaikumar J, et al. Chromosome 2 (2p16) abnormalities in Carney complex tumours. J Med Genet. 2003;40(4):268–77.
40. Rothenbuhler A, Stratakis CA. Clinical and molecular genetics of Carney complex. Best Pract Res Clin Endocrinol Metab. 2010;24(3):389–99.
41. Correa R, Salpea P, Stratakis CA. Carney complex: an update. Eur J Endocrinol. 2015;173(4):M85–97.
42. Bossis I, Voutetakis A, Bei T, Sandrini F, Griffin KJ, Stratakis CA. Protein kinase A and its role in human neoplasia: the Carney complex paradigm. Endocr Relat Cancer. 2004;11(2):265–80.
43. Siordia JA. Medical and surgical management of Carney complex. J Card Surg. 2015;30(7):560–7.
44. Rivkees SA, Mazzaferri EL, Verburg FA, Reiners C, Luster M, Breuer CK, et al. The treatment of differentiated thyroid cancer in children: emphasis on surgical approach and radioactive iodine therapy. Endocr Rev. 2011;32(6):798–826.
45. Ito Y, Fukushima M, Yabuta T, Inoue H, Uruno T, Kihara M, et al. Prevalence and prognosis of familial follicular thyroid carcinoma. Endocr J. 2008;55(5):847–52.
46. Bouys L, Bertherat J. MANAGEMENT OF ENDOCRINE DISEASE: Carney complex: clinical and genetic update 20 years after the identification of the CNC1 (PRKAR1A) gene. Eur J Endocrinol. 2021;184(3):R99–R109.
47. Stratakis CA, Raygada M. Carney complex. In: Adam MP, Ardinger HH, Pagon RA, Wallace SE, Bean LJH, Stephens K, et al., editors. GeneReviews(®). Seattle, WA: University of Washington, Seattle; 1993. Copyright © 1993-2020, University of Washington, Seattle. GeneReviews is a registered trademark of the University of Washington, Seattle. All rights reserved.
48. Stelmachowska-Banas M, Zgliczynski W, Tutka P, Carney JA, Korbonits M. Fatal Carney complex in siblings due to de novo large gene deletion. J Clin Endocrinol Metab. 2017;102(11):3924–7.
49. Stratakis CA, Carney JA, Lin JP, Papanicolaou DA, Karl M, Kastner DL, et al. Carney complex, a familial multiple neoplasia and lentiginosis syndrome. Analysis of 11 kindreds and linkage to the short arm of chromosome 2. J Clin Invest. 1996;97(3):699–705.
50. McConville CM, Stankovic T, Byrd PJ, McGuire GM, Yao QY, Lennox GG, et al. Mutations associated with variant phenotypes in ataxia-telangiectasia. Am J Hum Genet. 1996;59(2):320–30.
51. Gatti R, Perlman S. Ataxia-telangiectasia. In: Adam MP, Ardinger HH, Pagon RA, Wallace SE, Bean LJH, Mirzaa G, et al., editors. GeneReviews(®). Seattle, WA: University of Washington, Seattle; 1993. Copyright © 1993-2021, University of Washington, Seattle.

GeneReviews is a registered trademark of the University of Washington, Seattle. All rights reserved.

52. Xu L, Morari EC, Wei Q, Sturgis EM, Ward LS. Functional variations in the ATM gene and susceptibility to differentiated thyroid carcinoma. J Clin Endocrinol Metab. 2012;97(6):1913–21.

53. Zhang Q, Davis JC, Lamborn IT, Freeman AF, Jing H, Favreau AJ, et al. Combined immunodeficiency associated with DOCK8 mutations. N Engl J Med. 2009;361(21):2046–55.

54. Cavalieri S, Funaro A, Pappi P, Migone N, Gatti RA, Brusco A. Large genomic mutations within the ATM gene detected by MLPA, including a duplication of 41 kb from exon 4 to 20. Ann Hum Genet. 2008;72(Pt 1):10–8.

55. Telatar M, Wang S, Castellvi-Bel S, Tai LQ, Sheikhavandi S, Regueiro JR, et al. A model for ATM heterozygote identification in a large population: four founder-effect ATM mutations identify most of Costa Rican patients with ataxia telangiectasia. Mol Genet Metab. 1998;64(1):36–43.

56. Tavtigian SV, Oefner PJ, Babikyan D, Hartmann A, Healey S, Le Calvez-Kelm F, et al. Rare, evolutionarily unlikely missense substitutions in ATM confer increased risk of breast cancer. Am J Hum Genet. 2009;85(4):427–46.

57. Bernstein JL, Bernstein L, Thompson WD, Lynch CF, Malone KE, Teitelbaum SL, et al. ATM variants 7271T>G and IVS10-6T>G among women with unilateral and bilateral breast cancer. Br J Cancer. 2003;89(8):1513–6.

58. van Os NJ, Roeleveld N, Weemaes CM, Jongmans MC, Janssens GO, Taylor AM, et al. Health risks for ataxia-telangiectasia mutated heterozygotes: a systematic review, meta-analysis and evidence-based guideline. Clin Genet. 2016;90(2):105–17.

59. Sutton IJ, Last JI, Ritchie SJ, Harrington HJ, Byrd PJ, Taylor AM. Adult-onset ataxia telangiectasia due to ATM 5762ins137 mutation homozygosity. Ann Neurol. 2004;55(6):891–5.

60. Stankovic T, Kidd AM, Sutcliffe A, McGuire GM, Robinson P, Weber P, et al. ATM mutations and phenotypes in ataxia-telangiectasia families in the British Isles: expression of mutant ATM and the risk of leukemia, lymphoma, and breast cancer. Am J Hum Genet. 1998;62(2):334–45.

61. Verhagen MM, Abdo WF, Willemsen MA, Hogervorst FB, Smeets DF, Hiel JA, et al. Clinical spectrum of ataxia-telangiectasia in adulthood. Neurology. 2009;73(6):430–7.

62. Mitui M, Nahas SA, Du LT, Yang Z, Lai CH, Nakamura K, et al. Functional and computational assessment of missense variants in the ataxia-telangiectasia mutated (ATM) gene: mutations with increased cancer risk. Hum Mutat. 2009;30(1):12–21.

63. Byrd PJ, Srinivasan V, Last JI, Smith A, Biggs P, Carney EF, et al. Severe reaction to radiotherapy for breast cancer as the presenting feature of ataxia telangiectasia. Br J Cancer. 2012;106(2):262–8.

64. Swift M. Genetics and epidemiology of ataxia-telangiectasia. Kroc Found Ser. 1985;19:133–46.

65. Swift M, Morrell D, Cromartie E, Chamberlin AR, Skolnick MH, Bishop DT. The incidence and gene frequency of ataxia-telangiectasia in the United States. Am J Hum Genet. 1986;39(5):573–83.

66. Hadizadeh H, Salehi M, Khoramnejad S, Vosoughi K, Rezaei N. The association between parental consanguinity and primary immunodeficiency diseases: a systematic review and meta-analysis. Pediatr Allergy Immunol. 2017;28(3):280–7.

67. Ulusoy E, Edeer-Karaca N, Özen S, Ertan Y, Gökşen D, Aksu G, et al. An unusual manifestation: papillary thyroid carcinoma in a patient with ataxia-telengiectasia. Turk J Pediatr. 2016;58(4):442–5.

68. Savitsky K, Bar-Shira A, Gilad S, Rotman G, Ziv Y, Vanagaite L, et al. A single ataxia telangiectasia gene with a product similar to PI-3 kinase. Science. 1995;268(5218):1749–53.

69. Stray-Pedersen A, Borresen-Dale AL, Paus E, Lindman CR, Burgers T, Abrahamsen TG. Alpha fetoprotein is increasing with age in ataxia-telangiectasia. Eur J Paediatr Neurol. 2007;11(6):375–80.

70. Brasseur B, Beauloye V, Chantrain C, Daumerie C, Vermylen C, Waignein F, et al. Papillary thyroid carcinoma in a 9-year-old girl with ataxia-telangiectasia. Pediatr Blood Cancer. 2008;50(5):1058–60.
71. Wartofsky L, Van Nostrand D. Thyroid cancer: a comprehensive guide to clinical management. Berlin: Springer; 2016.
72. Klubo-Gwiezdzinska J, Van Nostrand D, Atkins F, Burman K, Jonklaas J, Mete M, et al. Efficacy of dosimetric versus empiric prescribed activity of 131I for therapy of differentiated thyroid cancer. J Clin Endocrinol Metab. 2011;96(10):3217–25.
73. Blom M, Schoenaker MHD, Hulst M, de Vries MC, Weemaes CMR, Willemsen M, et al. Dilemma of reporting incidental findings in newborn screening programs for SCID: parents' perspective on ataxia telangiectasia. Front Immunol. 2019;10:2438.
74. Bauer AJ. Clinical behavior and genetics of nonsyndromic, familial nonmedullary thyroid cancer. Front Horm Res. 2013;41:141–8.
75. Charkes ND. On the prevalence of familial nonmedullary thyroid cancer in multiply affected kindreds. Thyroid. 2006;16(2):181–6.
76. Ríos A, Rodríguez JM, Navas D, Cepero A, Torregrosa NM, Balsalobre MD, et al. Family screening in familial papillary carcinoma: the early detection of thyroid disease. Ann Surg Oncol. 2016;23(8):2564–70.
77. Moses W, Weng J, Kebebew E. Prevalence, clinicopathologic features, and somatic genetic mutation profile in familial versus sporadic nonmedullary thyroid cancer. Thyroid. 2011;21(4):367–71.
78. Capezzone M, Robenshtok E, Cantara S, Castagna MG. Familial non-medullary thyroid cancer: a critical review. J Endocrinol Investig. 2021;44(5):943–50.
79. Canzian F, Amati P, Harach HR, Kraimps JL, Lesueur F, Barbier J, et al. A gene predisposing to familial thyroid tumors with cell oxyphilia maps to chromosome 19p13.2. Am J Hum Genet. 1998;63(6):1743–8.
80. Bevan S, Pal T, Greenberg CR, Green H, Wixey J, Bignell G, et al. A comprehensive analysis of MNG1, TCO1, fPTC, PTEN, TSHR, and TRKA in familial nonmedullary thyroid cancer: confirmation of linkage to TCO1. J Clin Endocrinol Metab. 2001;86(8):3701–4.
81. Malchoff CD, Sarfarazi M, Tendler B, Forouhar F, Whalen G, Joshi V, et al. Papillary thyroid carcinoma associated with papillary renal neoplasia: genetic linkage analysis of a distinct heritable tumor syndrome. J Clin Endocrinol Metab. 2000;85(5):1758–64.
82. McKay JD, Thompson D, Lesueur F, Stankov K, Pastore A, Watfah C, et al. Evidence for interaction between the TCO and NMTC1 loci in familial non-medullary thyroid cancer. J Med Genet. 2004;41(6):407–12.
83. Peiling Yang S, Ngeow J. Familial non-medullary thyroid cancer: unraveling the genetic maze. Endocr Relat Cancer. 2016;23(12):R577–95.
84. Gara SK, Jia L, Merino MJ, Agarwal SK, Zhang L, Cam M, et al. Germline HABP2 mutation causing familial nonmedullary thyroid cancer. N Engl J Med. 2015;373(5):448–55.
85. He H, Bronisz A, Liyanarachchi S, Nagy R, Li W, Huang Y, et al. SRGAP1 is a candidate gene for papillary thyroid carcinoma susceptibility. J Clin Endocrinol Metab. 2013;98(5):E973–80.
86. Pereira JS, da Silva JG, Tomaz RA, Pinto AE, Bugalho MJ, Leite V, et al. Identification of a novel germline FOXE1 variant in patients with familial non-medullary thyroid carcinoma (FNMTC). Endocrine. 2015;49(1):204–14.
87. Ngan ES, Lang BH, Liu T, Shum CK, So MT, Lau DK, et al. A germline mutation (A339V) in thyroid transcription factor-1 (TITF-1/NKX2.1) in patients with multinodular goiter and papillary thyroid carcinoma. J Natl Cancer Inst. 2009;101(3):162–75.
88. Ye F, Gao H, Xiao L, Zuo Z, Liu Y, Zhao Q, et al. Whole exome and target sequencing identifies MAP2K5 as novel susceptibility gene for familial non-medullary thyroid carcinoma. Int J Cancer. 2019;144(6):1321–30.
89. Spinelli C, Piccolotti I, Bertocchini A, Morganti R, Materazzi G, Tonacchera M, et al. Familial non-medullary thyroid carcinoma in pediatric age: our surgical experience. World J Surg. 2021;45(8):2473–9.

90. Cirello V. Familial non-medullary thyroid carcinoma: clinico-pathological features, current knowledge and novelty regarding genetic risk factors. Minerva Endocrinol. 2021;46:5–20.
91. Klubo-Gwiezdzinska J, Kushchayeva Y, Gara SK, Kebebew E. Familial non-medullary thyroid cancer. In: Mallick UK, Harmer C, editors. Practical management of thyroid cancer: a multidisciplinary approach. Cham: Springer International Publishing; 2018. p. 241–70.
92. Sturgeon C, Clark OH. Familial nonmedullary thyroid cancer. Thyroid. 2005;15(6):588–93.
93. Byun SH, Min C, Choi HG, Hong SJ. Association between family histories of thyroid cancer and thyroid cancer incidence: a cross-sectional study using the Korean Genome and Epidemiology Study Data. Genes. 2020;11(9).
94. Raue F, Frank-Raue K. Genotype-phenotype correlation in multiple endocrine neoplasia type 2. Clinics (Sao Paulo). 2012;67(Suppl 1):69–75.
95. Goudie C, Hannah-Shmouni F, Kavak M, Stratakis CA, Foulkes WD. 65 YEARS OF THE DOUBLE HELIX: endocrine tumour syndromes in children and adolescents. Endocr Relat Cancer. 2018;25(8):T221–44.
96. Eng C. Multiple endocrine neoplasia type 2. In: Adam MP, Ardinger HH, Pagon RA, Wallace SE, Bean LJH, Mirzaa G, et al., editors. GeneReviews(®). Seattle, WA: University of Washington, Seattle; 1993. Copyright © 1993-2021, University of Washington, Seattle. GeneReviews is a registered trademark of the University of Washington, Seattle. All rights reserved.
97. Magalhaes PK, Antonini SR, de Paula FJ, de Freitas LC, Maciel LM. Primary hyperparathyroidism as the first clinical manifestation of multiple endocrine neoplasia type 2A in a 5-year-old child. Thyroid. 2011;21(5):547–50.
98. Roizen J, Levine MA. Primary hyperparathyroidism in children and adolescents. J Chin Med Assoc. 2012;75(9):425–34.
99. Rowland KJ, Chernock RD, Moley JF. Pheochromocytoma in an 8-year-old patient with multiple endocrine neoplasia type 2A: implications for screening. J Surg Oncol. 2013;108(4):203–6.
100. Klubo-Gwiezdzinska J. Targeting RET-mutated thyroid and lung cancer in the personalised medicine era. Lancet Diabetes Endocrinol. 2021;9:473.
101. Kraft IL, Akshintala S, Zhu Y, Lei H, Derse-Anthony C, Dombi E, et al. Outcomes of children and adolescents with advanced hereditary medullary thyroid carcinoma treated with Vandetanib. Clin Cancer Res. 2018;24(4):753–65.
102. Wells SA Jr, Robinson BG, Gagel RF, Dralle H, Fagin JA, Santoro M, et al. Vandetanib in patients with locally advanced or metastatic medullary thyroid cancer: a randomized, double-blind phase III trial. J Clin Oncol. 2012;30(2):134–41.
103. Elisei R, Schlumberger MJ, Müller SP, Schöffski P, Brose MS, Shah MH, et al. Cabozantinib in progressive medullary thyroid cancer. J Clin Oncol. 2013;31(29):3639.
104. Mathiesen JS, Kroustrup JP, Vestergaard P, Madsen M, Stochholm K, Poulsen PL, et al. Incidence and prevalence of multiple endocrine neoplasia 2B in Denmark: a nationwide study. Endocr Relat Cancer. 2017;24(7):L39–42.
105. Zenaty D, Aigrain Y, Peuchmaur M, Philippe-Chomette P, Baumann C, Cornelis F, et al. Medullary thyroid carcinoma identified within the first year of life in children with hereditary multiple endocrine neoplasia type 2A (codon 634) and 2B. Eur J Endocrinol. 2009;160(5):807–13.
106. Wray CJ, Rich TA, Waguespack SG, Lee JE, Perrier ND, Evans DB. Failure to recognize multiple endocrine neoplasia 2B: more common than we think? Ann Surg Oncol. 2008;15(1):293–301.
107. Wells SA Jr, Chi DD, Toshima K, Dehner LP, Coffin CM, Dowton SB, et al. Predictive DNA testing and prophylactic thyroidectomy in patients at risk for multiple endocrine neoplasia type 2A. Ann Surg. 1994;220(3):237–47; discussion 47–50.
108. Brauckhoff M, Gimm O, Weiss CL, Ukkat J, Sekulla C, Brauckhoff K, et al. Multiple endocrine neoplasia 2B syndrome due to codon 918 mutation: clinical manifestation and course in early and late onset disease. World J Surg. 2004;28(12):1305–11.
109. Moo-Young TA, Traugott AL, Moley JF. Sporadic and familial medullary thyroid carcinoma: state of the art. Surg Clin North Am. 2009;89(5):1193–204.

Chapter 6
Genetics, Biology, Clinical Presentation, Laboratory Diagnostics, and Management of Pediatric and Adolescent Pheochromocytoma and Paraganglioma

Graeme Eisenhofer, Christina Pamporaki, Michaela Kuhlen, and Antje Redlich

Age at Diagnosis and Prevalence

Pheochromocytoma and paraganglioma (PPGL) which respectively arise from intra-adrenal chromaffin cells and extra-adrenal sympathetic or parasympathetic paraganglia, exhibit numerous differences when they present in childhood through to early adulthood compared to later ages [1–3]. Many of these differences relate to underlying pathogenic variants of specific tumor susceptibility genes that are associated with a relatively early age of disease onset and contribute to disease prevalence in childhood. Prevalence of PPGL among children with hypertension is higher than in adults, reaching up to 1.7% [4] compared to 0.2% in adults. This presumably reflects the higher proportion of secondary forms of hypertension in children and adolescents than adults.

Among different pediatric series, the average age at which PPGL are diagnosed varies between 11 and 15 years [3, 5–15]. Among the larger series of patients, the youngest age at diagnosis is generally reported at 4–5 years [3, 8, 11, 13, 15, 16], but some isolated cases of the tumor have been reported as early as 2 years [14] or

G. Eisenhofer (✉) · C. Pamporaki
Department of Medicine III, University Hospital Carl Gustav Carus, Technische Universität Dresden, Dresden, Germany
e-mail: Graeme.Eisenhofer@ukdd.de; Christina.Pamporaki@ukdd.de

M. Kuhlen
Swabian Children's Cancer Center, Pediatrics and Adolescent Medicine, University Medical Center, Augsburg, Germany
e-mail: Michaela.Kuhlen@uk-augsburg.de

A. Redlich
Pediatric Hematology/Oncology, Department of Pediatrics, Otto von Guericke University Children's Hospital, Magdeburg, Germany
e-mail: Antje.Redlich@med.ovgu.de

© The Author(s), under exclusive license to Springer Nature Switzerland AG 2023
F. Hannah-Shmouni (ed.), *Familial Endocrine Cancer Syndromes*,
https://doi.org/10.1007/978-3-031-37275-9_6

even younger [17]. Several studies have reported a male predominance [6, 11, 13, 15, 16, 18], but this has not been corroborated by other studies [5, 7, 12].

Among the limited numbers of studies that have included data from both pediatric and adult patients with PPGL, about 8–10% are usually described to present during childhood and through adolescence [10, 11, 18]. However, in a series of 255 patients with PPGL, Barontini et al. reported 58 (23%) cases of the tumor detected before the age of 20 [16]. In another more recent series of 748 patients with PPGL, 95 cases (12.7%) were first diagnosed ≤18 years of age [3].

When interpreting data about childhood prevalence of PPGL it is important to recognize that for most cases of the tumor there is considerable delay from the time a tumor first appears to initial presentation of signs and symptoms and then to final diagnosis [19, 20]. Olson and colleagues clarified this delay using measurements of plasma metanephrines in serum collected and banked from 30 US Department of Defense active military service members for up to 20 years before diagnosis of PPGL [21]. Elevated serum metanephrines of more than two-fold above upper cut-offs of reference intervals were found at a medium of 6.6 years before diagnosis. The study also indicated an average doubling time for increases in plasma metanephrines of 3 years, which is in line with the slow growing nature of these tumors [22]. Since plasma concentrations of metanephrines directly relate to tumor volume [23], and assuming a doubling time of 2–3 years, it can be determined that it would take 6–9 years for a 1 cm diameter tumor to reach 2 cm in diameter and another 6–9 years to reach 3 cm (i.e., overall a 27-fold increase in volume). Since the average diameter of most chromaffin cell tumors at diagnosis is between 3 and 4 cm it can be appreciated that most PPGL that are diagnosed in young adults must first develop during childhood. Thus, the true prevalence of childhood PPGL is likely much higher than the 8–13% observed in population-based studies [3, 10, 11, 18], and is more likely to reach or even exceed the 23% prevalence indicated by Barontini et al. [16].

Based on a tumor doubling time of 2 years, it can be estimated from the data of Pamporaki et al. [3] that the 12.7% prevalence of childhood PPGL increases to 29.8% when tumor size at diagnosis is considered (Fig. 6.1). Of course, at a starting diameter of 1 cm, most tumors are unlikely to produce signs and symptoms of catecholamine excess. The only possibility for detecting such tumors would be as part of surveillance programs based on hereditary risk. Nevertheless, the likelihood of a larger proportion of PPGL arising during childhood than is widely appreciated raises the importance of these tumors for pediatricians. With this there is also a need for improved coordination and communication among various pediatric and adult care specialties, particularly since most of the clinical expertise for these tumors resides with the latter.

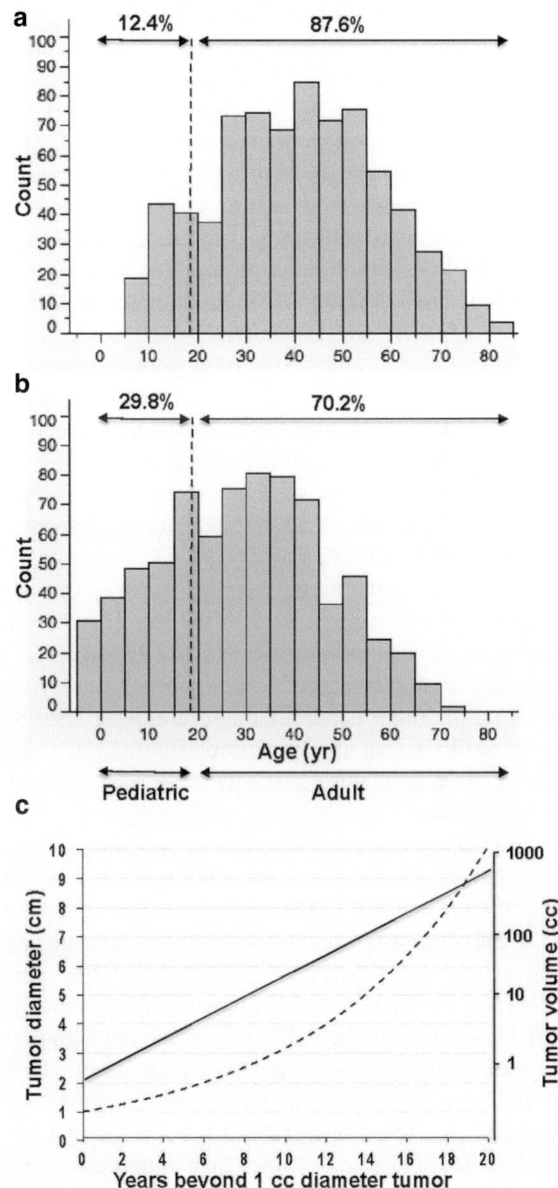

Fig. 6.1 Age distributions for patients with PPGL at first diagnosis (**a**) versus likely initial occurrence of tumors at an initial diameter of 1 cm (**b**), the latter according to calculations based on a tumor volume doubling time of 2 years as clarified in panel (**c**) for both tumor diameter (dashed line) and volume (solid line drawn according to logarithmic scale for tumor volume). Corrections of most likely age for presentations of tumors at a 1 cm diameter in panel (**b**) were based on tumor size at diagnosis and subtractions for estimated numbers of years to reach that size. Proportions of patients below 19 years (pediatric presentation) and above 19 years (adult presentation) are shown in panels (**a**) and (**b**) according to distributions. Data are from the 748 patients described by Pamporaki et al. [3]

Genetics and Biology

Although the importance of hereditary causes of PPGL has only truly become established over the past 20 years, the familial association in pediatric cases of the tumor was already recognized as far back as in the 1960s and early 1970s when

Knudson proposed the two-hit hypothesis for involvement of tumor suppressor genes in cancer [2]. As more and more genetic causes of PPGL were identified, the prevalence of germline pathogenic variants in tumor susceptibility genes in pediatric cases of the tumor has increased from 40% in studies of 2005–2010 [7, 16] to estimates that now reach or even exceed 80% [3, 11, 14, 15]. In keeping with early observations [1], the prevalence of germline variants of tumor susceptibility genes in children remains about two-fold higher than in adults.

Most common pathogenic variants in tumor susceptibility genes in pediatric cases of PPGL are observed in pseudohypoxic genes, particularly those encoding the von Hippel-Lindau (*VHL*) tumor suppressor and succinate dehydrogenase subunits B (*SDHB*) and D (*SDHD*); these variants respectively account for up to 27–50%, 20–47%, and 2–10% of all pediatric cases of the tumor [3, 10, 11, 14, 15]. Pathogenic variants have also been observed for succinate dehydrogenase subunit C (*SDHC*), MYC-associated factor X (MAX), and endothelial PAS domain-containing protein 1 (*EPAS1*), but at lower frequencies of 1–3% [10, 14, 15]. Apart from *MAX*, all aforementioned genes encode components of the pseudohypoxic pathway and involve mutations that lead to stabilization of hypoxia-inducible factors (HIFs), particularly HIF2α, encoded by *EPAS1*.

In contrast to the pseudohypoxic pathway genes, pathogenic variants in kinase signaling pathway genes, such as the rearranged during transfection (*RET*) pseudo-oncogene and neurofibromatosis 1 (*NF1*) gene, account for relatively low proportions of pediatric compared to adult pheochromocytomas [3]. Pathogenic variants in *MAX* on the other hand, although rare, have been described not only in pediatric cases of PPGL, but also in neuroblastoma [24]. This gene may, however, occupy a pivotal place as a convergence pathway point for upstream mutations of both pseudohypoxic and kinase signaling pathway genes [25].

A characteristic of PPGLs due to mutations of pseudohypoxic pathway genes is that the tumors do not express appreciable amounts of phenylethanolamine-N-methyltransferase (PNMT), the enzyme that converts norepinephrine to epinephrine [25]. This contrasts with tumors due to pathogenic variants in kinase signaling pathway genes, such as *RET*, *NF1*, *TMEM127*, *HRAS*, and *FGFR1*, all of which express PNMT and produce variable amounts of both epinephrine and norepinephrine [23, 26]. Consequent to these differences and the high prevalence of variants in pseudohypoxic pathway genes in pediatric cases of PPGL, these tumors are characterized by predominant production, storage and secretion of norepinephrine with little epinephrine [3]. These observations are also consistent with findings that PPGL that produce norepinephrine rather than mixtures of epinephrine and norepinephrine occur at earlier ages in both hereditary and sporadic cases of the tumors [27].

Although there are ethnic differences in the genomic landscape of presentation of PPGL, tumors that occur in Caucasians due to mutations of kinase signaling pathways and that produce epinephrine almost always have adrenal locations [23, 26]. In contrast, tumors due to pathogenic variants in pseudohypoxic genes occur at both adrenal and extra-adrenal sites, with the latter particularly characteristic of tumors due to mutations of *SDHB* and *SDHD*. This, therefore, accounts for differences in presentations of paragangliomas and adrenal pheochromocytomas in

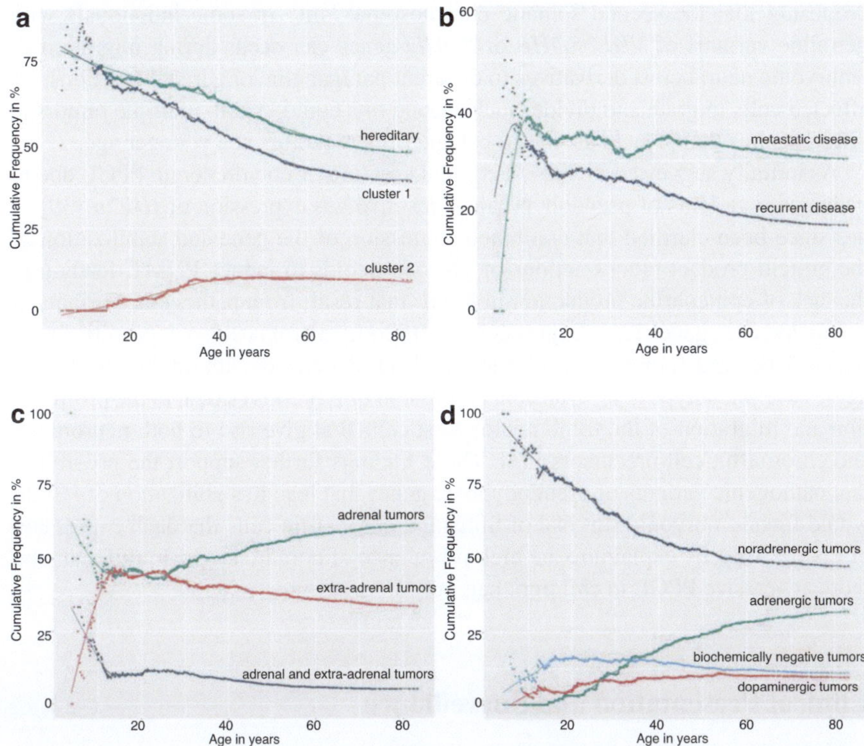

Fig. 6.2 Cumulative frequencies as a function of age, including (**a**) hereditary disease due to cluster 1 and cluster 2 mutations, (**b**) metastatic and recurrent disease, (**c**) adrenal, extra-adrenal, and synchronous adrenal and extra-adrenal first tumors, and (**d**) according to the catecholamines predominantly produced by the tumor. Results based on merged datasets of Pamporaki et al. [3] and Redlich et al. [15]

children compared to adults (Fig. 6.2), including a higher proportion of adrenal than extra-adrenal tumors in adults than children [3]. Other related characteristic features of pediatric compared to adult cases of PPGL involve predominance in the former of multifocal tumors, bilateral adrenal tumors, and recurrent disease [1–3, 10]. Some studies have also indicated that in addition to recurrent disease, childhood cases of PPGL tend to metastasize more often than those detected at later ages [3, 14, 28].

The aforementioned features of pediatric PPGL can be partially ascribed to the predominance of pathogenic variants in pseudohypoxic genes, which carry a higher risk of metastatic disease than variants in genes involved in kinase signaling [29]. Nevertheless, analyses restricted to tumors from such patients have indicated that multifocal PPGL occur at significantly younger ages than solitary tumors [27]. This suggests other contributing factors for the high prevalence of multifocal and recurrent PPGL in children than adults, including possible origins from single tumor precursor cells. This idea builds on the Knudson two-hit hypothesis [2], by proposing that the second somatic chromosomal "hit" in some individuals with germline variants of *VHL*, *SDHB* or *SDHD* genes can occur during migration of embryonic neural crest derivatives to different paraganglial or adrenal locations. As affected cells migrate and divide, such second hits could lead to multiple tumors at different sites that present as multifocal and/or new tumors at a younger age.

As initially suggested in 2004, a common feature of noradrenergic PPGL due to pathogenic variants of pseudohypoxia genes involves expression of *HIF2α* [30]. It has since been clarified that combined expression of the gene and stabilization of the protein product blocks actions of glucocorticoids to induce PNMT, leading to the lack of epinephrine production in PPGL that result from pathogenic variants in pseudohypoxia genes [25]. Expression of HIF2α in neuroblastoma, a primitive neural crest derived tumor of early childhood, is associated with an immature and aggressive phenotype [31]. Transient expression of HIF2α is critical to the proliferation and migration of the trunk neural crest cells that give rise to both neuroblasts and chromaffin cell precursors [32]. These findings further support the possibility that pathogenic variants of pseudohypoxic genes that lead to stabilization of HIF2α would favor embryonic survival of immature chromaffin cells that lack expression of PNMT, thereby explaining the high prevalence of noradrenergic, multifocal, and more aggressive PPGL in children than in adults.

Clinical Presentation and Surveillance

The clinical presentation of PPGLs in children as in adults is, in general, dominated by manifestations of catecholamines secreted by the tumors, which can result in hypertension and numerous signs and symptoms of catecholamine excess (Table 6.1). These signs and symptoms often have a recurrent paroxysmal nature, but can also occur unexpectedly and in isolation after provocation by various stimuli or pharmacological agents. Although hypertension is less common in children than in adults, this alone is not usually sufficient to justify a search for PPGL until other more common forms of secondary hypertension are excluded. Nevertheless, when hypertension is paroxysmal or accompanied by other signs or symptoms of catecholamine excess, then the possibility of PPGL should be considered. Signs and symptoms that are particularly important to consider include palpitations, inappropriate sweating, tremor, pallor, and nausea or vomiting [33]. Although, there is no clear distinction for the presentation of signs and symptoms in children versus adults [5, 7, 13, 16], nighttime sweatiness, polyuria, and disturbances of vision or mental status have been described in children that might warrant attention [6, 8, 16, 18]. Since hypertension may be intermittent and not always present at clinical evaluation [5], it is important not to discount a catecholamine-producing tumor in apparently normotensive children who nevertheless present with other signs and symptoms of catecholamine excess.

Table 6.1 Clinical manifestations of catecholamine-producing chromaffin cell tumors in children

	Signs and symptoms	Frequency
Cardiovascular	Hypertension[a]	60–90%
	Tachycardia (heart rate above 80 bpm)	40–60%
	Palpitations	45–55%
Neurologic	Headache[b]	60–70%
	Alterations in mental status/decline in school performance	40%
Gastrointestinal	Nausea/vomiting	45–55%
Dermatologic	Diaphoresis (sweating)	45–55%
	Pallor	45–55%
	Red puffy hands and feet	10–20%
Urologic	Polyuria/polydipsia	10–20%
Ophthalmologic	Visual disturbances	20%
Metabolic	Weight loss	20%

[a] Hypertension in children up to 12 years is assessed according to blood pressures beyond the 95th percentile of age, height and sex normative data in normal weight children; for adolescents' hypertension is defined by a systolic blood pressure > 130 and/or diastolic blood pressure > 80 mmHg. Importantly children with PPGL may be normotensive or only present with intermittent hypertension, best assessed by ambulatory blood pressure monitoring
[b] Headache is a relatively non-specific symptom, but when throbbing in nature and combined with other symptoms may be useful

It is the signs and symptoms of presumed catecholamine excess that have historically provided the basis for clinical suspicion of underlying PPGL. Significant proportions of PPGL are now, however, being discovered for other reasons, including findings of an incidental mass during imaging studies for unrelated conditions (i.e., incidentaloma) as well as during routine screening associated with familial tumor syndromes or variants in tumor susceptibility genes. At some specialist referral centers more than 50% of PPGL are now being discovered as incidentalomas [34], but this is mainly in adult patients.

Despite the changing nature in how PPGL are being discovered, the primary reason for clinical suspicion and laboratory testing in children, as in adults, remains based on presentation of signs and symptoms of presumed catecholamine excess. In children, incidentalomas are more rarely encountered than in adults, particularly older adults, and accordingly represent a relatively minor reason for testing. On the other hand, germline variants in tumor susceptibility genes are twice as common in pediatric than adult patients with PPGL; accordingly, biochemical testing as part of routine surveillance in carriers of pathogenic variants of tumor susceptibility genes is becoming increasingly important for disease discovery; there is a particular need for this in children, though it must also be recognized that in many children the variants are de novo and not present in their parents [10].

To meet the need for PPGL surveillance programs in at-risk children, there are now recommendations and even guidelines proposed for screening that allow for specific tumor susceptibility genes [35–37]. These recommendations and guidelines build on an accumulating wealth of natural history and genotype–phenotype data related to the presentation of childhood cases of PPGL according to not only affected genes, but also specific pathogenic variants in tumor susceptibility genes [3, 28, 37–39].

Recognizing the high proportion of childhood cases of PPGL due to *VHL* pathogenic variants, it is well established that screening for PPGL in *VHL* variant carriers should be initiated in childhood [35, 40]. Furthermore, since PPGL in *VHL* variant carriers can present at a young age, the emerging consensus is to initiate screening for the tumors at an age of 5 years. Because the penetrance of different tumors in *VHL* syndrome is impacted by whether gene variants involve missense versus truncating or deletion variants [41–43], there are possibilities that surveillance for PPGL in *VHL* variant carriers may be initiated at later ages or relaxed for some patients. As yet, however, there are no clear recommendations related to variant-specific screening and all patients with *VHL* variants should undergo periodic surveillance.

For pathogenic variants of genes encoding succinate dehydrogenase subunits, the most clear recommendations for surveillance concern children with *SDHB* variants, which are associated with a significant proportion of childhood cases and carry a high risk for multifocal, recurrent and metastatic disease [28]. Although disease penetrance is not high in *SDHB* variant carriers, the young age at which PPGLs can develop combined with the aggressiveness of disease has determined recommendations that routine screening should start at 5–6 years of age [36, 38]. For *SDHA, SDHC,* and *SDHD* pathogenic variant carriers, current recommendations are for screening to commence at 10 years of age and as in other patients to be repeated every 2–3 years if earlier screening returns negative results [36].

Although most pheochromocytomas in patients with *RET* pathogenic variants occur in adults, the tumors can also occur in children, so that screening beginning in childhood is recommended. However, the risk for pheochromocytoma and age distributions of incidence vary according to specific variants and their associated activating strength [44]. Associated refinements to screening guidelines indicate a start for PPGL screening at 11 years for high-risk variant carriers and at 16 or 26 years for others, and with intensity of screening varying from 1 to 3-year intervals dependent on age [44].

For patients with NF1, past recommendations for screening were based on whether patients present with hypertension. Recommendations now indicate that screening for pheochromocytoma in patients with NF1 be carried out once every 3 years starting at an age between 10 and 14 years [45].

In carriers of *MAX, FH, MDH2, TMEM127,* and pathogenic variants of other tumor susceptibility genes, the rare nature of PPGL due to these variants precludes any evidence-based recommendations for surveillance programs specific for these genes. Nevertheless, since all carriers are at risk for PPGL, they should undergo some form of periodic surveillance that probably should begin at least in adolescence or early adulthood. Although PPGL due to *EPAS1* pathogenic variants do occur during childhood [14, 15, 46], these invariably are somatic in nature and when involving the Pacak-Zhuang syndrome involve mosaicism due to post-zygotic pathogenic variants in early development [47]. Thus, for any patient found to have an *EPAS1* mutation whether in childhood or adulthood, there is the possibility of additional new or different neoplasms that should be considered under some form or a surveillance program.

As in adults, testing for an underlying pathogenic variant in a tumor susceptibility gene is recommended in all children with PPGL, but even more so because of the higher proportion of hereditary cases in children than adults. Even if a variant is not found it is important that opportunities for routine surveillance are provided postoperatively in order to check recurrent disease, which can present many years after apparently successful resection of a primary tumor [3].

Laboratory Diagnostics

The first step in all patients in whom PPGL is suspected, including children, is biochemical testing. This also applies to patients who undergo periodic surveillance due to past history of PPGL or hereditary predisposition, though in these cases surveillance may also include imaging studies. As outlined in the 2014 Endocrine Society guideline [48], biochemical testing should be initiated using measurements of either plasma or urinary normetanephrine and metanephrine, which together are referred to as metanephrines. Over the years since publication of that guideline, there have been further developments such as addition of methoxytyramine to the plasma test panel [49, 50], which may be particularly important in certain patient groups. Other developments relevant to pediatrics include use of the same plasma test panel for neuroblastoma and PPGL [51, 52] and formulation of age-specific reference intervals for children [53–55]. Development of advanced mass spectrometric methods of analyses and new testing strategies such as measurements of free metanephrines in spot or first morning collections of urine [56], dried blood spots [57], and saliva [58] represent further developments relevant to the pediatric field. More recent technological advances that involve in situ derivatization before sample purification and mass spectrometry provide for high analytical sensitivity and measurements of multiple analytes in single small volume samples [59]. This new technology looks to be particularly important for pediatrics where specimen volume can be a limiting factor.

When selecting plasma or urinary measurements of metanephrines for diagnosis of PPGL, it is of foremost importance for interpretation of test results to understand the sources and different forms of these metabolites in different matrices. Also important is how the metabolites are impacted by different pre-analytical factors or physiological or pharmacological influences and according to different methods of measurement.

Of primary importance to the above is recognition that increases in the metabolites due to a catecholamine-producing tumor do not in any significant manner reflect or depend on secretion of catecholamines from tumors. As such, measurements of the metabolites cannot be used to assess secretory activity, including whether a tumor is secretory or not. As originally indicated by Crout and Sjoerdsma in 1964 [60], the catecholamine metabolites produced by pheochromocytoma are mainly derived from metabolism within tumor cells. At the same time Irwin J Kopin described how the leakage of catecholamines from vesicular stores led to metabolism of the catecholamines within the same cells of catecholamine synthesis; in sympathetic nerves this involves deamination catalyzed by monoamine oxidase (MAO), which converts both norepinephrine and epinephrine to dihydroxyphanylglycol [61]. The importance of metabolism of catecholamines within cells of their synthesis, including in sympathetic neurons, adrenal chromaffin cells and tumor derivatives, was further clarified in subsequent publications by Kopin and colleagues [62–65].

In brief, compared to intraneuronal deamination of norepinephrine, extraneuronal O-methylation of catecholamines after secretion from sympathetic nerves and adrenal chromaffin cells makes only a minor contribution to total catecholamine metabolism [66]. Catechol-O-methyltransferase (COMT), the enzyme that, respectively, converts norepinephrine and epinephrine to normetanephrine and metanephrine, is not present within sympathetic neurons, but is present within chromaffin cells and at extraneuronal sites of metabolism. Thus, the O-methylated metabolites are normally minor catecholamine metabolites that circulate at low concentrations and are derived from metabolism of catecholamines either in extraneuronal tissues following release from neurons or the adrenal medulla and within adrenal medullary cells after leakage of catecholamines into the chromaffin cell cytoplasm. The latter pathway, however, predominates for metanephrine, over 90% of which is derived from intra-chromaffin cell metabolism of epinephrine; by contrast the amounts of circulating metanephrine derived from epinephrine after release by adrenal chromaffin cells are negligible. The same applies to normetanephrine, at least 24% of which is derived from O-methylation of norepinephrine within chromaffin cells; most normetanephrine, however, is derived from extraneuronal metabolism of norepinephrine after release by sympathetic nerves.

As a consequence of the above pathways of catecholamine metabolism, tumors that derive from adrenal and extra-adrenal chromaffin cells produce large amounts of metanephrines from metabolism of catecholamines within tumor cells, a process that is independent of catecholamine secretion. This then provides the basis for the importance of measuring the metanephrines versus the catecholamines and their deaminated metabolites, such as dihydroxyphenylglycol and vanillylmandelic acid.

When considering the choice of plasma or urinary metanephrines it should be appreciated that urinary metanephrines are usually measured after an acid hydrolysis step and represent mainly sulfate-conjugated metabolites, which are produced in gastro-intestinal tissues. For metanephrine this makes little difference since the sulfate-conjugated metabolite is produced from the free metabolite, almost all of which is derived from chromaffin cells or their tumor derivatives. However, for normetanephrine and methoxytyramine there are differences, particularly for the latter metabolite. Substantial amounts of these metabolites are derived from metabolism of norepinephrine and dopamine locally synthesized within gastrointestinal tissues and it is largely only the sulfate conjugates that escape from the hepato-portal circulation to reach the systemic circulation. Substantial amounts of dietary dopamine are also converted to sulfate-conjugated methoxytyramine, but dietary dopamine can also impact the free metabolite [67]. For this reason measurements of plasma free methoxytyramine for assessing tumoral dopamine production should be performed after an overnight fast. This additional source of sulfate conjugates acts to dilute the signal strength of the sulfate-conjugated normetanephrine and methoxytyramine derived from PPGLs. Consequently, the measurements of plasma free metanephrines offer superior performance for diagnosis of PPGLs than measurements of acid-hydrolyzed urinary metanephrines [50]. Urinary free methoxytyramine, similar to urinary dopamine, is mainly derived from renal uptake and decarboxylation of L-dopa and also shows little utility for assessing tumoral dopamine production.

Although measurements of the O-methylated catecholamine metabolites offer superior diagnostic performance over urinary measurements, blood draws should be carried out under stress-free conditions and after resting supine for at least 20 min (Box 6.1). These requirements can be troublesome in younger children or any child with needle phobia. For children, blood sampling via and indwelling intravenous line and after recovery from the venipuncture may be especially important to minimize false-positive results due to the stress of venipuncture associated sympathetic stimulation [68]. It is also important that the laboratory responsible for measurements can provide age-appropriate reference intervals for children [54, 55, 69]. Under these circumstances the plasma test can provide close to 100% sensitivity at a specificity that can be expected to exceed 90% [69].

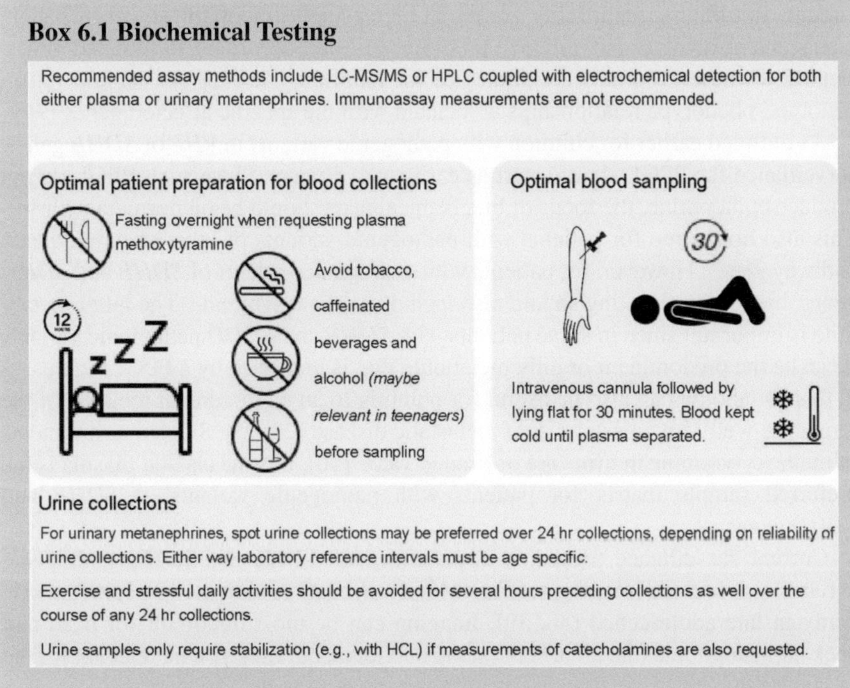

Box 6.1 Biochemical Testing

Recommended assay methods include LC-MS/MS or HPLC coupled with electrochemical detection for both either plasma or urinary metanephrines. Immunoassay measurements are not recommended.

Urine collections

For urinary metanephrines, spot urine collections may be preferred over 24 hr collections, depending on reliability of urine collections. Either way laboratory reference intervals must be age specific.

Exercise and stressful daily activities should be avoided for several hours preceding collections as well over the course of any 24 hr collections.

Urine samples only require stabilization (e.g., with HCL) if measurements of catecholamines are also requested.

Because of difficulties of blood sampling in children, as well as limited availability of laboratories that can offer mass spectrometric based measurements of plasma metabolites for children, the most commonly employed testing strategy in pediatrics remains measurements of urinary fractionated metanephrines (Box 6.1). Difficulties in the collection of 24 h urine specimens and poor reliability of complete collections in children make spot urine collections the more practical approach for children. In this case concentrations of metabolites are usually normalized to creatinine. Reference intervals for both 24-h and spot urine collections vary considerably over wide ranges from younger children to adolescents and there are also sex differences that should be considered. For 24 h urine collections, urinary outputs of normetanephrine and metanephrine increase by as much as four-fold from young children to older adolescents [70]. In contrast, for spot urines, normalization to creatinine leads to ratios that show profound decreases from younger through to older ages [53, 71–73]. The need for age-partitioning or age-adjusted reference intervals as well need to consider sex pose difficulties for laboratories to establish pediatric reference appropriate according to the methods they employ. Usually, reference intervals are set up according values reported in the literature, but this may not be ideal for methods that are not well standardized or harmonized.

Surveillance and Disease Management

Due to the increasing numbers of families and children identified with pathogenic variants in tumor susceptibility genes, an increasingly important aspect of patient management involves surveillance programs tailored according to mutated genes. Central to these programs are strategies for laboratory testing that should reflect genotype-phenotype relationships associated with the specific affected genes [74].

As outlined earlier for children with pathogenic variants in *VHL* or *SDHB* genes, surveillance for PPGL should start as early as 4–5 years. Since such PPGL do not produce epinephrine, the focus of biochemical tests should be on normetanephrine. This also holds true for patients with pathogenic variants of other pseudohypoxia pathway genes. However, for patients with pathogenic variants of *SDHB* and *SDHD* genes, biochemical testing should also include methoxytyramine. The latter metabolite is important since in some patients with *SDHB* and *SDHD* pathogenic variants it can be the predominant or only metabolite that is increased by a PPGL. Increases in this metabolite can also be useful for pointing to an extra-adrenal location of the tumors as well as increased risk of metastatic disease [23, 75]. Since measurements of methoxytyramine in urine are of limited value [50], this means that plasma is the preferred sample matrix for patients with pathogenic variants of *SDHB* and *SDHD* genes.

Current surveillance programs in patients with *SDHB* and *SDHD* pathogenic variants also include imaging studies, which may start as early as 10 years, but certainly in late adolescence [36, 39]. Imaging can be most important for head and neck paraganglioma that are usually non-functional, but may also be relevant for the abdomen and thorax for centers without access to mass spectrometric measurements of plasma normetanephrine and methoxytyramine. Tufton et al. have suggested that for *SDHB* variant carriers, such imaging could begin as early as 5 years [39].

For patients with *VHL* pathogenic variants, imaging for PPGL is not required until biochemical testing returns positive test results. Nevertheless, imaging in children with VHL variants beginning in adolescence is indicated for other tumors, such as clear cell renal carcinoma [76, 77].

Since pheochromocytoma due to pathogenic variants in *RET, NF1,* and other genes that involve kinase-signaling pathways invariable produce epinephrine, the focus of biochemical screening in patients affected by these variants should be on metanephrine and normetanephrine. Interpretation of test results should include appreciation that tumors for most patients are characterized by increases in both metabolites, but that on occasion only metanephrine may be increased. As in patients with VHL syndrome, imaging studies need not be initiated until biochemical testing returns a positive result.

For children, the decision for imaging studies and choice of imaging modalities has to be carefully considered according to the likelihood of a PPGL and radiation exposure. To avoid radiation exposure, magnetic resonance imaging is usually the preferred modality in children, but may not be tolerated in some children without sedation. For younger children ultrasound may be the preferred modality, but this is not particularly sensitive and can be non-informative for smaller tumors. Nevertheless, it may be considered during initial screening for most children with suspected PPGL. For children in whom there is no hereditary syndrome and in whom the pre-test probability of PPGL is low, the decision after a positive biochemical test to immediately proceed to imaging studies should consider the magnitude of increases in test results above reference intervals and thereby the post-test probability of a tumor. With increases of metabolites less than two-fold above reference intervals and only involving one metabolite, a wait and retest approach may be preferable to immediately moving to imaging studies. Alternatively, a clonidine suppression test can be considered, but only when positive test results involve increases of plasma normetanephrine [78].

Any decision to progress to functional imaging studies for tumor localization in children should be made on the basis of several considerations; a first consideration is that PPGL is highly likely but not clearly defined by conventional imaging in terms of location and possible metastatic involvement. Large extra-adrenal tumors, particularly those due to *SDHB* pathogenic variants or associated with increases in plasma methoxytyramine, are those most likely to feature metastatic involvement [75]. As in adults, the children with this presentation are those in whom functional imaging studies can be immediately considered. In others, functional imaging may be considered if after surgical resection there remains biochemical evidence of residual disease. Similar to adult series, ^{68}Ga-DOTATATE PET/CT appears to be superior to other available functional imaging modalities for characterizing metastatic involvement in children with PPGL due to *SDHB* variants [79]. This has been subsequently extended to a larger series of pediatric patients that confirmed the utility of ^{68}Ga-DOTATATE PET/CT not only for PPGL due to *SDHB* variants, but also *VHL* variants [80].

Once PPGL is diagnosed, as in adults, there is preoperative need for pharmacological blockade of the actions of catecholamines. Apart from body size or age-adjusted doses for medications, the principles of peri-operative and anesthesiologic management are similar in children and adults. Minimally invasive laparoscopy, via either the transperitoneal or retroperitoneal approach, is preferred for surgery [81]. Cortical sparing partial adrenalectomies should be considered for children with bilateral pheochromocytoma or in whom presence of a germline variant carries a high risk of additional adrenal tumors. Post-operatively there should be follow-up within 3 months after recovery from surgery to check that presurgical elevation of tumor biomarkers have returned to within age-appropriate reference intervals.

As outlined earlier, children with PPGL carry a higher risk than adults of carrying a pathogenic variant in a tumor susceptibility gene. Thus, unless a variant is already established, all children with a PPGL confirmed by postoperative histopathological examination should be provided with the opportunity of genetic counseling and testing for variants [14]. Clearly for children counseling must involve parents and if a variant is found, genetic counseling and testing should be extended to other family members. Similarly, if a pathogenic variant in a PPGL susceptibility gene is found in a parent, then genetic counseling and testing should also be extended to first degree relatives, including children.

Even if a germline pathogenic variant in a tumor susceptibility gene is not identified, there remains considerable risk in children with PPGL of recurrent or metastatic disease that may develop many years after resection of the original tumor [14]. Post-surgical normalization of pre-surgically elevated biomarkers cannot be assumed to equate with cure, so follow-up disease surveillance at periodic intervals for at least 20 years remains mandatory. In children with PPGL, most recurrent or metastatic disease appears in adulthood [3]. This makes it crucial that there is appropriate transition of pediatric to adult care, since earlier diagnosis and treatment of such disease can be expected to result in improved therapeutic outcomes.

Future Perspective

The need for appropriate transition of pediatric to adult care for childhood cases of PPGL remains important irrespective of the presence or absence of an identified germline pathogenic variant in a tumor susceptibility gene. Also, as has become clear over the first two decades of the twenty-first century, new genetic causes of PPGL have been increasingly identified and as a consequence the prevalence of hereditary childhood PPGL now reaches 80%. Associated with discoveries of new genetic causes of PPGL, there has been an explosion in knowledge concerning the underlying biology of the tumors and genotype phenotype relationships that can assist in personalized disease management according to mutated genes. PPGL, however, remains a rare tumor and management of affected patients now requires a depth of knowledge that is out of reach for most pediatricians who might first encounter children with a suspected PPGL. It has, therefore, become increasingly apparent that appropriate management of all patients with PPGL requires a multidisciplinary approach that involves centers of excellence staffed by personnel with experience and wide-ranging expertise in these tumors. This need is now being recognized by organizations with a focus on genetic syndromes or rare endocrine disorders who are now establishing procedures for review and accreditation of centers with appropriate resources and expertise. Through these and other efforts it is possible that the true prevalence of childhood PPGL will be clarified and clinical outcomes will improve.

References

1. Hume DM. Pheochromocytoma in the adult and in the child. Am J Surg. 1960;99:458–96.
2. Knudson AG Jr, Strong LC. Mutation and cancer: neuroblastoma and pheochromocytoma. Am J Hum Genet. 1972;24(5):514–32.
3. Pamporaki C, Hamplova B, Peitzsch M, Prejbisz A, Beuschlein F, Timmers HJ, et al. Characteristics of pediatric vs adult pheochromocytomas and paragangliomas. J Clin Endocrinol Metab. 2017;102:1122–32.
4. Wyszynska T, Cichocka E, Wieteska-Klimczak A, Jobs K, Januszewicz P. A single pediatric center experience with 1025 children with hypertension. Acta Paediatr. 1992;81:244–6.
5. Reddy VS, O'Neill JA Jr, Holcomb GW 3rd, Neblett WW 3rd, Pietsch JB, Morgan WM 3rd, et al. Twenty-five-year surgical experience with pheochromocytoma in children. Am Surg. 2000;66:1085–91; discussion 92.
6. Ciftci AO, Tanyel FC, Senocak ME, Buyukpamukcu N. Pheochromocytoma in children. J Ped Surg. 2001;36:447–52.
7. Ludwig AD, Feig DI, Brandt ML, Hicks MJ, Fitch ME, Cass DL. Recent advances in the diagnosis and treatment of pheochromocytoma in children. Am J Surg. 2007;194:792–6.
8. Bissada NK, Safwat AS, Seyam RM, Al Sobhi S, Hanash KA, Jackson RJ, et al. Pheochromocytoma in children and adolescents: a clinical spectrum. J Ped Surg. 2008;43:540–3.
9. Hammond PJ, Murphy D, Carachi R, Davidson DF, McIntosh D. Childhood phaeochromocytoma and paraganglioma: 100% incidence of genetic mutations and 100% survival. J Ped Surg. 2010;45(2):383–6.
10. Cascon A, Inglada-Perez L, Comino-Mendez I, de Cubas AA, Leton R, Mora J, et al. Genetics of pheochromocytoma and paraganglioma in Spanish pediatric patients. Endocr Relat Cancer. 2013;20:L1–6.
11. Bausch B, Wellner U, Bausch D, Schiavi F, Barontini M, Sanso G, et al. Long-term prognosis of patients with pediatric pheochromocytoma. Endocr Relat Cancer. 2014;21:17–25.
12. Khadilkar K, Sarathi V, Kasaliwal R, Pandit R, Goroshi M, Shivane V, et al. Genotype-phenotype correlation in paediatric pheochromocytoma and paraganglioma: a single centre experience from India. J Pediatr Endocrinol Metab. 2017;30:575.
13. Virgone C, Andreetta M, Avanzini S, Chiaravalli S, De Pasquale D, Crocoli A, et al. Pheochromocytomas and paragangliomas in children: data from the Italian cooperative study (TREP). Pediatr Blood Cancer. 2020;67(8):e28332.
14. de Tersant M, Genere L, Freycon C, Villebasse S, Abbas R, Barlier A, et al. Pheochromocytoma and paraganglioma in children and adolescents: experience of the French Society of Pediatric Oncology (SFCE). J Endocr Soc. 2020;4(5):bvaa039.
15. Redlich A, Pamporaki C, Lessel L, Fruhwald MC, Vorwerk P, Kuhlen M. Pseudohypoxic pheochromocytomas and paragangliomas dominate in children. Pediatr Blood Cancer. 2021;68:e28981.

16. Barontini M, Levin G, Sanso G. Characteristics of pheochromocytoma in a 4- to 20-year-old population. Ann N Y Acad Sci. 2006;1073:30–7.
17. Kaufman BH, Telander RL, van Heerden JA, Zimmerman D, Sheps SG, Dawson B. Pheochromocytoma in the pediatric age group: current status. J Ped Surg. 1983;18(6):879–84.
18. Sullivan J, Groshong T, Tobias JD. Presenting signs and symptoms of pheochromocytoma in pediatric-aged patients. Clin Pediatr. 2005;44(8):715–9.
19. Rogowski-Lehmann N, Geroula A, Prejbisz A, Timmers H, Megerle F, Robledo M, et al. Missed clinical clues in patients with pheochromocytoma/paraganglioma discovered by imaging. Endocr Connect. 2018;7(11):1168–77.
20. Ilias I, Thomopoulos C. Addressing delays in the diagnosis of pheochromocytoma/paraganglioma. Expert Rev Endocrinol Metab. 2019;14(5):359–63.
21. Olson SW, Yoon S, Baker T, Prince LK, Oliver D, Abbott KC. Longitudinal plasma metanephrines preceding pheochromocytoma diagnosis: a retrospective case-control serum repository study. Eur J Endocrinol. 2016;174:289–95.
22. Powers JF, Pacak K, Tischler AS. Pathology of human pheochromocytoma and paraganglioma xenografts in NSG mice. Endocr Pathol. 2017;28:2–6.
23. Eisenhofer G, Deutschbein T, Constantinescu G, Langton K, Pamporaki C, Calsina B, et al. Plasma metanephrines and prospective prediction of tumor location, size and mutation type in patients with pheochromocytoma and paraganglioma. Clin Chem Lab Med. 2020;59:353–63.
24. Seabrook AJ, Harris JE, Velosa SB, Kim E, McInerney-Leo AM, Dwight T, et al. Multiple endocrine tumors associated with germline MAX mutations: multiple endocrine neoplasia type 5? J Clin Endocr Metab. 2021;106:1163–82.
25. Qin N, de Cubas AA, Garcia-Martin R, Richter S, Peitzsch M, Menschikowski M, et al. Opposing effects of HIF1alpha and HIF2alpha on chromaffin cell phenotypic features and tumor cell proliferation: insights from MYC-associated factor X. Int J Cancer. 2014;135(9):2054–64.
26. Jiang J, Zhang J, Pang Y, Bechmann N, Li M, Monteagudo M, et al. Sino-European differences in the genetic landscape and clinical presentation of pheochromocytoma and paraganglioma. J Clin Endocrinol Metab. 2020;105:3295–307.
27. Eisenhofer G, Timmers HJ, Lenders JW, Bornstein SR, Tiebel O, Mannelli M, et al. Age at diagnosis of pheochromocytoma differs according to catecholamine phenotype and tumor location. J Clin Endocrinol Metab. 2011;96:375–84.
28. King KS, Prodanov T, Kantorovich V, Fojo T, Hewitt JK, Zacharin M, et al. Metastatic pheochromocytoma/paraganglioma related to primary tumor development in childhood or adolescence: significant link to SDHB mutations. J Clin Oncol. 2011;29:4137–42.
29. Bechmann N, Moskopp ML, Ullrich M, Calsina B, Wallace PW, Richter S, et al. HIF2α supports pro-metastatic behavior in pseudohypoxic pheochromocytomas/paragangliomas. Endocr Relat Cancer. 2020;27:625–40.
30. Eisenhofer G, Huynh TT, Pacak K, Brouwers FM, Walther MM, Linehan WM, et al. Distinct gene expression profiles in norepinephrine- and epinephrine-producing hereditary and sporadic pheochromocytomas: activation of hypoxia-driven angiogenic pathways in von Hippel-Lindau syndrome. Endocr Relat Cancer. 2004;11:897–911.
31. Pietras A, Hansford LM, Johnsson AS, Bridges E, Sjolund J, Gisselsson D, et al. HIF-2alpha maintains an undifferentiated state in neural crest-like human neuroblastoma tumor-initiating cells. Proc Natl Acad Sci. 2009;106:16805–10.
32. Niklasson CU, Fredlund E, Monni E, Lindvall JM, Kokaia Z, Hammarlund EU, et al. Hypoxia inducible factor-2alpha importance for migration, proliferation, and self-renewal of trunk neural crest cells. Dev Dyn. 2021;250:191–236.
33. Geroula A, Deutschbein T, Langton K, Masjkur J, Pamporaki C, Peitzsch M, et al. Pheochromocytoma and paraganglioma: clinical feature-based disease probability in relation to catecholamine biochemistry and reason for disease suspicion. Eur J Endocrinol. 2019;181:409–20.
34. Gruber LM, Hartman RP, Thompson GB, McKenzie TJ, Lyden ML, Dy BM, et al. Pheochromocytoma characteristics and behavior differ depending on method of discovery. J Clin Endocrinol Metab. 2019;104:1386–93.

35. Rednam SP, Erez A, Druker H, Janeway KA, Kamihara J, Kohlmann WK, et al. Von Hippel-Lindau and hereditary pheochromocytoma/paraganglioma syndromes: clinical features, genetics, and surveillance recommendations in childhood. Clin Cancer Res. 2017;23:e68–75.
36. Wong MY, Andrews KA, Challis BG, Park SM, Acerini CL, Maher ER, et al. Clinical practice guidance: surveillance for phaeochromocytoma and paraganglioma in paediatric succinate dehydrogenase gene mutation carriers. Clin Endocrinol. 2019;90(4):499–505.
37. Makri A, Akshintala S, Derse-Anthony C, Del Rivero J, Widemann B, Stratakis CA, et al. Pheochromocytoma in children and adolescents with multiple endocrine neoplasia type 2B. J Clin Endocrinol Metab. 2019;104:7–12.
38. Jochmanova I, Abcede AMT, Guerrero RJS, Malong CLP, Wesley R, Huynh T, et al. Clinical characteristics and outcomes of SDHB-related pheochromocytoma and paraganglioma in children and adolescents. J Cancer Res Clin Oncol. 2020;146:1051–63.
39. Tufton N, Shapiro L, Sahdev A, Kumar AV, Martin L, Drake WM, et al. An analysis of surveillance screening for SDHB-related disease in childhood and adolescence. Endocr Connect. 2019;8:162–72.
40. Aufforth RD, Ramakant P, Sadowski SM, Mehta A, Trebska-McGowan K, Nilubol N, et al. Pheochromocytoma screening initiation and frequency in von Hippel-Lindau syndrome. J Clin Endocrinol Metab. 2015;100:4498–504.
41. Lonser RR, Glenn GM, Walther M, Chew EY, Libutti SK, Linehan WM, et al. von Hippel-Lindau disease. Lancet. 2003;361(9374):2059–67.
42. McNeill A, Rattenberry E, Barber R, Killick P, MacDonald F, Maher ER. Genotype-phenotype correlations in VHL exon deletions. Am J Med Genet A. 2009;149A:2147–51.
43. Fagundes GFC, Petenuci J, Lourenco DM Jr, Trarbach EB, Pereira MAA, Correa D'Eur JE, et al. New insights into pheochromocytoma surveillance of young patients with VHL missense mutations. J Endocr Soc. 2019;3(9):1682–92.
44. Machens A, Lorenz K, Dralle H. Peak incidence of pheochromocytoma and primary hyperparathyroidism in multiple endocrine neoplasia 2: need for age-adjusted biochemical screening. J Clin Endocrinol Metab. 2013;98:E336–45.
45. Gruber LM, Erickson D, Babovic-Vuksanovic D, Thompson GB, Young WF Jr, Bancos I. Pheochromocytoma and paraganglioma in patients with neurofibromatosis type 1. Clin Endocrinol. 2017;86(1):141–9.
46. Abdallah A, Pappo A, Reiss U, Shulkin BL, Zhuang Z, Pacak K, et al. Clinical manifestations of Pacak-Zhuang syndrome in a male pediatric patient. Pediatr Blood Cancer. 2020;67(4):e28096.
47. Yang C, Hong CS, Prchal JT, Balint MT, Pacak K, Zhuang Z. Somatic mosaicism of EPAS1 mutations in the syndrome of paraganglioma and somatostatinoma associated with polycythemia. Hum Genome Var. 2015;2:15053.
48. Lenders JWM, Duh QY, Eisenhofer G, Gimenez-Roqueplo AP, Grebe SK, Murad MH, et al. Pheochromocytoma and paraganglioma: an endocrine society clinical practice guideline. J Clin Endocrinol Metab. 2014;99:1915–42.
49. Rao D, Peitzsch M, Prejbisz A, Hanus K, Fassnacht M, Beuschlein F, et al. Plasma methoxytyramine: clinical utility with metanephrines for diagnosis of pheochromocytoma and paraganglioma. Eur J Endocrinol. 2017;177:103–13.
50. Eisenhofer G, Prejbisz A, Peitzsch M, Pamporaki C, Masjkur J, Rogowski-Lehmann N, et al. Biochemical diagnosis of chromaffin cell tumors in patients at high and low risk of disease: plasma versus urinary free or deconjugated O-methylated catecholamine metabolites. Clin Chem. 2018;64:1646–56.
51. Barco S, Verly I, Corrias MV, Sorrentino S, Conte M, Tripodi G, et al. Plasma free metanephrines for diagnosis of neuroblastoma patients. Clin Biochem. 2019;66:57–62.
52. Peitzsch M, Butch ER, Lovorn E, Mangelis A, Furman WL, Santana VM, et al. Biochemical testing for neuroblastoma using plasma free 3-O-methyldopa, 3-methoxytyramine, and normetanephrine. Pediatr Blood Cancer. 2020;67(2):e28081.
53. Griffin A, O'Shea P, FitzGerald R, O'Connor G, Tormey W. Establishment of a paediatric age-related reference interval for the measurement of urinary total fractionated metanephrines. Ann Clin Biochem. 2011;48(Pt 1):41–4.

54. Franscini LC, Vazquez-Montes M, Buclin T, Perera R, Dunand M, Grouzmann E, et al. Pediatric reference intervals for plasma free and total metanephrines established with a parametric approach: relevance to the diagnosis of neuroblastoma. Pediatr Blood Cancer. 2015;62(4):587–93.

55. Peitzsch M, Mangelis A, Eisenhofer G, Huebner A. Age-specific pediatric reference intervals for plasma free normetanephrine, metanephrine, 3-methoxytyramine and 3-O-methyldopa: particular importance for early infancy. Clin Chim Acta. 2019;494:100–5.

56. Peitzsch M, Kaden D, Pamporaki C, Langton K, Constantinescu G, Conrad C, et al. Overnight/first-morning urine free metanephrines and methoxytyramine for diagnosis of pheochromocytoma and paraganglioma: is this an option? Eur J Endocrinol. 2020;182(5):499–509.

57. Richard VR, Zahedi RP, Eintracht S, Borchers CH. An LC-MRM assay for the quantification of metanephrines from dried blood spots for the diagnosis of pheochromocytomas and paragangliomas. Anal Chim Acta. 2020;1128:140–8.

58. Osinga TE, van der Horst-Schrivers AN, van Faassen M, Kerstens MN, Dullaart RP, Pacak K, et al. Mass spectrometric quantification of salivary metanephrines-a study in healthy subjects. Clin Biochem. 2016;49:983–8.

59. van Faassen M, Bischoff R, Eijkelenkamp K, de Jong WHA, van der Ley CP, Kema IP. In matrix derivatization combined with LC-MS/MS results in ultrasensitive quantification of plasma free metanephrines and catecholamines. Anal Chem. 2020;92:9072–8.

60. Crout JR, Sjoerdsma A. Turnover and metabolism of catecholamines in patients with pheochromocytoma. J Clin Invest. 1964;43:94–102.

61. Kopin IJ. Storage and metabolism of catecholamines: the role of monoamine oxidase. Pharmacol Rev. 1964;16:179–91.

62. Goldstein DS, Eisenhofer G, Stull R, Folio CJ, Keiser HR, Kopin IJ. Plasma dihydroxyphenylglycol and the intraneuronal disposition of norepinephrine in humans. J Clin Invest. 1988;81:213–20.

63. Eisenhofer G, Rundquist B, Aneman A, Friberg P, Dakak N, Kopin IJ, et al. Regional release and removal of catecholamines and extraneuronal metabolism to metanephrines. J Clin Endocrinol Metab. 1995;80:3009–17.

64. Eisenhofer G, Keiser H, Friberg P, Mezey E, Huynh TT, Hiremagalur B, et al. Plasma metanephrines are markers of pheochromocytoma produced by catechol-O-methyltransferase within tumors. J Clin Endocrinol Metab. 1998;83:2175–85.

65. Eisenhofer G, Goldstein DS, Kopin IJ, Crout JR. Pheochromocytoma: rediscovery as a catecholamine-metabolizing tumor. Endocr Pathol. 2003;14:193–212.

66. Eisenhofer G, Kopin IJ, Goldstein DS. Catecholamine metabolism: a contemporary view with implications for physiology and medicine. Pharmacol Rev. 2004;56(3):331–49.

67. de Jong WH, Eisenhofer G, Post WJ, Muskiet FA, de Vries EG, Kema IP. Dietary influences on plasma and urinary metanephrines: implications for diagnosis of catecholamine-producing tumors. J Clin Endocrinol Metab. 2009;94(8):2841–9.

68. Eijkelenkamp K, van Geel EH, Kerstens MN, van Faassen M, Kema IP, Links TP, et al. Blood sampling for metanephrines comparing venipuncture vs. indwelling intravenous cannula in healthy subjects. Clin Chem Lab Med. 2020;58(10):1681–6.

69. Weise M, Merke DP, Pacak K, Walther MM, Eisenhofer G. Utility of plasma free metanephrines for detecting childhood pheochromocytoma. J Clin Endocrinol Metab. 2002;87(5):1955–60.

70. Fitzgibbon MC, Tormey WP. Paediatric reference ranges for urinary catecholamines/metabolites and their relevance in neuroblastoma diagnosis. Ann Clin Biochem. 1994;31(Pt 1):1–11.

71. Davidson DF, Hammond PJ, Murphy DL, Carachi R. Age-related medical decision limits for urinary free (unconjugated) metadrenalines, catecholamines and metabolites in random urine specimens from children. Ann Clin Biochem. 2011;48:358–6.

72. Pussard E, Neveux M, Guigueno N. Reference intervals for urinary catecholamines and metabolites from birth to adulthood. Clin Biochem. 2009;42(6):536–9.

73. Roli L, Veronesi A, De Santis MC, Baraldi E. Pediatric total fractionated metanephrine. Age-related reference intervals in spot urine. Minerva Pediatr. 2018; https://doi.org/10.23736/S0026-4946.18.05319-7.
74. Eisenhofer G, Klink B, Richter S, Lenders JW, Robledo M. Metabologenomics of Phaeochromocytoma and Paraganglioma: an integrated approach for personalised biochemical and genetic testing. Clin Biochem Rev. 2017;38(2):69–100.
75. Eisenhofer G, Lenders JW, Siegert G, Bornstein SR, Friberg P, Milosevic D, et al. Plasma methoxytyramine: a novel biomarker of metastatic pheochromocytoma and paraganglioma in relation to established risk factors of tumour size, location and SDHB mutation status. Eur J Cancer. 2012;48:1739–49.
76. Chahoud J, McGettigan M, Parikh N, Boris RS, Iliopoulos O, Rathmell WK, et al. Evaluation, diagnosis and surveillance of renal masses in the setting of VHL disease. World J Urol. 2020;39:2409.
77. Binderup ML, Bisgaard ML, Harbud V, Moller HU, Gimsing S, Friis-Hansen L, et al. Von Hippel-Lindau disease (vHL). National clinical guideline for diagnosis and surveillance in Denmark. 3rd edition. Dan Med J. 2013;60(12):B4763.
78. Eisenhofer G, Goldstein DS, Walther MM, Friberg P, Lenders JW, Keiser HR, et al. Biochemical diagnosis of pheochromocytoma: how to distinguish true- from false-positive test results. J Clin Endocrinol Metab. 2003;88:2656–66.
79. Jha A, Ling A, Millo C, Gupta G, Viana B, Lin FI, et al. Superiority of (68)Ga-DOTATATE over (18)F-FDG and anatomic imaging in the detection of succinate dehydrogenase mutation (SDHx)-related pheochromocytoma and paraganglioma in the pediatric population. Eur J Nucl Med Mol Imaging. 2018;45(5):787–97.
80. Jaiswal SK, Sarathi V, Malhotra G, Hira P, Shah R, Patil VA, et al. The utility of (68) Ga-DOTATATE PET/CT in localizing primary/metastatic pheochromocytoma and paraganglioma in children and adolescents—a single-center experience. J Pediatr Endocrinol Metab. 2021;34(1):109–19.
81. Walz MK, Iova LD, Deimel J, Neumann HPH, Bausch B, Zschiedrich S, et al. Minimally invasive surgery (MIS) in children and adolescents with pheochromocytomas and retroperitoneal paragangliomas: experiences in 42 patients. World J Surg. 2018;42(4):1024–30.

Chapter 7
Imaging Approach to Pediatric and Adolescent Familial Cancer Syndromes

Brandon K. K. Fields, Natalie L. Demirjian, Hojjat Ahmadzadehfar, Anna Yordanova, Iraj Nabipour, Narges Jokar, Majid Assadi, Peter Joyce, and Ali Gholamrezanezhad

Introduction

Recent advances in our understanding of the genetic and pathophysiologic mechanism of human malignancies have led to the recognition of frequent hereditary basis of many cancers. Hereditary cancer syndromes, which are now believed to cause up to 5% of human malignancies, are characterized by the early onset of various, multifocal, often advanced malignancies of usually more than one organ system.

B. K. K. Fields
Department of Radiology & Biomedical Imaging, University of California, San Francisco, San Francisco, CA, USA

N. L. Demirjian
College of Medicine—Tucson, University of Arizona, Tucson, AZ, USA

H. Ahmadzadehfar
Department of Nuclear Medicine, Klinikum Westfalen, Dortmund, Germany

A. Yordanova
Department of Radiology, Marienhospital Bonn, Bonn, Germany

I. Nabipour
Department of Internal Medicine (Division of Endocrinology), The Persian Gulf Tropical Medicine Research Center, The Persian Gulf Biomedical Sciences Research Institute, Bushehr Medical University Hospital, School of Medicine, Bushehr University of Medical Sciences, Bushehr, Iran

N. Jokar · M. Assadi
Department of Molecular Imaging and Radionuclide Therapy, The Persian Gulf Nuclear Medicine Research Center, Bushehr Medical University Hospital, Bushehr University of Medical Sciences, Bushehr, Iran

P. Joyce · A. Gholamrezanezhad (⊠)
Department of Radiology, University of Southern California, Los Angeles, CA, USA

© The Author(s), under exclusive license to Springer Nature Switzerland AG 2023
F. Hannah-Shmouni (ed.), *Familial Endocrine Cancer Syndromes*,
https://doi.org/10.1007/978-3-031-37275-9_7

Frequently multiple family members are involved. These hereditary cancer syndromes may pose specific diagnostic and therapeutic challenges, as they warrant contemporary paradigms for their screening protocols and targeted therapies. Here, we review imaging approaches to the most common hereditary cancer syndromes, including multiple endocrine neoplasia (MEN) syndromes, von Hippel-Lindau (VHL) syndrome, and Li-Fraumeni cancer syndrome.

Multiple Endocrine Neoplasia Syndromes

Multiple endocrine neoplasia (MEN) syndromes are heritable neoplastic disorders in which affected individuals characteristically develop two or more synchronous or metachronous endocrine tumors. Germline mutations affecting the *MEN1*, *RET* (MEN2), and *CDKN1B* (MEN4) genes have been identified in driving a collection of phenotypically distinct tumor syndromes [1–7]. Each syndrome is thought to occur infrequently in the general population, with an estimated 1 in 30,000 individuals affected [7]. Neoplastic processes in MEN1 most classically affect the parathyroid gland (95%), pancreas (30–80%), and pituitary gland (15–50%), though other associated neoplasms can include adrenal cortical tumors, collagenomas, angiofibromas, lipomas, facial ependymomas, meningiomas, and foregut carcinoid tumors [1–5, 7, 8]. Medullary thyroid carcinomas (MTCs) (95–99%) and pheochromocytomas (50%) are common manifestations of both MEN2A/2B, with parathyroid tumors and mucocutaneous neuromas serving as differentiating features between MEN2A and MEN2B, respectively [1–5, 7]. Familial medullary thyroid cancer (FMTC), a related MEN2 variant disorder, is characterized solely by the heritable development of MTC in the absence of pheochromocytoma or hyperparathyroidism [4, 6, 7]. A more recently described condition, MEN4 also predisposes patients for developing neoplasms of the parathyroid (80–81%) and anterior pituitary glands (42%), albeit arising from a different driver mutation than seen in patients with MEN1 [1, 2, 5]. While diagnosis primarily relies on a combination of genetic testing, clinical features, and biochemical screening, imaging nevertheless remains essential to staging and surgical planning [3, 4, 7]. The following section is focused on the optimal imaging modalities for investigating tumors of the major organs affected by the MEN syndrome disorders collectively (Table 7.1).

Table 7.1 Summary of organs affected by MEN syndrome disorders. *MEN* multiple endocrine neoplasia

Organ	MEN syndromes affected
Pancreas	MEN1
Pituitary	MEN1, MEN4
Thyroid	MEN2
Parathyroid	MEN1, MEN2, MEN4
Adrenal gland	MEN1, MEN2

Pancreas

Pancreatic neuroendocrine tumors (pNETs) are responsible for the majority of MEN1-related deaths [1, 2, 5, 9]. Greater than half of pNETs occurring in MEN patients are gastrinomas, with insulinomas the second most common occurring pNET, which comprise approximately one-third of cases. Less than 5% of pNETs secrete pancreatic polypeptide, vasoactive intestinal peptide or glucagon, which are commonly referred to as PPomas, VIPomas, and glucagonomas [2, 7]. Initial detection and staging investigations often begin with conventional cross-sectional imaging by computed tomography (CT) or magnetic resonance imaging (MRI), each of which has demonstrated reported sensitivities of 73% and 93%, respectively [3, 10–12]. While cross-sectional imaging has demonstrated superiority compared to transabdominal ultrasound in the detection of pNETs secondary to poor sensitivity, endoscopic and intraoperative sonographic evaluation has demonstrated great utility [1, 3]. Endoscopic ultrasound in particular boasts sensitivities approaching 100% and has demonstrated superiority over advanced imaging modalities in head-to-head comparisons [9, 13–15]. While some authors suggest that endoscopic ultrasound may be used with equal appropriateness in initial assessments of MEN1 patients, routine evaluation is constrained by limited availability, operator skill, and the invasive nature of the procedure [8, 10, 12].

Functional imaging techniques using somatostatin receptor scintigraphy are useful in assessing for the presence of hepatic and distant metastatic disease, as well as for identifying which patients will respond to therapeutic radionuclide administration [1, 3, 12, 16]. Historically, ^{111}In-pentetreotide was used in combination with single-photon emission computed tomography (SPECT)/CT [1, 3], however, there exists a growing body of literature supporting the use of positron emission tomography (PET)/CT in conjunction with ^{68}Ga-labeled radiotracers or amine precursors. Recent data suggest that ^{68}Ga-DOTA-SSA PET/CT (which utilizes gallium labeled somatostatin analogs) is more accurate, yields superior spatial resolution, and requires a lower radiation dose, in addition to allowing for shorter scanning times [16] (Fig. 7.1). Amine precursors such as ^{18}F-DOPA and ^{11}C-5-HTP, while not as widely available, may additionally serve a role in imaging tumors with minimal or absent somatostatin receptor expression [3, 12, 16]. ^{18}F-FDG PET/CT tends to be less helpful for imaging well-differentiated tumors, which often demonstrate a more indolent course and lower metabolic activity. However, poorly-differentiated pNETs are more readily imaged by ^{18}F-FDG PET, where increased radiotracer uptake has in more recent studies been shown to correlate with histopathologic grade and Ki-67 positivity [1, 3, 10, 12, 16].

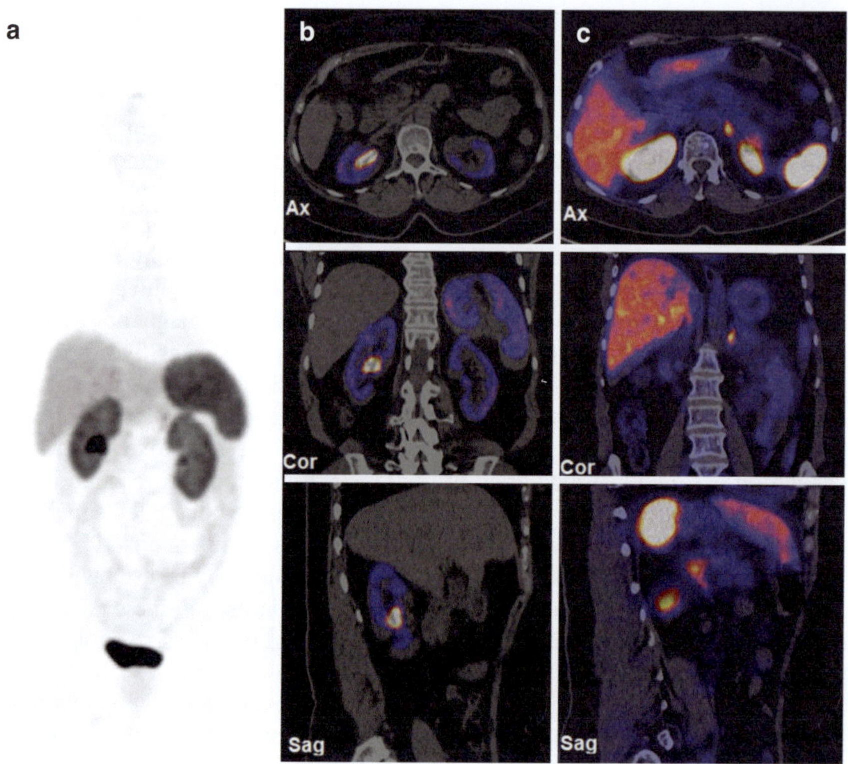

Fig. 7.1 Staging PET/CT in a 57-year-old woman with history of MEN2A 3 years status post-thyroidectomy for medullary thyroid carcinoma (MTC) who presented with elevated tumor markers and concern for MTC recurrence. (**a**) ⁶⁸Ga-DOTANOC whole-body maximum intensity projection (MIP) (**b**, **c**), transaxial, coronal, and sagittal images demonstrate heterogeneous hepatic uptake along with a DOTA-positive left adrenal nodule and focal DOTA activity in the pancreatic tail. Malignant pheochromocytoma with locoregional pancreatic and hepatic metastases was confirmed by histopathology. No abnormal DOTA activity was observed in the thyroid surgical bed or surrounding cervical regions to suggest recurrent MTC. *MTC* medullary thyroid carcinoma, *MIP* maximum intensity projection

Pituitary

The majority of MEN-associated pituitary tumors are prolactinomas (60–67%), followed by somatotrophinomas (25%), adrenocorticorphinomas (5%), and nonfunctioning adenomas (5%) [2, 3]. MRI is the standard-of-care imaging modality in patients with characteristic biochemical abnormalities and suspected pituitary gland pathology, as long as they have no contraindications to the imaging modality [3, 4, 17–19]. The anterior pituitary gland, also known as the adenohypophysis, normally appears homogeneously isointense to gray matter on T_1-weighted sequences whereas the posterior pituitary, also known as the neurohypophysis, typically appears as a small focus of hyperintense signal of T2-weighted sequences. On non-contrast enhanced sequences, the majority of microadenomas (≤10 mm) are often visualized as isointense to hypointense foci (relative to normal pituitary parenchyma) on T1-weighted imaging, while macroadenomas (>1 cm) tend to appear as isointense masses that fill the sella turcica [1, 2, 17–19]. Microadenomas are often hypovascular relative to the surrounding tissues and thus do not enhance as avidly as normal pituitary gland following intravenous contrast administration. By comparison, macroadenomas typically demonstrate appreciable post-contrast enhancement, likely owing to their increased size and vascularity [18–20]. T_2-weighted imaging is generally less helpful unless administration of intravenous contrast is contraindicated [17]. For patients in whom MRI is contraindicated, pituitary adenomas may be visualized as hypodense lesions on contrast-enhanced CT [3, 19]. Regardless of the imaging modality chosen, thin-section cuts in sagittal and coronal reformations are preferred for optimal detection of subtle lesions which may not overtly distort the surrounding bony or intra-axial architecture [1, 3, 17, 19].

Thyroid

Nearly all patients with MEN2 driver mutations go on to develop MTC [21]. MTC is an aggressive neoplasm of thyroid parafollicular C cells for which prophylactic thyroidectomy is recommended in early childhood in patients with MEN2A and as early as 6 months of age in patients with MEN2B [1, 2, 6, 22]. In contrast to the sporadic form, MTC in patients with MEN2 tends to present more commonly with bilateral, multicentric disease [1, 2]. Likewise, the American Thyroid Association recommends that all patients with newly diagnosed MTC receive DNA analysis for the presence of a germline *RET* mutation [6]. Ultrasound is the preferred imaging modality for initial investigations of suspected MTC, which characteristically reveals the presence of a hypoechoic mass with irregular or spiculated margins, calcifications, microlobulations, absence of a halo, taller-than-wide shape, and/or internal vascularity [6, 22–24]. Likewise, cross-sectional evaluation by CT or MRI may reveal a solid or cystic calcified mass [1, 3, 22]. Yet, no singular imaging modality provides absolute diagnostic certainty, as even ultrasound has only been shown to be 72% sensitive for diagnosing MTC [23, 25].

As MTC is frequently locally invasive or metastatic on presentation, advanced cross-sectional imaging by CT or MRI may also be of use for initial disease staging [3, 6, 22, 25]. Recent advances in whole-body diffusion-weighted imaging (WB-DWI) and dynamic contrast-enhanced (DCE) MRI have also shown applicability in detecting distant metastases and response to anti-angiogenic therapies, though molecular imaging still remains essential to evaluating overall oncologic burden [25]. Distant metastatic sites most frequently include the lungs, liver, and bone [3, 23]. In the case of bone metastases, Guidelines from the American Thyroid Association recommend use of both MRI combined with bone scintigraphy for optimal detection [6]. However, despite conflicting data on the reported sensitivities of many radiopharmaceuticals in detecting metastatic lesions [1, 3, 6, 22, 25–27], recent data do suggest that metastatic skeletal tumor burden evaluated using ^{18}F-NaF PET/CT correlates with overall survival in patients with MTC [28]. Additionally, somatostatin receptor scintigraphy may similarly serve a complementary role in identifying those patients whose tumors would be amenable to therapeutic radionuclide administration, especially in the setting of unresectable disease [22, 25].

Parathyroid

Historically, bilateral neck exploration was often pursued solely on the basis of biochemical diagnosis, though recent trends in parathyroid surgical practices recognize an increasingly prominent role for preoperative imaging localization to aid in surgical planning [3, 4, 29–31]. Imaging of the parathyroid glands is optimally done first using high-frequency ultrasonography, which is 82% sensitive for detecting parathyroid adenomas [1, 3, 29, 32]. Parathyroid adenomas are commonly located posterior to the thyroid gland and can typically be identified as discrete hypoechoic ovoid masses [3, 29, 32]. Additionally, office-based ultrasound confers the added advantage of incidentally detecting adjacent thyroid pathology that may warrant additional investigations [32]. However, many authors agree that the addition of thin-section CT does not provide any additional information except in localizing ectopic glandular foci that would otherwise be inaccessible to ultrasound, such as in the mediastinum and behind the trachea [1, 3, 29]. As such, localization by conventional CT scanning is most frequently employed in the setting of persistent hyperparathyroidism prior to re-operation [29]. Similarly, while MRI boasts a slightly higher sensitivity overall for localization of ectopic parathyroid tissue, its use is typically reserved for investigations preceding operative revision and not as a first-line modality [1, 3, 29].

Sctintigraphic localization using ^{99m}Tc-MIBI planar and SPECT imaging is highly sensitive in detection of parathyroid adenomas when used in conjunction with ultrasound [4, 30]. Dual-phase imaging obtained after 10–15 min and 2–3 h demonstrates sustained radiotracer uptake in adenomatous foci [3, 32]. As an imaging modality, hybrid SPECT/CT scanners have in recent years allowed for increasingly precise anatomic localization of metabolic activity [33]. Recent data have shown that early-phase SPECT/CT used in combination with delayed-phase imaging was superior for localization parathyroid adenomas [34, 35]. As such, recent guidelines from the American Head and Neck Society Endocrine Surgery Section support the use of early-phase SPECT/CT followed by delayed-phase planar imaging for optimal preoperative imaging and to aid in intraoperative localization [32]. Similarly, in cases of persistent postoperative hypercalcemia, the addition of fusion CT imaging to conventional SPECT acquisition may also further aid in localization of ectopic glandular tissue [3, 36].

Adrenal

Anywhere from 5 to 40% of MEN1 patients will develop adrenal cortical adenomas while approximately 50% of MEN2 patients will manifest pheochromocytomas, which can arise from the adrenal medulla. Most adrenal adenomas in MEN1 are nonfunctioning, though a minority of cases may present as Cushing's or Conn's Syndrome. As part of hereditary syndromes such as MEN2, pheochromocytoma occur in up to 25% of cases with additional syndromes including von Hippel-Lindau syndrome type 2, in which there is a mutation in the VHL gene; and neurofibromatosis type 1 (Recklinghausen's disease), in which the neurofibromatosis type 1 gene

Table 7.2 List of drugs to be withdrawn before testing metanephrines or normetanephrines in plasma

Drug	MN	NMN
Acetaminophen	N	Y
Buspirone	Y	N
Cocaine	N	Y
Levodopa	Y	Y
Mesalamine/sulfasalazine	N	Y
Monoamine oxidase inhibitors	Y	Y
Phenoxybenzamine	N	Y
Sympathomimetics	Y	Y
Tricyclic antidepressants	N	Y
α-Methyldopa	N	Y

MN metanephrine, *NMN* normetanephrine, *Y* consider withdrawing the drug before testing (if consistent with patient's clinical condition), *N* do not stop the medication

is mutated [37]. Bilateral disease in MEN2 is common and manifests about half of the time [1–5, 7]. Malignant transformation in the case of either cortical or medullary disease is uncommon [1, 3]. In either case, cross-sectional imaging with either CT or MRI is preferred for anatomic investigations, where observation of characteristic imaging findings in the appropriate clinical context may be helpful in narrowing the differential diagnosis [1, 3, 38, 39]. Specific to pheochromocytomas, as these lesions secrete catecholamines and their metabolites, measurement of serum metabolites is also utilized for detection. Measuring fractionated plasma metanephrine (the metabolite of epinephrine/adrenaline) is a highly sensitive method (97%) for diagnosing pheochromocytoma and paraganglioma, and it is the choice of laboratory diagnostics in particular for patients at high risk due to familial endocrine syndromes [40, 41]. Certain drugs, such as sulfasalazine, acetaminophen, antihypertensive drugs, and tricyclic antidepressants, can be responsible for false-positive test results and, if possible, should be withdrawn before testing (Table 7.2). Furthermore, caffeine, alcohol, nicotine, stress, and strenuous physical activity should be avoided for approximately 24 h prior to the blood test [42, 43]. A flow chart of baseline diagnostics and follow-up is provided below (Fig. 7.2).

The most sensitive method in the diagnosis of pheochromocytoma/paraganglioma is the CT, however, MRI can reach better specificity in the detection or differentiation of these tumors. Another reason to favor MRI might be the avoidance of radiation exposure. Ultrasound imaging can be useful in cases of superficially localized tumors [44]. Pheochromocytomas have a heterogeneous pattern in the US: from solid to partially cystic or necrotic and hemorrhagic lesions [45]. Most adrenal cortical adenomas are lipid-rich and appear hypoattenuating on CT [1, 3]. In a landmark study, Boland et al. found that maintaining an upper limit of 10 Hounsfield units (HU) to diagnose benign lesions on unenhanced CT yielded a test sensitivity of 71% for correctly identifying benign lesions while maintaining a specificity of 98% [46], a guideline which is still commonly used today [38, 39, 47]. In comparison to malignant lesions, adenomas tend to enhance avidly and exhibit much more rapid contrast washout [38, 39, 47, 48]. On dual-energy CT, decreased attenuation

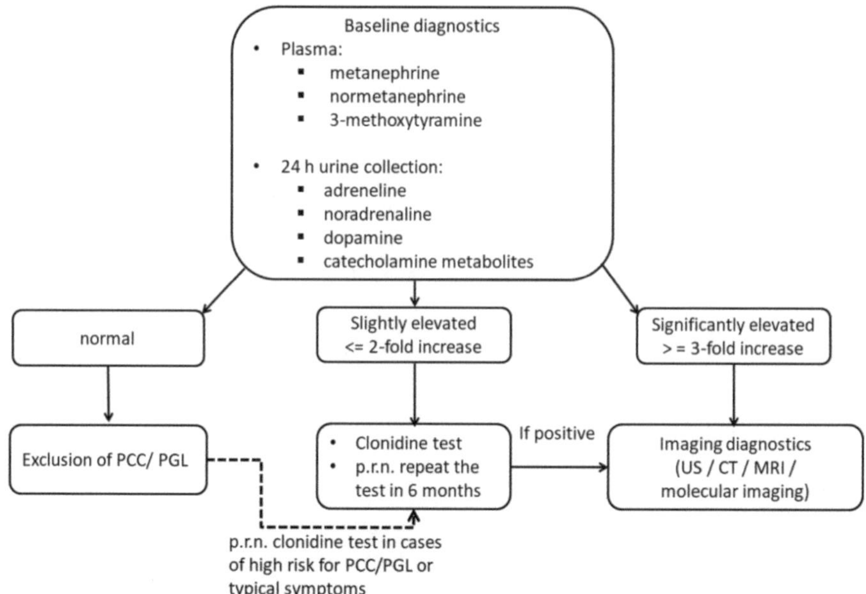

Fig. 7.2 Flow chart of baseline diagnostics in adrenal masses in patients with MEN. *PCC* pheochromocytoma, *PGL* paraganglioma, *US* ultrasound, *CT* computed tomography, *MRI* magnetic resonance imaging, *p.r.n.* "pro re nata," as the circumstances require

at 80 kVp as compared to 140 kVp is highly specific for the presence of intracellular lipid and thus consistent with a diagnosis of adenoma [39]. Similarly, signal drop on opposed-phase imaging on chemical shift (CS)-MRI, which is consistent with the presence of microscopic fat, is also suggestive of an adenomatous lesion [38, 39, 47, 48]. However, as both of these techniques rely on delineating characteristics specific to intracellular lipid, imaging of lipid-poor adenomas remains a diagnostic challenge [3, 38, 39, 47]. On the other hand, pheochromocytomas almost uniformly demonstrate avid enhancement on CT following intravenous contrast administration and characteristic "light bulb" brightness on T_2-weighted imaging [3, 38, 39, 47, 48]. Despite previous concerns of triggering a hypertensive crisis following administration of older iodinated contrast agents, administration of non-ionic iodinated contrast agents appears to be safe and may be helpful in differentiating between a cortical adenoma if there is diagnostic uncertainty [3, 47, 48].

The main indication for functional imaging is the search for metastatic disease or the identification of multiple chromaffin tumors [37]. While not typically considered first-line for imaging the adrenal glands, functional imaging using ^{18}F-FDG PET/CT may aid in differentiating between benign and malignant adrenal lesions. Qualitatively, increased ^{18}F-FDG adrenal uptake relative to hepatic uptake can be considered a positive finding [38, 39]. Quantitatively, Metser et al. found that maintaining a SUV_{max} threshold value of 3.1 was 100% sensitive and 98% specific for differentiating between benign and malignant lesions when combined with CT attenuation analysis [49]. For pheochromocytomas, functional scanning using MIBG-labeled radiotracers can be especially helpful in localizing disease [1, 38,

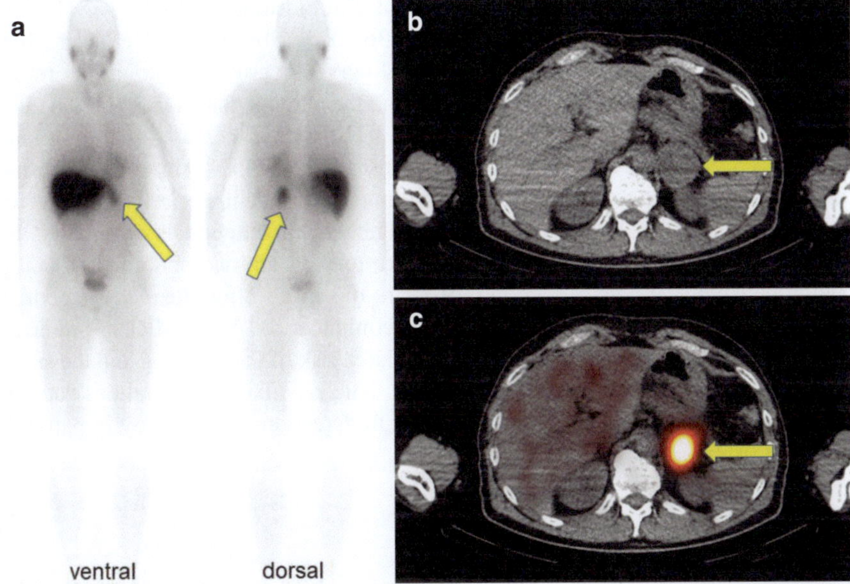

Fig. 7.3 A 55-year-old man with typical symptoms of pheochromocytoma demonstrated on ultrasound (not pictured) a left adrenal mass which was confirmed as pheochromocytoma with ^{123}I-MIBG SPECT/CT. (**a**) Planar whole-body scan demonstrates a focal region of avidity in the region of the left adrenal gland, suggesting pheochromocytoma. (**b** and **c**), Axial SPECT/CT and SPECT/CT of the abdomen demonstrates focal high MIBG uptake in an enlarged adrenal gland

39]. MIBG is a guanethidine analog which is actively taken up and stored in catecholamine-producing cells. ^{123}I-labeling is preferred over ^{131}I-labeling as ^{123}I is more amenable to high-quality SPECT imaging and offers a more favorable radiation-safety profile for the patient [47, 48, 50]. ^{123}I-MIBG scintigraphy can thus be used to visualize the adrenergic tissues of the adrenal medulla with greater sensitivity than ^{18}F-FDG PET [15, 38]. In patients with clinical or biochemical suspicion of pheochromocytoma, multimodal imaging using I^{131}MIBG SPECT/CT, compared to SPECT and planar imaging, has a significantly higher accuracy [51] (Fig. 7.3). For the minority of pheochromocytomas that are MIBG-negative, somatostatin scintigraphy using ^{111}In-octreotide provides an excellent alternative and has also been shown to be highly sensitive for detecting distant metastases [48].

Von Hippel-Lindau Syndrome

Von Hippel-Lindau (VHL) disease is an autosomal dominant familial syndrome affecting multiple organ systems and characterized by a variety of cystic lesions in addition to specific varieties of benign and malignant pathology [52, 53]. This syndrome is caused by a germline mutation in the coding sequence of the VHL tumor suppressor gene located on the short arm of chromosome 3 (3p25.5) [54]. This syndrome is rare, with an incidence of one in 36,000 live births [55]. VHL can affect multiple organ systems including the central nervous system including the retina and the inner ear, the pancreas, the kidneys and the adrenal glands [56]. Of the multiple organ systems affecting patient's with VHL, retinal hemangioblastoma and renal cell carcinoma are the most common causes of death [57]. Although confirmatory genetic testing is available, various imaging modalities are necessary for screening, diagnosis, monitoring, and management of individuals who carry the VHL gene [58]. Screening of the central nervous system and abdomen typically begins between the ages of 13 and 19 years old in an effort to readily identify pathology with potentially life-threatening complications [59]. MRI is preferred over multidetector CT due to the radiation related risk of CT imaging and the superior tissue characterization of MRI [60, 61]. Nuclear imaging modalities such as SPECT and PET also play a significant role in detection of pathology in patient's suffering from VHL (Fig. 7.4).

Central Nervous System

Common lesions which are seen within the central nervous system in patients with VHL including hemangioblastoma of the central nervous system (60–80%) and retina (45–60%), in addition to endolymphatic sac tumors (10–15%) [62]. Hemangioblastoma of the central nervous system can occur within the spinal cord, cerebellum, medulla, and supratentorial brain [52]. The standard imaging modality

Fig. 7.4 52-year-old female with Von Hippel-Lindau syndrome. Axial contrast enhanced CT (**a**) of abdomen demonstrates a large, intensely enhancing mass within the pancreatic body and tail (arrow) and multiple cysts of varying sizes (*) in addition to tortuous blood peripancreatic and perisplenic vessels. Axial PET (**b**) and PET-CT (**c**) demonstrate intense heterogeneous uptake of 68Ga-labeled-1-Nal3-Octreotide (68Ga-DOTANOC within the pancreatic mass [arrow]. Focal 68Ga-DOTANOC uptake was also seen in segment III of the liver (**b, c**, broken arrow) suggesting liver metastasis, confirmed at fine needle aspiration. Axial contrast enhanced CT (**d**) of the abdomen also demonstrates another enhancing mass arising from the interpolar region of the left kidney (arrow) suggestive of renal cell carcinoma. PET (**e**) and PET-CT (**f**) images reveal mild 68Ga-DOTANOC uptake within the renal mass (arrow). Axial PET (**g**) and PET-CT (**h**) images of the brain show a focal area of 68Ga-DOTANOC uptake within a hypoattenuating cerebellar lesion (arrow). Subsequent T2 weighted gadolinium enhanced MRI (**i**) of the brain reveals a nodular lesion in the left cerebellar hemisphere with intense post contrast enhancement (arrow), suggestive of hemangioblastoma. Transaxial PET (**j**) and PET-CT (**k**) images also revealed focal 68Ga-DOTANOC uptake in the left globe, corresponding to a heterogeneous nodular lesion (arrow). Axial T2 weighted gadolinium enhanced MRI (**l**) demonstrates an eccentric, enhancing nodule in the left globe, suggesting retinal hemangioblastoma (arrow). (Adopted from Sharma P, et al. Von Hippel-Lindau syndrome: demonstration of the entire disease spectrum with (68) Ga-DOTANOC PET-CT. Korean J Radiol. 2014 Jan-Feb;15(1):169–72)

for early diagnosis and monitoring of central nervous system hemangioblastoma is gadolinium-enhanced MRI, with annual screening suggested in patients older than 10 years old [63]. Cerebellar hemangioblastoma typically appears as a well-defined relatively homogeneous cystic lesion with avid peripheral and septal post-contrast enhancement or a solid mass with internal cystic components. Spinal hemangioblastoma typically appears as cord expansion associated with a syrinx, avidly enhancing solid components and flow voids [64–66]. Retinal hemangioblastoma

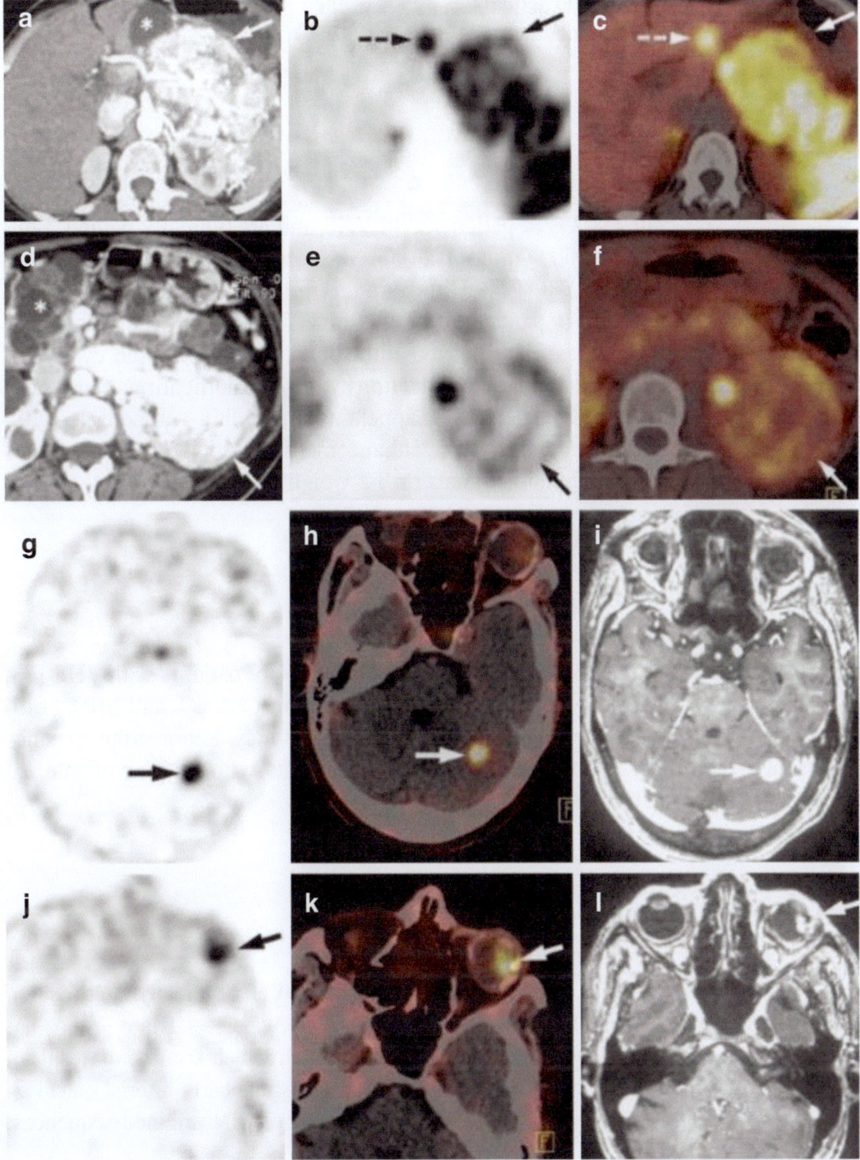

typically occurs between the ages of 10 and 30 years old, resulting in blindness in 6% of patients [66, 67]. On MRI, retinal lesions are hyperintense to normal vitreous on T1-weighted sequences, with contrast typically demonstrated in more severe cases [68]. Endolymphatic sac tumors are typically slow growing and locally invasive, typically located within the dorsal petrous bone, usually characterized as a destructive or "moth eaten" mass. On CT images lesions typically demonstrate a spiculated or reticular pattern of intratumoral bone growth, while on MRI lesions demonstrate heterogeneity on T1-weighted sequences, hyperintense solid components on T2/FLAIR-weighted sequences and "stippled" or "paintbrush" like heterogeneous post-contrast enhancement [59, 62, 64, 69, 70].

Pancreatic Cysts

Pancreatic cysts occur in 42% of patients with VHL and are typically benign, typically yielding the patient mild symptoms or absent symptoms and commonly characterized as simple cysts [70, 71]. Ultrasound is typically used as a first-line screening tool for detection of pancreatic cysts, with CT reserved for further clarification of suspicious features identified on ultrasound. On CT, simple cysts will appear as thin-walled fluid attenuation collections without calcification, mural nodularity or post-contrast enhancement make appear as simple thin-walled cysts without calcification, mural nodularity or enhancement. On MRI, simple cysts demonstrate intrinsic hyperintense signals on T2-weighted sequences [72].

Pancreatic Serous Cystadenoma

Pancreatic serous cystadenomas will occur in 9% to 17% of patients with VHL [73, 74]. These lesions will appear as a multi-cystic mass on both CT and MRI, commonly characterized as a "bunch of grapes." Ultrasound may demonstrate an echogenic mass, with or without small or multilocular cysts with regions of internal heterogeneity [74, 75].

Pancreatic Neuroendocrine Tumors (pNET)

pNET will develop in approximately 15% of patients with VHL, typically multifocal in nature and occurring in any anatomical region within the pancreas. These lesions are typically asymptomatic, slow growing, and nonfunctional, which commonly result in large in size on initial diagnosis [73, 76]. Lesions demonstrate early arterial enhancement on post-contrast sequences, appearing hypointense on T1-weighted sequences, and hyperintense on T2-weighted sequences. Metastatic disease is most common to the liver, which will also demonstrate hypervascularity on post-contrast sequences. Studies report the sensitivity of CT in the identification of pancreatic NETs to range between 29% and 94%, with this high variation favored secondary to the occurrence of lesions <1 cm which may elude detection [62, 66, 74]. PET imaging also plays a role in treatment and screening, as well-differentiated lesions will demonstrate increased ^{18}F-FDG avidity [77]. Many radiolabeled peptides such as somatostatin analogs like ^{68}Ga-DOTA peptide (DOTATATE, DOTANOC, DOTATOC) have been utilized in patients with NETs, in addition to various other malignancies which also overexpress the somatostatin receptor (SSR). Studies have demonstrated ^{68}Ga-DOTATOC PET/CT as a sensible screening tool when compared with CT and MRI, with a combination of abdominal MRI and ^{68}Ga-DOTATATE PET/CT recommended to identify pancreatic NET associated with VHL. Shamim et al. evaluated the role of ^{68}Ga-DOTANOC PET/CT in carriers with a germline mutation of the VHL gene and found that ^{68}Ga-DOTANOC PET/CT has potential as both a useful screening method and follow-up method for these particular demographics [78–83]. Furthermore, several case reports have demonstrated the advantages of ^{68}Ga-DOTA-conjugated peptides in the detection and follow-up of VHL patients [84–90]. pNETs can also be diagnosed with high sensitivity via octreotide SPECT [60] and while small size tumors are not well visualized with this modality, PET imaging with 5-hydroxytryptophan (5-HTP) or L-dopa serve as alternatives [91, 92].

Renal Cysts

Renal cysts occur in 50–75% of patients with VHL, either simple or complex including a combination of solid and cystic components. Simple cysts appear as thin walled, ovoid, fluid density lesions, with solid components worrisome for malignant transformation. Ultrasound and CT are both recommended for periodic monitoring, with ultrasound recommended for initial evaluation and CT recommended in small lesions (< 2 cm) and in cases of multiplicity [66, 68, 93] (Fig. 7.5).

Clear Cell Renal Cell Carcinoma

Renal cell carcinomas (RCC) occur in 28–45% of patients with VHL, most commonly occurring in the third decade. Clear cell RCC is typically characterized by necrosis with hypervascular solid components which enhances greater than the adjacent cortex, with or without calcification [94, 95]. While contrast-enhanced CT is the most common screening and surveillance modality, MRI is growing in utilization secondary to lack of ionizing radiation exposure for young patients and lack of need for intravenous contrast in patient with diminished renal function [72, 75].

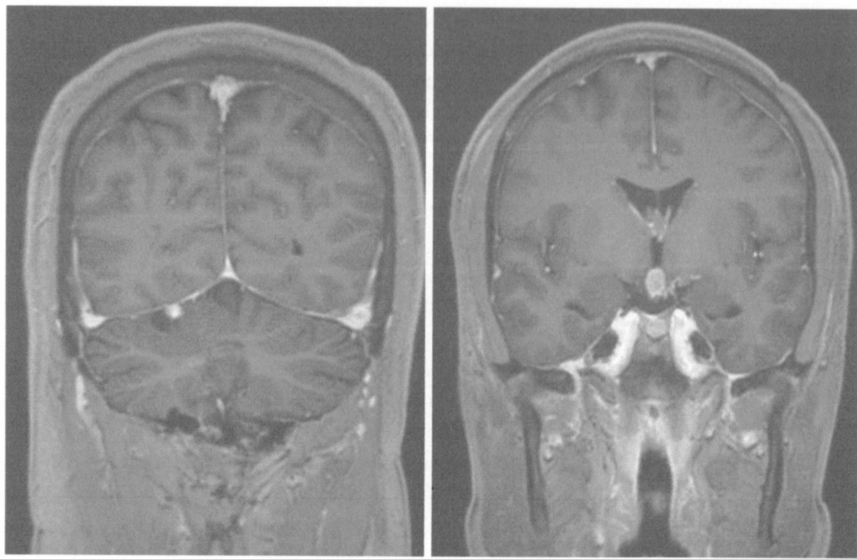

Fig. 7.5 42-year-old female with Von Hippel-Lindau syndrome. Brain images shows multiple subcentimeter enhancing nodules and cysts with enhancing moural nodularity in the right cerebellar hemisphere and vermis as well as inferior right tentorium cerebelli and obex with perilesional edema (FLAIR sequence), compatible with multiple hemangioblastomas

Pheochromocytoma

Pheochromocytomas are found in less than 30% of patients with VHL, occurring bilaterally in approximately 50% of patients. While many of these lesions occur within the adrenal glands, between 15% and 18% of cases are extra-adrenal in origin and are termed paragangliomas [75]. Pheochromocytomas are adrenal tumors which arise from chromaffin cells within the adrenal medulla, while paragangliomas arise from extra-adrenal paraganglia. The anatomical locations of these rare catecholamine-producing neuroendocrine tumors are used to distinguish between them because they cannot be differentiated based on histological findings [96]. The term *paraganglioma* is also used for tumors derived from parasympathetic tissue within the head and neck, most of which do not produce catecholamines [97]. Biochemical testing (serum and urinary catecholamines) and various imaging modalities are the main diagnostic tests utilized for pheochromocytomas [98]. On CT, pheochromocytomas appear as complex solid and cystic masses, occasionally with calcification, necrosis and hemorrhage. On MRI, lesions will appear isointense to hypointense on T1-weighted sequences, "light-bulb" bright on T2-weighted sequences and markedly hypervascular on post-contrast sequences. In larger tumors, there can be varying degrees of necrosis or cystic change [64, 72, 75]. In regard to nuclear imaging modalities common tumor-specific radiopharmaceuticals utilized in detection of pheochromocytoma include ^{11}C-hydroxyephedrine (^{11}C-HED), $^{123/131}$I-metaiodobenzylguanidine (MIBG), ^{18}F-Fluorodopamine (^{18}F-DA), 18F

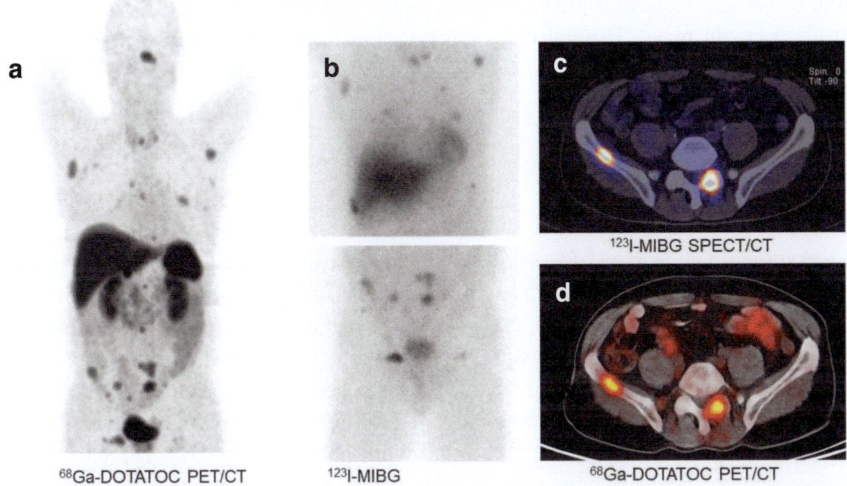

Fig. 7.6 A 62-year-old man with multiple metastases secondary to malignant pheochromocytoma evaluated for radionuclide therapy. The patient received both SSTR PET and MIBG scans. (**a**) Whole-body SSTR PET demonstrates multiple bone metastases. (**b**) Similar to the SSTR PET, MIBG planar scans demonstrates high MIBG uptake in the osseous lesions. (**c**) MIBG SPECT/CT and (**d**) SSTR PET/CT demonstrating similar uptake in two bone metastases. Both therapies could be effective in this case

dihydroxyphenylalanine (^{18}F-DOPA), and ^{18}F-FDG [69]. While $^{123/131}$I-MIBG radiotracers are approved as a method for localization of pheochromocytoma, this modality demonstrates low sensitivity in detection of pheochromocytoma associated with VHL. ^{18}F-DA using dopamine analog compared with [$^{123/131}$I]-MIBG scintigraphy has demonstrated favorable results in the diagnosis and localization of VHL-related adrenal pheochromocytoma [99–101]. Current guidelines recommend paragangliomas and pheochromocytomas in VHL patients should be initially assessed utilizing ^{18}F-DOPA PET/CT followed by ^{123}I-MIBG [100, 102]. Specific radiotracers such as SSTR-PET can be used to target radionuclide therapy in the setting of ^{177}Lu-DOTATOC/DOTATATE, which serves as a theranostic radioactive medication (Fig. 7.6) [103].

Epididymal and Broad Ligament Cystadenomas

Cystic and papillary cystadenomas of the epididymis occur in greater than 50% of males suffering from VHL [75]. Epididymal cystadenomas are commonly asymptomatic and are rarely reported as the first clinical manifestation of VHL. In a small number of cases, obstruction of efferent ducts and spermatic cords has been associated with infertility [76, 77]. On ultrasound, epididymal lesions demonstrate mixed echotexture and are commonly associated with ductal ectasia of the rete testes and testicular atrophy [104]. In the papillary subtype, CT may demonstrate a cystic mass. Typically, no intervention is planned unless it is associated with acute local pain [64, 105, 106].

Li-Fraumeni Syndrome

Li-Fraumeni syndrome (LFS) is a rare syndrome caused by a germline mutation in the tumor suppressor gene TP53 (chromosome 17p13), resulting in early onset of malignancy including sarcoma, breast cancers, leukemia, brain tumors, and adrenal tumors [107, 108]. Due to the variety of tumors associated with LFS, whole-body imaging serves as a main form of surveillance. For example, many asymptomatic aggressive carcinomas and sarcomas, in addition to many other premalignant lesions, are successfully detected through whole-body MRI [107]. Typical surveillance protocol includes annual brain MRI and rapid whole-body MRI at all ages, annual ultrasound of abdomen and pelvis in patients older than 18 years old, and annual mammography/breast MRI screening for patients between 35 and 70 years old. In patients aged from birth to 18 years old, ultrasound of abdomen and pelvis is suggested every 3 to 4 months to detect adenoid cystic carcinoma [107, 109]. One meta-analysis determined that whole-body MRI yielded a 7% detection rate for unrecognized new, localized malignant lesions and a 42.5% false-positive rate in asymptomatic early stage malignancy [110]. ^{18}F-FDG PET-CT has been evaluated for surveillance of patients with LFS, however its use has been limited due the risk of false-positives and radiation exposure. Nevertheless FDG-PET/CT provides unique opportunity to provide information on different cancer types at potentially treatable stages, with some studies even demonstrating validity of an early diagnostic and follow-up role of ^{18}F-FDG PET/CT in patients with LFS [108, 111, 112].

References

1. Grajo JR, Paspulati RM, Sahani DV, Kambadakone A. Multiple endocrine neoplasia syndromes: a comprehensive imaging review. Radiol Clin N Am. 2016;54(3):441–51. https://doi.org/10.1016/j.rcl.2015.12.001.
2. Walls GV. Multiple endocrine neoplasia (MEN) syndromes. Semin Pediatr Surg. 2014;23(2):96–101. https://doi.org/10.1053/j.sempedsurg.2014.03.008.
3. Scarsbrook AF, Thakker RV, Wass JA, Gleeson FV, Phillips RR. Multiple endocrine neoplasia: spectrum of radiologic appearances and discussion of a multitechnique imaging approach. Radiographics. 2006;26(2):433–51. https://doi.org/10.1148/rg.262055073.
4. Brandi ML, Gagel RF, Angeli A, Bilezikian JP, Beck-Peccoz P, Bordi C, Conte-Devolx B, Falchetti A, Gheri RG, Libroia A, Lips CJ, Lombardi G, Mannelli M, Pacini F, Ponder BA, Raue F, Skogseid B, Tamburrano G, Thakker RV, Thompson NW, Tomassetti P, Tonelli F, Wells SA Jr, Marx SJ. Guidelines for diagnosis and therapy of MEN type 1 and type 2. J Clin Endocrinol Metab. 2001;86(12):5658–71. https://doi.org/10.1210/jcem.86.12.8070.
5. McDonnell JE, Gild ML, Clifton-Bligh RJ, Robinson BG. Multiple endocrine neoplasia: an update. Intern Med J. 2019;49(8):954–61. https://doi.org/10.1111/imj.14394.

6. Wells SA Jr, Asa SL, Dralle H, Elisei R, Evans DB, Gagel RF, Lee N, Machens A, Moley JF, Pacini F, Raue F, Frank-Raue K, Robinson B, Rosenthal MS, Santoro M, Schlumberger M, Shah M, Waguespack SG, American Thyroid Association Guidelines Task Force on Medullary Thyroid C. Revised American Thyroid Association guidelines for the management of medullary thyroid carcinoma. Thyroid. 2015;25(6):567–610. https://doi.org/10.1089/thy.2014.0335.

7. Lakhani VT, You YN, Wells SA. The multiple endocrine neoplasia syndromes. Annu Rev Med. 2007;58:253–65. https://doi.org/10.1146/annurev.med.58.100305.115303.

8. Daskalakis K, Tsoli M, Alexandraki KI, Angelousi A, Chatzellis E, Tsolakis AV, Karoumpalis I, Kolomodi D, Kassi E, Kaltsas G. Magnetic resonance imaging or endoscopic ultrasonography for detection and surveillance of pancreatic neuroendocrine neoplasms in patients with multiple endocrine neoplasia type 1? Horm Metab Res. 2019;51(9):580–5. https://doi.org/10.1055/a-0931-7005.

9. Langer P, Kann PH, Fendrich V, Richter G, Diehl S, Rothmund M, Bartsch DK. Prospective evaluation of imaging procedures for the detection of pancreaticoduodenal endocrine tumors in patients with multiple endocrine neoplasia type 1. World J Surg. 2004;28(12):1317–22. https://doi.org/10.1007/s00268-004-7642-7.

10. Tamm EP, Bhosale P, Lee JH, Rohren EM. State-of-the-art imaging of pancreatic neuroendocrine tumors. Surg Oncol Clin N Am. 2016;25(2):375–400. https://doi.org/10.1016/j.soc.2015.11.007.

11. Sundin A, Vullierme MP, Kaltsas G, Plockinger U, Mallorca Consensus Conference P, European Neuroendocrine Tumor S. ENETS consensus guidelines for the standards of care in neuroendocrine tumors: radiological examinations. Neuroendocrinology. 2009;90(2):167–83. https://doi.org/10.1159/000184855.

12. Kartalis N, Mucelli RM, Sundin A. Recent developments in imaging of pancreatic neuroendocrine tumors. Ann Gastroenterol. 2015;28(2):193–202.

13. van Asselt SJ, Brouwers AH, van Dullemen HM, van der Jagt EJ, Bongaerts AH, Kema IP, Koopmans KP, Valk GD, Timmers HJ, de Herder WW, Feelders RA, Fockens P, Sluiter WJ, de Vries EG, Links TP. EUS is superior for detection of pancreatic lesions compared with standard imaging in patients with multiple endocrine neoplasia type 1. Gastrointest Endosc. 2015;81(1):159–167 e152. https://doi.org/10.1016/j.gie.2014.09.037.

14. Power N, Reznek RH. Imaging pancreatic islet cell tumours. Imaging. 2002;14(2):147–59. https://doi.org/10.1259/img.14.2.140147.

15. Anderson MA, Carpenter S, Thompson NW, Nostrant TT, Elta GH, Scheiman JM. Endoscopic ultrasound is highly accurate and directs management in patients with neuroendocrine tumors of the pancreas. Am J Gastroenterol. 2000;95(9):2271–7. https://doi.org/10.1111/j.1572-0241.2000.02480.x.

16. Lee L, Ito T, Jensen RT. Imaging of pancreatic neuroendocrine tumors: recent advances, current status, and controversies. Expert Rev Anticancer Ther. 2018;18(9):837–60. https://doi.org/10.1080/14737140.2018.1496822.

17. Pressman BD. Pituitary Imaging. Endocrinol Metab Clin N Am. 2017;46(3):713–40. https://doi.org/10.1016/j.ecl.2017.04.012.

18. Johnsen DE, Woodruff WW, Allen IS, Cera PJ, Funkhouser GR, Coleman LL. MR imaging of the sellar and juxtasellar regions. Radiographics. 1991;11(5):727–58. https://doi.org/10.1148/radiographics.11.5.1947311.

19. Evanson EJ. Imaging the pituitary gland. Imaging. 2002;14(2):93–102. https://doi.org/10.1259/img.14.2.140093.

20. Yuh WT, Fisher DJ, Nguyen HD, Tali ET, Gao F, Simonson TM, Schlechte JA. Sequential MR enhancement pattern in normal pituitary gland and in pituitary adenoma. AJNR Am J Neuroradiol. 1994;15(1):101–8.

21. Frank-Raue K, Rondot S, Raue F. Molecular genetics and phenomics of RET mutations: impact on prognosis of MTC. Mol Cell Endocrinol. 2010;322(1–2):2–7. https://doi.org/10.1016/j.mce.2010.01.012.

22. Ganeshan D, Paulson E, Duran C, Cabanillas ME, Busaidy NL, Charnsangavej C. Current update on medullary thyroid carcinoma. AJR Am J Roentgenol. 2013;201(6):W867–76. https://doi.org/10.2214/AJR.12.10370.
23. Lee S, Shin JH, Han BK, Ko EY. Medullary thyroid carcinoma: comparison with papillary thyroid carcinoma and application of current sonographic criteria. AJR Am J Roentgenol. 2010;194(4):1090–4. https://doi.org/10.2214/AJR.09.3276.
24. Yun G, Kim YK, Choi SI, Kim JH. Medullary thyroid carcinoma: application of thyroid imaging reporting and data system (TI-RADS) classification. Endocrine. 2018;61(2):285–92. https://doi.org/10.1007/s12020-018-1594-4.
25. Kushchayev SV, Kushchayeva YS, Tella SH, Glushko T, Pacak K, Teytelboym OM. Medullary thyroid carcinoma: an update on imaging. J Thyroid Res. 2019;2019:1893047. https://doi.org/10.1155/2019/1893047.
26. Giovanella L, Treglia G, Iakovou I, Mihailovic J, Verburg FA, Luster M. EANM practice guideline for PET/CT imaging in medullary thyroid carcinoma. Eur J Nucl Med Mol Imaging. 2020;47(1):61–77. https://doi.org/10.1007/s00259-019-04458-6.
27. Giraudet AL, Vanel D, Leboulleux S, Auperin A, Dromain C, Chami L, Ny Tovo N, Lumbroso J, Lassau N, Bonniaud G, Hartl D, Travagli JP, Baudin E, Schlumberger M. Imaging medullary thyroid carcinoma with persistent elevated calcitonin levels. J Clin Endocrinol Metab. 2007;92(11):4185–90. https://doi.org/10.1210/jc.2007-1211.
28. Ueda CE, Duarte PS, de Castroneves LA, Flavio J, Marin G, Sado HN, Sapienza MT, Hoff AO, Buchpiguel CA. Burden of metastatic bone disease measured on 18F-NaF PET/computed tomography studies as a prognostic indicator in patients with medullary thyroid cancer. Nucl Med Commun. 2020;41(5):469–76. https://doi.org/10.1097/MNM.0000000000001175.
29. Sohaib SA, Cook G. The parathyroid glands. Imaging. 2002;14(2):115–21. https://doi.org/10.1259/img.14.2.140115.
30. De Feo ML, Colagrande S, Biagini C, Tonarelli A, Bisi G, Vaggelli L, Borrelli D, Cicchi P, Tonelli F, Amorosi A, Serio M, Brandi ML. Parathyroid glands: combination of (99m)Tc MIBI scintigraphy and US for demonstration of parathyroid glands and nodules. Radiology. 2000;214(2):393–402. https://doi.org/10.1148/radiology.214.2.r00fe04393.
31. Greene AB, Butler RS, McIntyre S, Barbosa GF, Mitchell J, Berber E, Siperstein A, Milas M. National trends in parathyroid surgery from 1998 to 2008: a decade of change. J Am Coll Surg. 2009;209(3):332–43. https://doi.org/10.1016/j.jamcollsurg.2009.05.029.
32. Zafereo M, Yu J, Angelos P, Brumund K, Chuang HH, Goldenberg D, Lango M, Perrier N, Randolph G, Shindo ML, Singer M, Smith R, Stack BC Jr, Steward D, Terris DJ, Vu T, Yao M, Tufano RP. American head and neck society endocrine surgery section update on parathyroid imaging for surgical candidates with primary hyperparathyroidism. Head Neck. 2019;41(7):2398–409. https://doi.org/10.1002/hed.25781.
33. Buck AK, Nekolla S, Ziegler S, Beer A, Krause BJ, Herrmann K, Scheidhauer K, Wester HJ, Rummeny EJ, Schwaiger M, Drzezga A. Spect/Ct. J Nucl Med. 2008;49(8):1305–19. https://doi.org/10.2967/jnumed.107.050195.
34. Lavely WC, Goetze S, Friedman KP, Leal JP, Zhang Z, Garret-Mayer E, Dackiw AP, Tufano RP, Zeiger MA, Ziessman HA. Comparison of SPECT/CT, SPECT, and planar imaging with single- and dual-phase (99m)Tc-sestamibi parathyroid scintigraphy. J Nucl Med. 2007;48(7):1084–9. https://doi.org/10.2967/jnumed.107.040428.
35. Wong KK, Fig LM, Gross MD, Dwamena BA. Parathyroid adenoma localization with 99mTc-sestamibi SPECT/CT: a meta-analysis. Nucl Med Commun. 2015;36(4):363–75. https://doi.org/10.1097/MNM.0000000000000262.
36. Gayed IW, Kim EE, Broussard WF, Evans D, Lee J, Broemeling LD, Ochoa BB, Moxley DM, Erwin WD, Podoloff DA. The value of 99mTc-sestamibi SPECT/CT over conventional SPECT in the evaluation of parathyroid adenomas or hyperplasia. J Nucl Med. 2005;46(2):248–52.
37. Neumann HPH, Young WF Jr, Eng C. Pheochromocytoma and paraganglioma. N Engl J Med. 2019;381(6):552–65.

38. Blake MA, Cronin CG, Boland GW. Adrenal imaging. AJR Am J Roentgenol. 2010;194(6):1450–60. https://doi.org/10.2214/AJR.10.4547.
39. Elsayes KM, Emad-Eldin S, Morani AC, Jensen CT. Practical approach to adrenal imaging. Radiol Clin N Am. 2017;55(2):279–301. https://doi.org/10.1016/j.rcl.2016.10.005.
40. Peaston RT, Weinkove C. Measurement of catecholamines and their metabolites. Ann Clin Biochem. 2004;41(Pt 1):17–38.
41. Sawka AM, Jaeschke R, Singh RJ, Young WF Jr. A comparison of biochemical tests for pheochromocytoma: measurement of fractionated plasma metanephrines compared with the combination of 24-hour urinary metanephrines and catecholamines. J Clin Endocrinol Metab. 2003;88(2):553–8.
42. Pacak K, Tella SH. Pheochromocytoma and paraganglioma. In: Feingold KR, Anawalt B, Boyce A, Chrousos G, de Herder WW, Dungan K, et al. Endotext. South Dartmouth, MA, 2000.
43. Lenders JW, Duh QY, Eisenhofer G, Gimenez-Roqueplo AP, Grebe SK, Murad MH, et al. Pheochromocytoma and paraganglioma: an endocrine society clinical practice guideline. J Clin Endocrinol Metab. 2014;99(6):1915–42.
44. Katabathina VS, Rajebi H, Chen M, Restrepo CS, Salman U, Vikram R, et al. Genetics and imaging of pheochromocytomas and paragangliomas: current update. Abdom Radiol (NY). 2020;45(4):928–44.
45. Leung K, Stamm M, Raja A, Low G. Pheochromocytoma: the range of appearances on ultrasound, CT, MRI, and functional imaging. AJR Am J Roentgenol. 2013;200(2):370–8.
46. Boland GW, Lee MJ, Gazelle GS, Halpern EF, McNicholas MM, Mueller PR. Characterization of adrenal masses using unenhanced CT: an analysis of the CT literature. AJR Am J Roentgenol. 1998;171(1):201–4. https://doi.org/10.2214/ajr.171.1.9648789.
47. Taffel M, Haji-Momenian S, Nikolaidis P, Miller FH. Adrenal imaging: a comprehensive review. Radiol Clin N Am. 2012;50(2):219–43. https://doi.org/10.1016/j.rcl.2012.02.009.
48. Baez JC, Jagannathan JP, Krajewski K, O'Regan K, Zukotynski K, Kulke M, Ramaiya NH. Pheochromocytoma and paraganglioma: imaging characteristics. Cancer Imaging. 2012;12:153–62. https://doi.org/10.1102/1470-7330.2012.0016.
49. Metser U, Miller E, Lerman H, Lievshitz G, Avital S, Even-Sapir E. 18F-FDG PET/CT in the evaluation of adrenal masses. J Nucl Med. 2006;47(1):32–7.
50. Intenzo CM, Jabbour S, Lin HC, Miller JL, Kim SM, Capuzzi DM, Mitchell EP. Scintigraphic imaging of body neuroendocrine tumors. Radiographics. 2007;27(5):1355–69. https://doi.org/10.1148/rg.275065729.
51. Sharma P, Dhull VS, Jeph S, Reddy RM, Singh H, Naswa N, et al. Can hybrid SPECT-CT overcome the limitations associated with poor imaging properties of 131I-MIBG?: comparison with planar scintigraphy and SPECT in pheochromocytoma. Clin Nucl Med. 2013;38:e346.
52. Lonser RR, Glenn GM, Walther M, Chew EY, Libutti SK, Linehan WM, et al. von Hippel-Lindau disease. Lancet. 2003;361(9374):2059–67.
53. Maher ER. Von Hippel-Lindau disease. Eur J Cancer. 1994;30:1987.
54. Seizinger B, Rouleau G, Ozelius L, Lane A, Farmer G, Lamiell J, et al. Von Hippel–Lindau disease maps to the region of chromosome 3 associated with renal cell carcinoma. Nature. 1988;332(6161):268–9.
55. Latif F, Tory K, Gnarra J, Yao M, Duh F-M, Orcutt ML, et al. Identification of the von Hippel-Lindau disease tumor suppressor gene. Science. 1993;260(5112):1317–20.
56. Gläsker S, Neumann HP, Koch CA, Vortmeyer A. Von Hippel-Lindau Disease. Endotext: MDText.com, Inc.; 2018.
57. Katabathina V, Vinu-Nair S. Cross-sectional imaging spectrum of von Hippel-Lindau disease. J Transl Med Epidemiol. 2014;2(1):1021.
58. Linehan WM, Walther MM, Zbar B. The genetic basis of cancer of the kidney. J Urol. 2003;170(6):2163–72.
59. Choyke P, Filling-Katz M, Shawker T, Gorin M, Travis W, Chang R, et al. von Hippel-Lindau disease: radiologic screening for visceral manifestations. Radiology. 1990;174(3):815–20.

60. Linet MS, Slovis TL, Miller DL, Kleinerman R, Lee C, Rajaraman P, et al. Cancer risks associated with external radiation from diagnostic imaging procedures. CA Cancer J Clin. 2012;62(2):75–100.
61. Ballinger ML, Ferris NJ, Moodie K, Mitchell G, Shanley S, James PA, et al. Surveillance in germline TP53 mutation carriers utilizing whole-body magnetic resonance imaging. JAMA Oncol. 2017;3(12):1735–6.
62. Ganeshan D, Menias CO, Pickhardt PJ, Sandrasegaran K, Lubner MG, Ramalingam P, et al. Tumors in von Hippel–Lindau syndrome: from head to toe—comprehensive state-of-the-art review. Radiographics. 2018;38(3):849–66.
63. Anupindi SA, Bedoya MA, Lindell RB, Rambhatla SJ, Zelley K, Nichols KE, et al. Diagnostic performance of whole-body MRI as a tool for cancer screening in children with genetic cancer-predisposing conditions. Am J Roentgenol. 2015;205(2):400–8.
64. Leung RS, Biswas SV, Duncan M, Rankin S. Imaging features of von Hippel–Lindau disease. Radiographics. 2008;28(1):65–79.
65. Shuin T, Yamasaki I, Tamura K, Okuda H, Furihata M, Ashida S. Von Hippel–Lindau disease: molecular pathological basis, clinical criteria, genetic testing, clinical features of tumors and treatment. Jpn J Clin Oncol. 2006;36(6):337–43.
66. Malik A, Misra R, Chawla AS, Chandra R, Bajaj SK, Thukral BB. Imaging spectrum of von Hippel–Lindau disease. Astrocyte. 2015;2(3):136.
67. Tootee A, Hasani-Ranjbar S. Von Hippel-Lindau disease: a new approach to an old problem. Int J Endocrinol Metabol. 2012;10(4):619.
68. Choyke PL, Glenn GM, Walther M, Patronas NJ, Linehan WM, Zbar B. von Hippel-Lindau disease: genetic, clinical, and imaging features. Radiology. 1995;194(3):629–42.
69. Manski TJ, Heffner DK, Glenn GM, Patronas NJ, Pikus AT, Katz D, et al. Endolymphatic sac tumors: a source of morbid hearing loss in von Hippel-Lindau disease. JAMA. 1997;277(18):1461–6.
70. Ayadi K, Ben Mahfoudh K, Khannous M, Mnif J. Endolymphatic sac tumor and von Hippel-Lindau disease: imaging features. Am J Roentgenol. 2000;175(3):925–6.
71. Hough DM, Stephens DH, Johnson CD, Binkovitz L. Pancreatic lesions in von Hippel-Lindau disease: prevalence, clinical significance, and CT findings. AJR Am J Roentgenol. 1994;162(5):1091–4.
72. Shanbhogue KP, Hoch M, Fatterpaker G, Chandarana H. von Hippel-Lindau disease: review of genetics and imaging. Radiol Clin North Am. 2016;54(3):409–22.
73. Charlesworth M, Verbeke CS, Falk GA, Walsh M, Smith AM, Morris-Stiff G. Pancreatic lesions in von Hippel–Lindau disease? A systematic review and meta-synthesis of the literature. J Gastrointest Surg. 2012;16(7):1422–8.
74. Keutgen XM, Hammel P, Choyke PL, Libutti SK, Jonasch E, Kebebew E. Evaluation and management of pancreatic lesions in patients with von Hippel–Lindau disease. Nat Rev Clin Oncol. 2016;13(9):537.
75. Taouli B, Ghouadni M, Corréas J-M, Hammel P, Couvelard A, Richard S, et al. Spectrum of abdominal imaging findings in von Hippel-Lindau disease. Am J Roentgenol. 2003;181(4):1049–54.
76. Marcos HB, Libutti SK, Alexander HR, Lubensky IA, Bartlett DL, Walther MM, et al. Neuroendocrine tumors of the pancreas in von Hippel–Lindau disease: spectrum of appearances at CT and MR imaging with histopathologic comparison. Radiology. 2002;225(3):751–8.
77. Kok J, Lin M, Wong V, Campbell P, Lin P. [18F] FDG PET/CT in pancreatic neuroendocrine tumours associated with von Hippel Lindau syndrome. Clin Endocrinol. 2009;70(4):657–9.
78. De Jong M, Breeman WA, Kwekkeboom DJ, Valkema R, Krenning EP. Tumor imaging and therapy using radiolabeled somatostatin analogues. Acc Chem Res. 2009;42(7):873–80.
79. Haug AR, Auernhammer CJ, Wängler B, Schmidt GP, Uebleis C, Göke B, et al. 68Ga-DOTATATE PET/CT for the early prediction of response to somatostatin receptor–mediated radionuclide therapy in patients with well-differentiated neuroendocrine tumors. J Nucl Med. 2010;51(9):1349–56.

80. Prasad V, Tiling N, Denecke T, Brenner W, Plöckinger U. Potential role of 68 Ga-DOTATOC PET/CT in screening for pancreatic neuroendocrine tumour in patients with von Hippel-Lindau disease. Eur J Nucl Med Mol Imaging. 2016;43(11):2014–20.
81. Shell J, Tirosh A, Millo C, Sadowski SM, Assadipour Y, Green P, et al. The utility of 68Gallium-DOTATATE PET/CT in the detection of von Hippel-Lindau disease associated tumors. Eur J Radiol. 2019;112:130–5.
82. Hopp AC, Collins JM, Nguyen CC, Yang M. Radiopathological correlation of a von Hippel-Lindau syndrome associated pancreatic neuroendocrine tumour with clear cell features. BMJ Case Rep. 2019;12(2):bcr-2018-227891.
83. Shamim SA, Arora G, Arunraj S, Shankar K, Hussain J, Kumar D, et al. Role of 68Ga-DOTANOC PET/CT scan in von Hippel-Lindau disease. J Nucl Med. 2020;61(supplement 1):127.
84. Papadakis GZ, Millo C, Sadowski Veuthey MSD, Bagci U, Patronas NJ. Kidney tumor in a von Hippel-Lindau (VHL) patient with intensely increased activity on 68Ga-DOTA-TATE PET/CT. Clin Nucl Med. 2016;41(12):970–1.
85. Liberini V, Nicolotti DG, Maccario M, Finessi M, Deandreis D. 68Ga-DOTA-TOC PET/CT of von Hippel–Lindau disease. Clin Nucl Med. 2019;44(2):125–6.
86. Papadakis GZ, Millo C, Jassel IS, Bagci U, Sadowski SM, Karantanas AH, et al. 18F-FDG and 68Ga-DOTATATE PET/CT in von Hippel-Lindau disease-associated retinal hemangioblastoma. Clin Nucl Med. 2017;42(3):189–90.
87. Ambrosini V, Campana D, Allegri V, Opocher G, Fanti S. 68Ga-DOTA-NOC PET/CT detects somatostatin receptors expression in von Hippel-Lindau cerebellar disease. Clin Nucl Med. 2011;36(1):64–5.
88. Banezhad F, Kiamanesh Z, Emami F, Sadeghi R. 68Ga DOTATATE PET/CT versus 18F-FDG PET/CT for detecting intramedullary hemangioblastoma in a patient with von Hippel-Lindau disease. Clin Nucl Med. 2019;44(6):e385–e7.
89. Meneret P, Girard A, Pagenault M, Riffaud L, Palard-Novello X. Different manifestations detected with 68Ga-DOTATOC PET/CT in patients with von Hippel-Lindau disease: a case report. Nuklearmedizin. 2020;59(04):332–4.
90. Papadakis GZ, Millo C, Sadowski Veuthey MSD, Bagci U, Patronas NJ. Epididymal cystadenomas in von Hippel-Lindau disease showing increased activity on 68Ga DOTATATE PET/CT. Clin Nucl Med. 2016;41(10):781–2.
91. Tamura K, Nishimori I, Ito T, Yamasaki I, Igarashi H, Shuin T. Diagnosis and management of pancreatic neuroendocrine tumor in von Hippel-Lindau disease. World J Gastroenterol: WJG. 2010;16(36):4515.
92. Plöckinger U, Rindi G, Arnold R, Eriksson B, Krenning E, De Herder W, et al. Guidelines for the diagnosis and treatment of neuroendocrine gastrointestinal tumours. Neuroendocrinology. 2004;80(6):394–424.
93. Lamiell JM, Salazar FG, Hsia YE. von Hippel-Lindau disease affecting 43 members of a single kindred. Medicine. 1989;68(1):1–29.
94. Choyke PL, Glenn GM, Walther MM, Zbar B, Linehan WM. Hereditary renal cancers. Radiology. 2003;226(1):33–46.
95. Chauveau D, Duvic C, Chrétien Y, Paraf F, Droz D, Melki P, et al. Renal involvement in von Hippel-Lindau disease. Kidney Int. 1996;50(3):944–51.
96. Lam AK. Update on adrenal tumours in 2017 World Health Organization (WHO) of endocrine tumours. Endocr Pathol. 2017;28(3):213–27.
97. Lenders JW, Eisenhofer G, Mannelli M, Pacak K. Phaeochromocytoma. Lancet. 2005;366(9486):665–75.
98. Neumann HP, Bender BU, Berger DP, Laubenberger J, Schultze-Seemann W, Wetterauer U, et al. Prevalence, morphology and biology of renal cell carcinoma in von Hippel-Lindau disease compared to sporadic renal cell carcinoma. J Urol. 1998;160(4):1248–54.
99. Kaji P, Carrasquillo JA, Linehan WM, Chen CC, Eisenhofer G, Pinto PA, et al. The role of 6-[18F] fluorodopamine positron emission tomography in the localization of adre-

nal pheochromocytoma associated with von Hippel–Lindau syndrome. Eur J Endocrinol. 2007;156(4):483–7.
100. Ilias I, Pacak K. Current approaches and recommended algorithm for the diagnostic localization of pheochromocytoma. J Clin Endocrinol Metabol. 2004;89(2):479–91.
101. Taieb D, Sebag F, Hubbard J, Mundler O, Henry J, Conte-Devolx B. Does iodine-131 meta-iodobenzylguanidine (MIBG) scintigraphy have an impact on the management of sporadic and familial phaeochromocytoma? Clin Endocrinol. 2004;61(1):102–8.
102. Timmers HJ, Kozupa A, Chen CC, Carrasquillo JA, Ling A, Eisenhofer G, et al. Superiority of fluorodeoxyglucose positron emission tomography to other functional imaging techniques in the evaluation of metastatic SDHB-associated pheochromocytoma and paraganglioma. J Clin Oncol. 2007;25(16):2262–9.
103. Vyakaranam AR, Crona J, Norlen O, Granberg D, Garske-Roman U, Sandstrom M, et al. Favorable outcome in patients with pheochromocytoma and paraganglioma treated with (177)Lu-DOTATATE. Cancers (Basel). 2019;11(7):909.
104. Choyke PL, Glenn GM, Wagner JP, Lubensky IA, Thakore K, Zbar B, et al. Epididymal cystadenomas in von Hippel-Lindau disease. Urology. 1997;49(6):926–31.
105. Gläsker S, Tran M, Shively S, Ikejiri B, Lonser R, Maxwell P, et al. Epididymal cystadenomas and epithelial tumourlets: effects of VHL deficiency on the human epididymis. J Pathol. 2006;210(1):32–41.
106. Mehta GU, Shively SB, Duong H, Tran MG, Moncrief TJ, Smith JH, et al. Progression of epididymal maldevelopment into hamartoma-like neoplasia in VHL disease. Neoplasia. 2008;10(10):1146–53.
107. Villani A, Shore A, Wasserman JD, Stephens D, Kim RH, Druker H, et al. Biochemical and imaging surveillance in germline TP53 mutation carriers with li-Fraumeni syndrome: 11 year follow-up of a prospective observational study. Lancet Oncol. 2016;17(9):1295–305.
108. Masciari S, Van den Abbeele AD, Diller LR, Rastarhuyeva I, Yap J, Schneider K, et al. F18-fluorodeoxyglucose–positron emission tomography/computed tomography screening in li-Fraumeni syndrome. JAMA. 2008;299(11):1315–9.
109. Schneider K, Zelley K, Nichols KE, Garber J. Li-fraumeni syndrome. In: GeneReviews®. Seattle, WA: University of Washington; 2013.
110. Ballinger ML, Best A, Mai PL, Khincha PP, Loud JT, Peters JA, et al. Baseline surveillance in li-Fraumeni syndrome using whole-body magnetic resonance imaging: a meta-analysis. JAMA Oncol. 2017;3(12):1634–9.
111. Nogueira STS, Lima ENP, Nóbrega AF, Torres IDCG, Cavicchioli M, Hainaut P, et al. 18F-FDG PET-CT for surveillance of Brazilian patients with li-Fraumeni syndrome. Front Oncol. 2015;5:38.
112. Chadaz T, Hobbs SK, Son H. Chest wall sarcoma: 18F-FDG PET/CT in a patient with li-Fraumeni syndrome. Clin Nucl Med. 2013;38(10):818–20.

Chapter 8
Pharmacokinetics and Pharmacodynamics in Adolescents Receiving Cancer Therapies

Amal Ayyoub

Pharmacokinetics and Pharmacodynamics in Adolescents Compared to Adults

Age-associated changes in body composition and organ function are dynamic; nonetheless, developmental changes in physiologic factors that influence drug disposition (absorption, distribution, metabolism, and excretion) approximate adult levels by 12 years of age leading to common physiologic characteristics between adolescents and adults [1]. Gastrointestinal structure and function represented by hydrochloric acid production, bile acid secretion, intestinal length, and glutathione conjugation capacity reach full activity between 5 and 10 years of age [2]. Expressed as a percentage of total body weight, adolescents have the same levels of total body water, extracellular fluid, and body fat compared to adults suggesting that the apparent volume of distribution of drugs will be similar for children 12 years of age and older compared with adults [2]. The drug metabolic capacity facilitated by phase I cytochrome P-450 isoenzymes and phase II conjugation enzymes in the liver and intestine also reach full maturation by adolescence leading to similar metabolic drug clearance. The renal glomerular filtration rate and tubular secretion rise until adult levels are reached at approximately 12 months of age suggesting similar renal clearance compared to adults. Collectively, from a pharmacokinetic perspective, differences would not be expected between adolescents, 12 years of age and older, compared to adults. Indeed, apparent drug clearance, a fundamental parameter in pharmacokinetics, in adolescents averaged 93% of adult values indicating that the same adult dosage can often be used in adolescents [3, 4].

Unlike age-related physiologic factors that impact pharmacokinetics, the ontogeny of pharmacodynamics is not clearly understood. Little information exists on the

A. Ayyoub (✉)
Division of Cancer Pharmacology II, Office of Clinical Pharmacology, Food and Drug Administration, Silver Spring, MD, USA

149

F. Hannah-Shmouni (ed.), *Familial Endocrine Cancer Syndromes*,
https://doi.org/10.1007/978-3-031-37275-9_8

age-related differences in the interaction of a drug with its specific receptor or in the relation between the drug concentration in the plasma or site of action with the pharmacologic effect or toxicity. Nonetheless, based on pharmacokinetic-pharmacodynamic analyses for drugs administered to adolescents and adults, developmental changes that can alter the action and response to a drug are expected to reach maturation by adolescence, and patient-specific factors such as pharmacogenetic factors are thought to potentially contribute to the individual variability of the response. The latter is exemplified in altered sensitivity to the ototoxic effects of cisplatin associated with variants in the thiopurine S-methyltransferase (TPMT) gene [5, 6].

Considerations for Drug Development of Oncology Therapeutics in Adolescents

Cancers in pediatric patients are often distinct from those in adult patients and require unique treatment strategies; however, some cancer types found in adolescent patients, including familial endocrine cancer syndromes, are similar in histology and biologic behavior to those in adults. To expedite drug development of cancer products in adolescents, inclusion of children 12 years of age and older in adult oncology trials at all stages of drug development is encouraged by the American Society of Clinical Oncology/Friends of Cancer Research, ACCELERATE, the Innovative Therapies for Children with Cancer, and the U.S. Food and Drug Administration [7–10]. Combined adolescent-adult trials are recommended when the histology and biologic behavior of the cancer under investigation is the same in, or the molecular target of the drug is relevant to, cancers in both adult and adolescent patients. Indeed, an analysis of combined pediatric and adult trials between 2012 and 2018 performed by Tanaudommongkon et al. shows that a substantial number of adult clinical trials across various therapeutic areas (56 trials in 24 products) included children between 12 and 18 years of age [11]. As described in FDA's 2019 Guidance for Industry, titled, *"Considerations for the inclusion of adolescent patients in adult oncology clinical trials"* for drugs with body size-adjusted dosing for adults, adolescent patients should receive the same body size-adjusted dose (mg/kg or mg/m^2) that is administered in adults. However, for drugs administered as a fixed dose in adults, based on the lack of clinically meaningful body size effect on drug exposure and toxicity in adults, a minimum body weight threshold should be defined to prevent adolescent patients who have a lower body weight than average from exceeding adult exposures. In general, a minimum body weight threshold of 40 kg, as the approximate median body weight value corresponding to a 12 year old, is suggested. The Guidance document further specifies that adolescents weighing less than 40 kg should be administered body weight or surface area adjusted dosages [11].

In conclusion, considering that pediatric patients 12 years of age and older share common physiologic characteristics between adolescents and adults, and inclusion of adolescents in adult oncology trials, specifically, is a successful strategy to accelerate access to potentially efficacious therapies to adolescents.

References

1. Shebley M, Menon RM, Gibbs JP, Dave N, Kim SY, Marroum PJ. Accelerating drug development in pediatriconcology with the clinical pharmacology storehouse. J Clin Pharmacol. 2019;59(5):625–37.
2. Kearns GL, Abdel-Rahman SM, Alander SW, Blowey DL, Leeder JS, Kauffman RE. Developmental pharmacology—drug disposition, action, and therapy in infants and children. N Engl J Med. 2003;349(12):1157–67.
3. Leong R, Zhao H, Reaman G, Liu Q, Wang Y, Stewart CF, Burckart G. Bridging adult experience to pediatrics in oncology drug development. J Clin Pharmacol. 2017;57:S129–35. https://doi.org/10.1002/jcph.910.
4. Momper JD, Mulugeta Y, Green DJ, et al. Adolescent dosing and labeling since the Food and Drug Administration amendments act of 2007. JAMA Pediatr. 2013;167(10):926–32.
5. Ross CJ, Katzov-Eckert H, Dube MP, et al. Genetic variants in TPMT and COMT are associated with hearing loss in children receiving cisplatin chemotherapy. Nat Genet. 2009;41:1345–9.
6. Green D. Ontogeny and the application of pharmacogenomics to pediatric drug development. J Clin Pharmacol. 2019;59(Suppl 1):S82–6. https://doi.org/10.1002/jcph.1488. PMID: 31502695.
7. Gore L, Ivy SP, Balis FM, et al. Modernizing clinical trial eligibility: recommendations of the American Society of Clinical Oncology–Friends of Cancer Research Minimum Age Working Group. J Clin Oncol. 2017;35(33):3781–7.
8. Gaspar N, Marshall LV, Binner D, et al. Joint adolescent adult early phase clinical trials to improve access to new drugs for adolescents with cancer proposals from the multistakeholder platform—ACCELERATE. Ann Oncol. 2018;29(3):766–71.
9. Moreno L, Pearson ADJ, Paoletti X, et al. Early phase clinical trials of anticancer agents in children and adolescents—an ITCC perspective. Nat Rev Clin Oncol. 2017;14(8):497–507.
10. FDA. https://www.fda.gov/regulatory-information/search-fda-guidance-documents/considerations-inclusion-adolescent-patients-adult-oncology-clinical-trials.
11. Tanaudommongkon I, Miyagi SJ, Green DJ, Burnham JM, van den Anker JN, Park K, Wu J, McCune SK, Yao L, Burckart GJ. Combined pediatric and adult trials submitted to the US Food and Drug Administration 2012–2018. Clin Pharmacol Ther. 2020;108(5):1018.

Chapter 9
Surgical Indications for Pediatric and Adolescent Familial Cancer Syndromes: Thyroid Surgery

Areeba Saif and Samira Mercedes Sadowski

Introduction

Familial thyroid cancers are broadly characterized into two groups based on the cells of origin in the thyroid gland. The first group, familial medullary thyroid cancer (FMTC), arises from the calcitonin-producing parafollicular C cells of the thyroid gland (Fig. 9.1), whereas cancers arising from the follicular cells are assigned the nomenclature familial non-medullary thyroid cancer (FNMTC). FNMTC is further divided into syndromic and non-syndromic types based on whether the thyroid malignancy is a predominant feature (non-syndromic) or occurs as part of a constellation of other nonthyroidal malignancies (syndromic) in syndromes such as Cowden syndrome, Werner syndrome, Carney complex, familial adenomatous polyposis, Pendred syndrome, Ataxia-telangiectasia, Bannayan-Riley-Ruvalcaba syndrome, Peutz-Jeghers syndrome, and PTEN hamartoma tumor syndrome [1]. While there are clear American Thyroid Association (ATA) guidelines on the management of hereditary MTC, the optimal clinical approach to FNMTC, given its rarity, is yet to be established [2]. This chapter will review the surgical management of FMTC.

A. Saif
Surgical Oncology Program, National Cancer Institute, National Institutes of Health, Bethesda, MD, USA
e-mail: areeba.saif@uth.tmc.edu

S. M. Sadowski (✉)
Surgical Oncology Program, National Cancer Institute, National Institutes of Health, Bethesda, MD, USA

Surgical Oncology Program, Endocrine Surgery Section, National Cancer Institute, NIH, Bethesda, MD, USA
e-mail: Samira.sadowski@nih.gov

F. Hannah-Shmouni (ed.), *Familial Endocrine Cancer Syndromes*,
https://doi.org/10.1007/978-3-031-37275-9_9

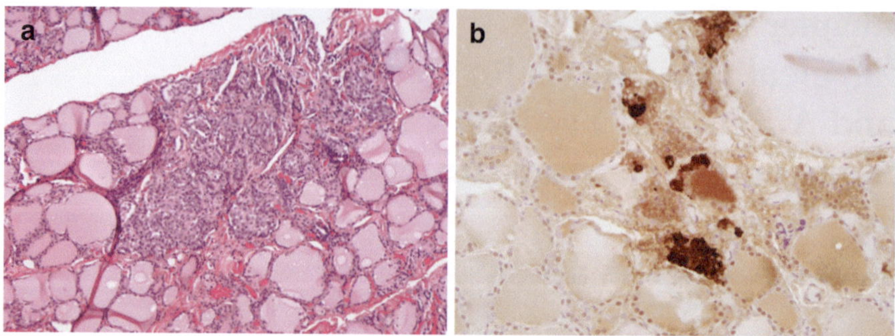

Fig. 9.1 Pediatric Medullary Hyperplasia. (**a**) Focus of medullary hyperplasia in a 8 year old patient with MEN2A (H&E). (**b**) Nests of C cells stained for Calcitonin. (Courtesy of Dr. Maria Merino (National Institutes of Health, Bethesda, Maryland, USA))

Surgical Management of Hereditary Medullary Thyroid Cancer

Medullary thyroid cancer, which accounts for 1–2% of all thyroid cancers in the USA, occurs sporadically or in the hereditary form in 20–25% of cases as part of syndromes associated with an activating RET-proto-oncogene mutation including type 2 multiple endocrine neoplasia (MEN) syndromes, MEN2A and MEN2B, and the familial MTC syndrome [2, 3]. MTC is extremely rare in the pediatric population with an estimated incidence of 0.03 cases per 100,000 population years [4]. In the USA, between 1998 and 2016, based on the results from Surveillance, Epidemiology, and End Results (SEER) database, there were 110 pediatric cases (<20 years) of MTC [4]. In a comparison of pediatric and adult MTC based on the SEER database, Zhao et al. reported that the pediatric population was more likely to have localized disease and a lack of regional lymph node involvement when compared to adults [4]. Pediatric patients were also more likely to undergo a total/subtotal thyroidectomy [4]. In this section, we will review the evidence-based approach to surgical management of hereditary MTC in the pediatric population.

Indications for a Prophylactic Thyroidectomy

In the past, the term "prophylactic thyroidectomy" was defined as the early removal of the thyroid gland in children with an inherited RET proto-oncogene mutation. However, given that there is evidence of C-cell hyperplasia (CCH) or frank MTC in most of these cases, the term has been re-defined by the ATA. The term "prophylactic" thyroidectomy is now defined as the removal of the thyroid gland either before MTC develops or while it is still intrathyroidal and consequently clinically unapparent [2].

The diagnosis of hereditary MTC has evolved from using serum calcitonin levels to the use of direct DNA analysis to detect a RET mutation. However, the substantial variations in aggressiveness and age of onset of hereditary MTC within families with the same RET mutation have led to the realization that direct DNA analysis alone is not sufficient to determine the age of prophylactic thyroidectomy. Several studies have recommended the use of basal and stimulated serum calcitonin levels in RET gene mutation carriers to determine the timing of a total thyroidectomy [5, 6]. Elisei et al. reported that the timing of thyroidectomy in carriers of the RET germline mutation with negative calcitonin could be personalized and planned independently of the type of RET mutation and patient's age when stimulated calcitonin becomes positive [5]. However, there is a lack of established guidelines on the specific values of basal and stimulated calcitonin, due to which the ATA recommends clinicians become familiar with the reference ranges in their institutions and develop institution-based criteria for recommending prophylactic thyroidectomy in children who are carriers of the mutated RET allele.

The ATA guidelines for the management of MTC in MEN2 patients differ based on the perceived clinical behavior of the specific RET proto-oncogene mutation causing MTC. There are at present three categories of RET mutations based on their phenotypical patterns of aggressiveness and age of onset: highest risk (HST), high risk (H), and moderate risk (MOD) [2].

While all patients with MEN2 syndrome ultimately require a thyroidectomy, the timing differs based on the RET proto-oncogene mutation the patient carries (Table 9.1). For carriers of the RET codon 634 and 883 mutations (ATA-H), it is recommended that annual physical examination, cervical ultrasound, and measurement of serum calcitonin levels are initiated at 3 years of age, as these patients develop MTC during the early years of life. While serum calcitonin levels guide the exact timing and extent of surgery, these patients should undergo a prophylactic thyroidectomy at/or before 5 years of age. For patients with MEN2B and the RET codon M918T mutation (ATA-HST), MTC is highly aggressive and a thyroidectomy is recommended in the first year, perhaps even the first few months of life. Conversely, children in the ATA-MOD category develop a less aggressive form of MTC and at a later stage. For example, in a study investigating the role of prophylactic thyroidectomy in patients with the RET codon 609 mutation, Calva et al. reported that the youngest patient with a C609Y RET mutation and MTC was 21 years old while the youngest patient with C-cell hyperplasia was 15 years old [7]. The study concluded that in patients with RET C609Y mutations a prophylactic thyroidectomy can be deferred until 10–15 years of age, with annual calcitonin screening prior to surgery.

In summary, all children who are carriers of the RET codon M918T mutation (ATA-HST) should undergo a prophylactic thyroidectomy in the first year of life. For patients in the ATA-H category, a thyroidectomy should be performed at age 5 years or sooner based on the detection of elevated calcitonin levels. Finally, for patients in the ATA-MOD category, a 6 month or annual physical examination, ultrasound of the neck, and measurement of serum calcitonin levels should be started at age 5 years. While the timing of the thyroidectomy would be determined

Table 9.1 ATA-risk categories of *RET* mutations for development of MTC [2]

ATA risk level for MTC	*RET* mutation	Exon	Recommended age to begin screening for MTC	Recommended age for prophylactic thyroidectomy
Highest	M918T	16	N/A	≤ age 1 year
High	C634F/G/R/ S/W/Y	11	3 years	≤ age 5 years
	A883F	15		
Moderate	G533C	8	5 years	Childhood/adolescence
	C609F/G/R/ S/Y	10		
	C611F/G/S/ Y/W	10		
	C618F/R/S	10		
	C620F/R/S	10		
	C630R/Y	11		
	D631Y	11		
	K666E	11		
	E768D	13		
	L790F	13		
	V804L	14		
	V804M	14		
	S891A	15		
	R912P	16		

ATA American Thyroid Association, *MTC* Medullary Thyroid Cancer. (Data obtained from: *Wells SA, Jr., Asa SL, Dralle H, Elisei R, Evans DB, Gagel RF,* et al. *Revised American Thyroid Association guidelines for the management of medullary thyroid carcinoma. Thyroid: official journal of the American Thyroid Association. 2015;25 (6):567–610)*

by the detection of elevated serum calcitonin levels, parents may opt for a thyroidectomy for their children at around 5 years of age if there are concerns about adherence to the long-term follow-up plan [2].

The complications of a prophylactic thyroidectomy in children must be weighed against the risks associated with delaying a potentially curative intervention for MTC in patients with the RET proto-oncogene mutation.

Surgical Approach in Carriers of Germline RET Mutations

The preferred surgical intervention for patients with a RET proto-oncogene mutation is a total thyroidectomy with or without central compartment neck dissection (level VI dissection) [2]. All patients with MEN2 syndromes should be screened for a pheochromocytoma prior to surgery.

A prophylactic central neck dissection should include surgical excision of lymph nodes between the hyoid bone superiorly, the carotid arteries laterally, and the thoracic inlet inferiorly. This consists of removal of the prelaryngeal, pretracheal, and paratracheal lymph node basins, which requires meticulous dissection of the parathyroid glands, the external branch of the superior laryngeal nerves, and the recurrent laryngeal nerves [8, 9]. Central compartment neck dissection in children may be associated with a higher risk of injury to the recurrent laryngeal nerves and parathyroid glands as these structures are more difficult to delineate in young children [9].

In patients with a germline RET mutation undergoing a prophylactic thyroidectomy, there is a lack of consensus on the role of a prophylactic central neck dissection. Per ATA guidelines, the inclusion of central neck dissection should depend upon both the ATA-risk category and the basal serum calcitonin levels. In patients with ATA-MOD and ATA-H mutations, a central neck dissection may not be performed if basal calcitonin levels are <40 pg/mL and there is no evidence of lymph node involvement on direct observation or imaging [2, 10]. However, in a consensus statement on the timing and extent of thyroid surgery for carriers of the RET mutation, the European Society of Endocrine Surgeons (ESES) cautions against the use of ultrasonography (US) in guiding decision-making as US is insufficiently sensitive in detecting micrometastases in lymph nodes [11, 12]. Per ATA guidelines, in patients with the ATA-HST category mutation, in the absence of any suspicious lymph nodes, a central neck dissection should only be performed if parathyroid glands can be identified and left in situ or auto transplanted [2]. However, in a study including 387 carriers of the germline RET mutation, 201 of whom were node-negative and 186 were node-positive, Machens et al. reported that tumor progression to lymph node metastasis in MTC was independent of the underlying RET mutation [13]. Patients with low-moderate risk mutations had comparable time to lymph node involvement as those with high and highest risk mutations, leading the authors to conclude that following disease onset, the biologic behavior of MTC is the same irrespective of the underlying RET mutation [13]. This raises questions about the necessity of a central lymph node dissection in all patients undergoing a prophylactic thyroidectomy irrespective of their mutation status and serum calcitonin levels.

Auto-transplantation of the parathyroid gland should be performed if a parathyroid gland is devascularized. While in patients with FMTC or MEN2B syndrome, the parathyroid gland can be autotransplanted into the sternocleidomastoid muscle, in patients with MEN2A syndrome the parathyroid tissue should be autotransplanted into the non-dominant forearm due to the risk of development of primary hyperparathyroidism in the remnant tissue [14].

In addition to a traditional open prophylactic thyroidectomy, the use of a minimally invasive video-assisted approach for prophylactic thyroidectomy (MIVAT) in children with MEN2 syndromes has been reported in the literature. Glynn et al. published their experience of MIVAT in six children with the RET codon mutations 634, 620, 611, and 918 [15]. None of the children in the study underwent a central lymph node dissection. They reported similar outcomes compared to the traditional approach with possible benefits in terms of pain and cosmesis. There has also been a report of video-assisted central compartment lymphadenectomy in 15 carriers of RET proto-oncogene mutation [16]. The mean number of lymph nodes removed was 5.1 with the authors reporting a comparable complication rate with the open approach, better cosmesis, and reduced post-operative pain. However, further multi-institutional experiences with long-term follow-up are needed to establish the safety and feasibility of these approaches.

Post-Operative Management and Surveillance

In the immediate post-operative period, children should be closely monitored for the development of hypocalcemia secondary to hypoparathyroidism or signs of injury to the recurrent laryngeal and the superior laryngeal nerves. Patients may be admitted overnight for observation, pain control, and monitoring for neck hematoma formation. Long-term thyroid hormone replacement therapy is required to maintain euthyroid status; however, suppressive doses are not required as the parafollicular C cells are not thyroid-stimulating hormone (TSH) responsive [9]. Fluctuations in TSH levels are common in children secondary to growth and physiologic changes and potentially due to medication non-compliance, hence TSH should be routinely monitored to maintain a euthyroid state. However, there are no clear ATA guidelines on the frequency of TSH monitoring [17].

Seib et al. have recommended routine thyroglobulin measurements following prophylactic thyroidectomy in patients with germline RET mutations [17]. They postulate that even in experienced hands, there may be residual thyroid tissue left behind, especially in the posterolateral thyroid bed where there is an embryologic predominance of parafollicular C levels. The measurement of post-operative thyroglobulin levels may aid in the detection of residual thyroid tissue. However, the ATA guidelines at present do not include recommendations for routine post-operative measurement of thyroglobulin.

For patients with the MEN2B ATA-HST category and MEN2A-H category mutations, long-term follow-up should include a thorough physical exam, ultrasound of the neck, and measurement of serum calcitonin and CEA levels every 6 months for 1 year and then annually [2]. The patients should also begin undergoing screening for pheochromocytoma at 11 years of age. In patients with MEN2A ATA-MOD mutations, long-term follow-up should include evaluation every 6 months for 1 year and then annually if serum calcitonin levels remain undetectable or within the normal range [2]. These children should undergo screening for pheochromocytoma beginning at 16 years of age. If during the follow-up period, the serum calcitonin levels are found to be elevated but <150 pg/mL, they should be measured along with serum CEA levels every 3–6 months to determine doubling times, which is a prognostic indicator of the progression of MTC. However, if serum calcitonin levels are >150 pg/mL, a full metastatic workup with imaging including neck US, chest CT, contrast-enhanced CT/MRI of the liver, bone scintigraphy, and PET/CT/MRI of the pelvis and axial skeleton should be performed and the patient subsequently managed based on the site of metastasis [2, 6, 18].

Complications

The most significant complications following a thyroidectomy in children include hypocalcemia secondary to hypoparathyroidism, hoarseness, vocal cord paresis or paralysis, and wound seroma or hematoma formation [19, 20]. A single-center study including 464 patients undergoing prophylactic thyroidectomy, reported the incidence of post-operative transient hypoparathyroidism to be 37% while the incidence of persistent hypoparathyroidism was 0.6%. Young children have a much higher rate of complications following thyroid surgery compared to adults, especially the occurrence of hypoparathyroidism. This is because the parathyroid glands in younger children are small and translucent and much more challenging to identify [2]. For these reasons, several studies have established that prophylactic thyroidectomy for children is associated with better outcomes when performed at high-volume tertiary care centers [2, 10, 20, 21].

Long-Term Outcomes

Machens et al. published a study outlining the long-term outcomes of prophylactic thyroidectomy in a large cohort of 167 children with germline RET mutations [22]. They found that there was no increased surgical morbidity in younger children aged 3 years or less when compared to older children indicating a prophylactic thyroidectomy is a viable option in affected infants and small children once calcitonin serum levels have increased. In 114 of the 115 children with raised preoperative serum calcitonin levels, post-operative normalization of calcitonin serum levels was achieved. No residual structural disease or recurrence was observed in any patients. Several studies have reported similar 100% disease-free rates in children undergoing age-appropriate prophylactic thyroidectomy [23, 24].

Insufficient post-operative thyroxine replacement therapy leading to impaired normal growth, development, and intellectual function was found to be a significant problem in a study on the long-term outcomes of 46 gene carriers of the RET germline mutation following a prophylactic thyroidectomy [25]. Consequently, the authors recommend TSH monitoring every 3 months secondary to concerns regarding both optimal dosage and non-compliance.

References

1. Ammar SA, Alobuia WM, Kebebew E. An update on familial nonmedullary thyroid cancer. Endocrine. 2020;68(3):502–7.
2. Wells SA Jr, Asa SL, Dralle H, Elisei R, Evans DB, Gagel RF, et al. Revised american thyroid association guidelines for the management of medullary thyroid carcinoma. Thyroid. 2015;25(6):567–610.

3. Nosé V. Familial thyroid cancer: a review. Mod Pathol. 2011;24(2):S19–33.
4. Zhao Z, Yin XD, Zhang XH, Li ZW, Wang DW. Comparison of pediatric and adult medullary thyroid carcinoma based on SEER program. Sci Rep. 2020;10(1):13310.
5. Elisei R, Romei C, Renzini G, Bottici V, Cosci B, Molinaro E, et al. The timing of total thyroidectomy in RET gene mutation carriers could be personalized and safely planned on the basis of serum calcitonin: 18 years experience at one single center. J Clin Endocrinol Metab. 2012;97(2):426–35.
6. Li SY, Ding YQ, Si YL, Ye MJ, Xu CM, Qi XP. 5P strategies for management of multiple endocrine neoplasia type 2: a paradigm of precision medicine. Front Endocrinol. 2020;11:543246.
7. Calva D, O'Dorisio TM, Sue O'Dorisio M, Lal G, Sugg S, Weigel RJ, et al. When is prophylactic thyroidectomy indicated for patients with the RET codon 609 mutation? Ann Surg Oncol. 2009;16(8):2237–44.
8. Carty SE, Cooper DS, Doherty GM, Duh QY, Kloos RT, Mandel SJ, et al. Consensus statement on the terminology and classification of central neck dissection for thyroid cancer. Thyroid. 2009;19(11):1153–8.
9. Wang TS, Opoku-Boateng A, Roman SA, Sosa JA. Prophylactic thyroidectomy: who needs it, when, and why. J Surg Oncol. 2015;111(1):61–5.
10. Prete FP, Abdel-Aziz T, Morkane C, Brain C, Kurzawinski TR. Prophylactic thyroidectomy in children with multiple endocrine neoplasia type 2. Br J Surg. 2018;105(10):1319–27.
11. Niederle B, Sebag F, Brauckhoff M. Timing and extent of thyroid surgery for gene carriers of hereditary C cell disease—a consensus statement of the European Society of Endocrine Surgeons (ESES). Langenbeck's Arch Surg. 2014;399(2):185–97.
12. Morris LF, Waguespack SG, Edeiken-Monroe BS, Lee JE, Rich TA, Ying AK, et al. Ultrasonography should not guide the timing of thyroidectomy in pediatric patients diagnosed with multiple endocrine neoplasia syndrome 2A through genetic screening. Ann Surg Oncol. 2013;20(1):53–9.
13. Machens A, Lorenz K, Weber F, Dralle H. Lymph node metastasis in hereditary medullary thyroid cancer is independent of the underlying RET germline mutation. Eur J Surg Oncol. 2020;47:920.
14. Roy M, Chen H, Sippel RS. Current understanding and management of medullary thyroid cancer. Oncologist. 2013;18(10):1093–100.
15. Glynn RW, Cashman EC, Doody J, Phelan E, Russell JD, Timon C. Prophylactic total thyroidectomy using the minimally invasive video-assisted approach in children with multiple endocrine neoplasia type 2. Head Neck. 2014;36(6):768–71.
16. Miccoli P, Elisei R, Donatini G, Materazzi G, Berti P. Video-assisted central compartment lymphadenectomy in a patient with a positive RET oncogene: initial experience. Surg Endosc. 2007;21(1):120–3.
17. Seib CD, Harari A, Conte FA, Duh QY, Clark OH, Gosnell JE. Utility of serum thyroglobulin measurements after prophylactic thyroidectomy in patients with hereditary medullary thyroid cancer. Surgery. 2014;156(2):394–8.
18. Giovanella L, Treglia G, Iakovou I, Mihailovic J, Verburg FA, Luster M. EANM practice guideline for PET/CT imaging in medullary thyroid carcinoma. Eur J Nucl Med Mol Imaging. 2020;47(1):61–77.
19. Baumgarten HD, Bauer AJ, Isaza A, Mostoufi-Moab S, Kazahaya K, Adzick NS. Surgical management of pediatric thyroid disease: complication rates after thyroidectomy at the Children's Hospital of Philadelphia high-volume pediatric thyroid center. J Pediatr Surg. 2019;54(10):1969–75.
20. Kluijfhout WP, van Beek DJ, Verrijn Stuart AA, Lodewijk L, Valk GD, van der Zee DC, et al. Postoperative complications after prophylactic thyroidectomy for very young patients with multiple endocrine neoplasia type 2: retrospective cohort analysis. Medicine. 2015;94(29):e1108.
21. Breuer C, Tuggle C, Solomon D, Sosa JA. Pediatric thyroid disease: when is surgery necessary, and who should be operating on our children? J Clin Res Pediatr Endocrinol. 2013;5 Suppl 1(Suppl 1):79–85.

22. Machens A, Elwerr M, Lorenz K, Weber F, Dralle H. Long-term outcome of prophylactic thyroidectomy in children carrying RET germline mutations. Br J Surg. 2018;105(2):e150–e7.
23. Shepet K, Alhefdhi A, Lai N, Mazeh H, Sippel R, Chen H. Hereditary medullary thyroid cancer: age-appropriate thyroidectomy improves disease-free survival. Ann Surg Oncol. 2013;20(5):1451–5.
24. Machens A, Dralle H. Long-term outcome after DNA-based prophylactic neck surgery in children at risk of hereditary medullary thyroid cancer. Best Pract Res Clin Endocrinol Metab. 2019;33(4):101274.
25. Frank-Raue K, Buhr H, Dralle H, Klar E, Senninger N, Weber T, et al. Long-term outcome in 46 gene carriers of hereditary medullary thyroid carcinoma after prophylactic thyroidectomy: impact of individual RET genotype. Eur J Endocrinol. 2006;155(2):229–36.

Chapter 10
Long-Term Effects of Cancer Treatment

Kyle P. McNerney and Sina Jasim

Introduction

After the treatment of cancer, individuals still face the prospect of future complications and adverse health conditions. Survival after childhood cancer has continued to increase, and 5-year relative survival rates are 83–86% for children, adolescents, and young adults [1]. With longer expected survival, providers must be vigilant and monitor not only for recurrence or for complications from the underlying cancer or disease, but also monitor for side effects from treatments that can occur even years after therapy. Treatment complications typically fall into three broad categories: radiation-related side effects, surgery-related side effects, and medication-related side effects. Long-term outcome data from cohorts such as the Childhood Cancer Survivor Study (CCSS) demonstrate that survivors of childhood cancer have increased risk of adverse outcomes including second cancers, endocrine hormone deficiencies, pulmonary complications, obesity, and worse scholastic outcomes [2]. Cancer survivors require long-term multidisciplinary follow-up to monitor for the metabolic, neurocognitive, and psychosocial effects that can present or worsen even years after cancer treatment [1].

K. P. McNerney
Department of Pediatrics, School of Medicine, Washington University in St. Louis, St. Louis, MO, USA
e-mail: k.mcnerney@wustl.edu

S. Jasim (✉)
Division of Endocrinology, Metabolism and Lipid Research, School of Medicine, Washington University in St. Louis, St. Louis, MO, USA
e-mail: s.jasim@wustl.edu

© The Author(s), under exclusive license to Springer Nature Switzerland AG 2023
F. Hannah-Shmouni (ed.), *Familial Endocrine Cancer Syndromes*,
https://doi.org/10.1007/978-3-031-37275-9_10

Radiation Therapy

Radiation therapy causes complications through damage to healthy cells and tissues in proximity to the treatment area. The type, dose, and area of radiation treatment are critical for predicting the extent of complications. Younger children are more sensitive to the effects of radiation and have increased long-term complications [3]. Children exposed to therapeutic radiation may have different long-term effects due to continued cellular development and anatomic differences that can place more structures in close proximity to the radiation field. Short-term complications of radiation therapy include skin changes, nausea/vomiting, fatigue, hair loss, and hearing problems [4]. Long-term complications depend on the dose of radiation and can have unique effects depending on the site, the method of delivery, and the tissues involved.

Cranial Irradiation

Cranial irradiation has a broad spectrum of long-term complications that is more profound in children. Cranial or whole brain radiation therapy in an infant or very young child can have severe development sequelae, which impairs future cognitive function and development. Cranial radiation therapy overall is associated with increased cerebrovascular events and vascular damage, brain tissue necrosis, craniosynostosis due to premature growth arrest of the calvarium, eye changes including optic neuropathy or cataracts, and worsening cranial neuropathies [3]. The hypothalamus and pituitary gland are particularly sensitive to radiation, and patients can develop pituitary hormone deficiencies even years after cranial radiation. Long-term monitoring for pituitary hormone deficiencies is critical for survivors of cancer with cranial irradiation [5].

The development of pituitary hormone deficiencies after cranial radiation can range from a single hormone deficiency to complete hypopituitarism. Risk factors for pituitary hormone deficiencies include younger age at treatment, radiation fields involving the hypothalamus/pituitary, and the amount of time elapsed since treatment [6]. Additionally, the dose of radiation (Gy) is an important prognostic factor for the future risk of pituitary hormone deficiencies. Pituitary hormone deficiencies (e.g., growth hormone deficiency) and central precocious puberty can be seen with cranial irradiation of 18 Gy and greater. Multiple pituitary hormone deficiencies can be seen with a dose of 30 Gy or higher [7].

Growth hormone deficiency: Pituitary somatotrophs are highly vulnerable to radiation. Growth hormone deficiency is the most common pituitary hormone deficiency attributed to radiation therapy [6]. Growth hormone deficiency can occur with cranial irradiation with a dose of 18 Gy or higher, single fraction total body irradiation of 10 Gy or higher, or fractionated total body radiotherapy with 12 Gy or higher. Growth hormone deficiency is often identified in children due to impaired linear growth. Growth impairment due to growth hormone deficiency can initially be subtle, and longitudinal growth measurements at least every 6–12 months are essential to identify growth changes. Concurrent sex steroids hormone exposure due to puberty (precocious or otherwise) can mask growth deceleration due to growth hormone deficiency. Measurement of random or prolonged sampling of growth hormone levels over a 12–24 h period is not practical for the diagnosis of growth hormone deficiency due to its pulsatile secretion, diurnal rhythm favoring growth hormone secretion overnight, and substantial overlap in serial growth hormone measurements between healthy controls and patients with growth hormone deficiency [8]. IGF-1 levels, when adjusted for age and pubertal status, can help screen for growth hormone deficiency. A significantly low IGF-1 level (−2 SD) is highly suggestive of growth hormone deficiency, however, normal IGF-1 levels do not preclude possible growth hormone deficiency. Provocative growth hormone stimulation testing is recommended to diagnose growth hormone deficiency unless multiple other pituitary hormone deficiencies are already present. Growth hormone stimulation testing is performed with agents including glucagon, arginine, clonidine, or levodopa [8]. Insulin tolerance tests are reliable tests for the growth hormone axis, however, they are not used in many centers due to the risks associated with hypoglycemia [9]. Children with growth hormone deficiency can be retested for growth hormone deficiency during the transition to adulthood and therapy can be continued at a decreased, adult-appropriate dose if indicated.

Growth hormone therapy is given in injectable format usually daily. Longer-acting growth hormone therapies are in development, which will allow extended dosing intervals (e.g., once weekly). Treatment of growth hormone deficiency with growth hormone significantly improves linear growth [10]. Children and adults with growth hormone deficiency in general show increased muscle mass, decreased total body fat, and increased bone mineral density when treated with growth hormone therapy. Adverse effects of growth hormone therapy include insulin resistance, edema, arthralgia, slipped capital femoral epiphysis, pseudotumor cerebri, and carpal tunnel syndrome [11]. For survivors of cancer, there is a theoretical concern for recurrence of primary tumors or secondary tumor development with growth hormone therapy since growth hormone and IGF-1 drive cellular proliferation [12]. Due to this concern, growth hormone therapy has traditionally been deferred until 1 year of disease-free survival, although some studies have not found harm with earlier introduction of growth hormone, or treatment of growth hormone therapy in patients with stable but present disease [7].

Precocious puberty: Alterations in the hypothalamic-pituitary gonadal axis are common in survivors of childhood cancer. Precocious puberty (pubertal development before 8 years of age in females or 9 years of age in males) is the second most common manifestation of hypothalamic/pituitary dysfunction after growth hormone deficiency, seen in 15% of children with a history of central nervous system tumor or cranial radiation therapy [13]. Central precocious puberty can be seen after cranial radiation therapy with 18 Gy or higher. It is most commonly seen in patients with brain tumors near the hypothalamus/optic pathways, with a history of radiation to the hypothalamus/pituitary, or with a history of hydrocephalus [14]. Precocious puberty can lead to early height acceleration but later produces early cessation of growth leading to significant short stature in adulthood. Clinical monitoring of growth and pubertal staging support identification of precocious puberty; however, coexisting growth hormone deficiency or primary gonadal dysfunction due to cytotoxic chemotherapy can make interpretation of growth and pubertal development challenging. Due to this, biochemical tests of gonadotropins and sex steroids (Luteinizing hormone (LH), follicle-stimulating hormone (FSH), estradiol, and testosterone) or gonadotropin-releasing hormone (GnRH) suppression tests to evaluate for gonadotropin production are frequently used for the diagnosis of precocious puberty. Treatment with GnRH agonists can suppress gonadotropin production and delay pubertal progression, leading to improved adult height [13].

Hypogonadism: In addition to the increased risk of central precocious puberty, cancer survivors with a history of cranial irradiation are at increased risk for hypogonadotropic hypogonadism [15]. Hypogonadotropic hypogonadism may present as delayed or stalled puberty in children, or with symptoms of hypogonadism in adults. Clinical assessment of growth and puberty, and biochemical evaluation of gonadotropins and sex steroids are essential for diagnosis. Prolactin levels should be assessed concurrently since hyperprolactinemia can present as hypogonadotropic hypogonadism, and can occur with cranial irradiation, CNS tumors, or certain medications [7].

The testes and ovaries are highly sensitive to radiation. Gonadal dysfunction, subfertility, infertility, or primary hypogonadism are all known consequences of irradiation treatment. Testicular radiation of 0.3–0.5 Gy can induce temporary oligospermia, and oocytes are also highly sensitive to DNA damage from irradiation [16]. Depletion of oocyte count by ovarian irradiation can lead to decreased ovarian reserve and early menopause. The adverse effects of radiation on testicular and ovarian functions are most likely to occur with localized abdominal or pelvic radiation, but can also occur from total body radiation or internal scatter of radiation indirectly leading to exposure [16].

Hypogonadism and decreased sex steroid production has adverse effects on pubertal or post-pubertal survivors of cancer including alterations in mood, decreased quality of life, impaired fertility, and decreased bone mineral density [17]. Diagnosis of hypogonadism in males requires finding signs and symptoms of low testosterone (e.g., erectile dysfunction/low libido, decreased energy, reduced bone mass) along with biochemical testing including LH, FSH, and testosterone measured in the morning in the absence of illness. Diagnosis of hypogonadism in females is suspected based on oligomenorrhea or amenorrhea and is confirmed with measurement of LH, FSH, and estradiol in the absence of other causes of menstrual irregularities such as hyperprolactinemia, thyroid disease, or hyperandrogenism. Hypogonadism is treated with replacement of sex steroid hormones (testosterone or estrogen) to achieve a level appropriate for age, and in adolescents is titrated to their pubertal development [7]. Hormone replacement therapy in adult females can be discontinued around the age for menopause [18].

Children, adolescents, and adults undergoing radiation or cytotoxic chemotherapy with risk of gonadal dysfunction should receive counseling on the risk of future subfertility and infertility. The risks/benefits of treatment and potential options for future fertility should be addressed through the use of a shared decision-making framework between patients and providers, ideally with the involvement of subspecialists familiar with oncology related fertility issues [19]. Ovarian tissue cryopreservation is established as a method for fertility preservation in pre-menopausal females and is routinely offered to pubertal and post-pubertal females [15]. Data for ovarian tissue cryopreservation in pre-pubertal females is limited, but is considered an experimental option [20]. Use of GnRH agonists in females to suppress follicle activation during chemotherapy treatment and preserve ovarian function is used experimentally but currently lacks robust outcome data of efficacy and safety [21]. In pubertal and post-pubertal males, sperm banking with cryopreservation is effective and well established and should be considered prior to gonadotoxic therapy [15]. Pre-pubertal males have limited established options for fertility preservation, but ongoing research into cryopreservation of immature testicular tissue may offer an experimental approach for fertility preservation [22].

TSH deficiency: A decrease in hypothalamic thyrotropin-releasing hormone (TRH) or pituitary thyroid-stimulating hormone (TSH) can cause impaired production of thyroid hormone and central hypothyroidism. Patients with hypothyroidism may have symptoms including fatigue, cold intolerance, dry skin, constipation, or irregular menstrual cycles. Notably, the TSH level can appear inappropriately normal in patients with central hypothyroidism with a corresponding low free T4 level [23]. Therefore, the use of TSH only in screening for hypothyroidism may miss patients with central hypothyroidism. The free T4 level is not only useful in diagnosing but also monitoring patients with central hypothyroidism treated with thyroid hormone replacement, with treatment aimed to maintain high normal T4 levels.

ACTH deficiency: Cortisol production occurs through the hypothalamic-pituitary-adrenal axis, and relies on hypothalamic corticotropin-releasing hormone (CRH) and pituitary adrenocorticotropic hormone (ACTH) production. Adrenal insufficiency has an overall prevalence of ~4% in childhood cancer survivors that received cranial irradiation, though prevalence varies based on the type and location of tumor [24]. The development of adrenal insufficiency is more common in patients receiving 30 Gy or more of hypothalamic/pituitary irradiation [7]. Mild adrenal insufficiency may not be noted until a patient encounters severe stress such as illness, infection, or surgery. In patients at risk for pituitary hormone deficiency, a morning cortisol level can be used to assess for adrenal insufficiency. In a patient with equivocal cortisol levels, diagnosis of adrenal insufficiency can be made with ACTH stimulation tests. Patients with adrenal insufficiency may require daily glucocorticoids replacement (e.g., hydrocortisone or prednisone) along with instructions to give additional stress dose glucocorticoids during "stress" including fever, illness, or surgery. Long-term follow-up of children with hypothalamic-pituitary disorders shows a three–four fold increase in mortality compared to unaffected children, with 12–25% attributable to hypoglycemia and adrenal insufficiency [25]. The risk of increased mortality in patients with hypopituitarism continues into adulthood, though the attributable cause is often multifactorial. A meta-analysis of multiple studies on patients with hypopituitarism showed greater risk of death seen in patients diagnosed at a younger age, females, diagnosis of craniopharyngioma, treatment with radiation or surgery, or presence of diabetes insipidus or hypogonadism [26].

Diabetes Insipidus: Central diabetes insipidus occurs due to diminished or absent anti-diuretic hormone (ADH) production by neurons of the posterior pituitary. This leads to impaired urinary concentrating ability, which leads to characteristic polyuria, minimally concentrated urine, and rapid increases in serum osmolality and sodium concentration if a patient is not able to hydrate adequately [27]. Thirst is often significantly increased due to the hyperosmolality, but thirst may be impaired or absent in association with a patient's CNS disease. Diabetes insipidus is more common with CNS tumors with pituitary and hypothalamic extension such as craniopharyngiomas. Diabetes insipidus can be confirmed by fasting blood and urine samples or during a water deprivation test. Desmopressin (DDAVP) administered at the conclusion of the water deprivation restores urinary concentrating ability in patients with central diabetes insipidus, and is also the mainstay of treatment of central diabetes insipidus [28]. The circulating peptide Copeptin has recently been shown to be a reliable surrogate measure for arginine vasopressin, so many centers are now using measurement of osmotically-stimulated Copeptin levels to diagnose central diabetes insipidus [29].

Spinal Radiation

Radiation delivered elsewhere in the body can affect development of bone and muscle, leading to limb length discrepancy, atrophy, and predisposition to fracture. Radiation to the spine can cause scoliosis, impaired bone mineralization, or decreased height due to a relatively shorter trunk [30]. Increased risk of short stature is seen with children treated with spinal radiation at young ages, with larger areas of spine treated, and with doses >20 Gy [7]. Short stature arising from spine irradiation typically causes a disproportionate short stature from impaired spinal height but preserved extremity growth. This can be measured clinically by comparing arm span length to height (arm span may greatly exceed height in children with spinal growth impairment), measuring the sitting height, and monitoring for reduction in the upper-to-lower segment ratio [7].

Organ-Specific Adverse Effect of Radiation Therapy

Radiation effect on the lungs: Thoracic radiation therapy in adults and children can induce short- and long-term detrimental lung changes. Radiation pneumonitis is a well described short-term complication causing cough, shortness of breath, and sometimes fever, that can typically be managed conservatively [31]. However, children with a history of thoracic radiation have long-term pulmonary symptoms, with greater than 15% having shortness of breath with exercise at 25 years from treatment, and greater than 10% having chronic cough at 25 years from treatment [32]. Radiation fibrosis is a rarer long-term side effect that can occur years after radiation but can significantly compromise lung function. Treatment for acute inflammation such as in radiation pneumonitis may require glucocorticoids or immunosuppressive therapy, but radiation fibrosis is managed with pulmonary rehabilitation and oxygen supplementation if needed [32].

Radiation effect on the thyroid: Radiation to the head and neck can cause disruption of the hypothalamic-pituitary signaling (central hypothyroidism), or can cause direct damage to the thyroid gland itself (primary hypothyroidism). Increasing doses of radiation delivered to the hypothalamus/pituitary and to the thyroid gland itself cause an increased rate of hypothyroidism in survivors of childhood cancer [33]. The prevalence of hypothyroidism is increased in adult survivors of childhood cancer, with a 7% overall prevalence of hypothyroidism after 16 years of follow-up found in Britain [34]. Survivors of Hodgkin's lymphoma have rates of hypothyroidism as high as 32% by 30 years after diagnosis, with the majority attributable to primary hypothyroidism [33]. Continued monitoring for hypothyroidism in survivors of childhood cancer with a history of radiation is important, as the risk of developing hypothyroidism remains elevated even 25 years after exposure [33]. Furthermore, head and neck radiation exposure is identified as a well-known environmental risk factor for the development of papillary thyroid cancer.

Secondary Cancers: Ionizing radiation therapy is associated with increased diagnosis of a subsequent malignant cancer that can occur years after therapy is complete [35]. Childhood cancer survivors have a ten times greater risk of a new tumor than the general population [36]. Notably, the risk of a secondary tumor does not diminish with time, but actually continues to increase over the lifespan. Certain organs are at higher risk, including thyroid, skin, breast, and the brain. Increasing doses of radiation and younger age at radiation are frequently cited risk factors for development of a secondary tumor [37].

Future of Radiation: Newer techniques show promise for reducing the complications of radiation therapy. Conventional external beam radiotherapy delivers photon radiation to tissues but affects many surrounding structures. Photons deposit a burst of energy shortly after entering the body, and they continue to release energy as they travel to the target area and until exiting the body [38]. This can lead to substantial field radiation effect on surrounding structures upon entry and until exit of the photons. Newer techniques such as intensity modulated radiation therapy (IMRT) uses conformal radiotherapy to better target radiation to the tumor and minimize the effect on surrounding tissue. Additionally, proton therapy is a newer form of external beam radiotherapy that targets a specific depth with protons instead of photons [39]. This allows for intensified local therapy and decreased dose effect on surrounding tissues. Proton therapy is becoming more widely available, and clinical evidence suggests that it offers improved tumor control with reduced adverse effects compared to conventional external beam therapy [38].

Long-Term Effects of Surgery and Chemotherapy

Surgery: Resection or surgical treatment of a childhood cancer carries short- and long-term risks, mostly associated with the tissue and structures directly in the area of surgery. Organ-specific surgery such as thyroidectomy has known complications such as hypothyroidism and the possible risks of parathyroid dysfunction or vocal cord palsy. Treatment of papillary thyroid microcarcinoma with surgical lobectomy carries a risk of post-operative hypothyroidism as high as 64%, though a pre-operative TSH level can help predict which of these patients will later have spontaneous remission [40]. In children with tumor syndromes such as von-Hippel-Lindau, total adrenalectomy for pheochromocytoma can lead to adrenal insufficiency and lifelong glucocorticoids dependence [41]. This has led to the adoption of surgical techniques such as partial adrenalectomy or cortical-sparing adrenalectomy that may preserve endogenous adrenal function while carrying a small risk of recurrence of tumor [42]. The surgical resection of any CNS tumor carries risks of post-operative neurological deficits. CNS tumors located near the pituitary/hypothalamus such as craniopharyngiomas carry substantial risk of pre- and post-operative endocrine deficits including panhypopituitarism or hypothalamic obesity. Cancer treatment is frequently multi-modal, and the combination of surgical treatment with radiation or chemotherapy increases the risk of long-term complications [43].

Chemotherapy: Short-term endocrine effects of chemotherapy can cause increased morbidity and mortality. Multiple chemotherapeutic agents induce hyperglycemia, which is associated with a worse prognosis for tumors including colorectal cancer, glioblastoma, breast cancer, and prostate cancer [44]. Therapy with mammalian target of rapamycin (mTOR) inhibitors acutely impair insulin secretion while also worsening insulin resistance, and have an associated risk of new-onset diabetes of 13% to 50% [45]. Similarly, glucocorticoid therapy causes peripheral insulin resistance in skeletal muscle, and exposure to glucocorticoids has an associated increased odds ratio for the development of new-onset diabetes of 1.36–2.31 [44]. Immunotherapy with checkpoint inhibitors offer promising therapy for multiple cancers including melanoma, non-small cell lung cancer, breast cancer, and head and neck tumors, but has been found to increase the rate of immune-related side effects affecting the endocrine system [46]. Therapy with the anti-CTLA4 agent ipilimumab has been associated with hypophysitis in about 13% of patients, which can cause symptomatic pituitary changes and severely disrupt pituitary hormone production [47]. Organ-specific changes from immune checkpoint inhibitors can induce primary thyroid disease, adrenal insufficiency, hypoparathyroidism, and hyperglycemia or the development of type 1 diabetes [48].

Long-term late effects of chemotherapy are seen years after treatment and can cause life-limiting illnesses. Platinum based chemotherapy can cause sensorineural hearing loss, particularly in children treated at a younger age [49]. Cardiomyopathy and heart failure can occur with anthracycline chemotherapy, and some studies report it is more common in females treated at a younger age (<5 years of age) [50]. Secondary tumors can result from the cellular damage of chemotherapy, and alkylating agents have been found to increase the future risk of therapy-related leukemia [51]. Fertility and pubertal development can also be adversely affected by chemotherapy with gonadotoxic alkylating agents which can cause infertility or primary hypogonadism [52]. The assessment of primary hypogonadism in cancer survivors may be challenging, as the increased LH and FSH levels used to diagnose primary hypogonadism may not be present if the patient has coexisting CNS disease and hypogonadotropic hypogonadism [36].

Long-Term Outcomes Childhood Cancer

Chronic Diseases, Quality of Life, and Neurocognitive Outcomes

Two-thirds of survivors of childhood cancer have a chronic illness, which is increased compared to the general population due to the long-lasting adverse effects of cancer and cancer therapy with radiation, surgery, and/or chemotherapy [36]. Obesity affects 50% of survivors of childhood cancer, and illnesses such as osteoporosis and diabetes are increased as well [53]. Heart disease and cardiovascular complications are a leading cause of therapy-related morbidity and mortality in survivors of childhood cancer, with risk increased particularly for survivors who received anthracycline therapy [50]. Early identification and structured treatment of obesity, osteoporosis, diabetes, or heart disease can help modulate the substantial risk that these diseases confer on survivors of childhood cancer [54]. Unfortunately, the diagnosis of a chronic illness in survivors of childhood cancer is associated with impaired quality of life including impaired physical activity, increased pain, increased fatigue, and decreased perception of general health [36].

Neurocognitive sequelae can also be seen in survivors of childhood cancer and is more common after surgery/radiation to the brain or treatment with systemic or intrathecal methotrexate. The effect may initially be subtle, but children can develop academic difficulties and information-processing deficits within 1–2 years of cranial radiation [55]. Neurocognitive deficits can continue to progress into adulthood, affecting job performance, relationships, and the ability to perform activities of daily living. Neurocognitive testing of survivors of childhood cancers can identify individuals with subtle or profound impairments so that specific therapy and interventions can be provided.

Monitoring of long-term outcomes for survivors of childhood outcomes is challenging given the multidisciplinary, long-term, disease-specific care that is required. To address this, groups such as the Children's Oncology Group (COG) has developed tools and monitoring programs for medical professionals and resources for patients [56, 57]. These can help standardize care, however, many survivors still may face additional barriers to treatment such as lack of access to specialists or lack of insurance coverage, which has been shown to significantly decrease adolescent and young adult access to medical care [58]. Digital health delivery programs and mobile health interventions have shown that there are effective, novel ways to engage survivors of cancer and help them follow a survivorship care plan specific to them [59].

Conclusion

Long-term survival from childhood cancer continues to increase, but it remains critical to assess long-term health complications, which can develop or progress over time. Knowledge of specific treatment effects due to radiation, surgery, or chemotherapy helps guide monitoring. After treatment for childhood cancer, patients are faced with increased rates of both rarer disorders such as pituitary hormone deficiencies and more common but life-limiting illnesses such as obesity, osteoporosis, and heart disease. Cancer survivors require long-term multidisciplinary follow-up to recognize long-term complications after cancer treatment including endocrine deficiencies, recurrence of disease, development of second cancers, pulmonary complications, neurocognitive deficits, and metabolic disorders.

References

1. Siegel RL, Miller KD, Jemal A. Cancer statistics, 2020. CA Cancer J Clin. 2020;70(1):7–30.
2. Mitby PA, Robison LL, Whitton JA, Zevon MA, Gibbs IC, Tersak JM, et al. Utilization of special education services and educational attainment among long-term survivors of childhood cancer: a report from the childhood cancer survivor study. Cancer. 2003;97(4):1115–26.
3. Krasin MJ, Constine LS, Friedman DL, Marks LB. Radiation-related treatment effects across the age spectrum: differences and similarities or what the old and young can learn from each other. Semin Radiat Oncol. 2010;20(1):21–9.
4. Rowe LS, Krauze AV, Ning H, Camphausen KA, Kaushal A. Optimizing the benefit of CNS radiation therapy in the pediatric population-part 1: understanding and managing acute and late toxicities. Oncology (Williston Park). 2017;31(3):182–8.
5. van Iersel L, Li Z, Srivastava DK, Brinkman TM, Bjornard KL, Wilson CL, et al. Hypothalamic-pituitary disorders in childhood cancer survivors: prevalence, risk factors and long-term health outcomes. J Clin Endocrinol Metab. 2019;104(12):6101–15.
6. Vatner RE, Niemierko A, Misra M, Weyman EA, Goebel CP, Ebb DH, et al. Endocrine deficiency as a function of radiation dose to the hypothalamus and pituitary in pediatric and young adult patients with brain tumors. J Clin Oncol. 2018;36(28):2854–62.
7. Sklar CA, Antal Z, Chemaitilly W, Cohen LE, Follin C, Meacham LR, et al. Hypothalamic-pituitary and growth disorders in survivors of childhood cancer: an endocrine society clinical practice guideline. J Clin Endocrinol Metab. 2018;103(8):2761–84.
8. Sfeir JG, Kittah NEN, Tamhane SU, Jasim S, Chemaitilly W, Cohen LE, et al. Diagnosis of GH deficiency as a late effect of radiotherapy in survivors of childhood cancers. J Clin Endocrinol Metab. 2018;103(8):2785–93.
9. Lone SW, Khan YN, Qamar F, Atta I, Ibrahim MN, Raza J. Safety of insulin tolerance test for the assessment of growth hormone deficiency in children. JPMA J Pak Med Assoc. 2011;61(2):153–7.

10. Tamhane S, Sfeir JG, Kittah NEN, Jasim S, Chemaitilly W, Cohen LE, et al. GH therapy in childhood cancer survivors: a systematic review and meta-analysis. J Clin Endocrinol Metab. 2018;103(8):2794–801.
11. Richmond E, Rogol AD. Treatment of growth hormone deficiency in children, adolescents and at the transitional age. Best Pract Res Clin Endocrinol Metab. 2016;30(6):749–55.
12. Jasim S, Alahdab F, Ahmed AT, Tamhane SU, Sharma A, Donegan D, et al. The effect of growth hormone replacement in patients with hypopituitarism on pituitary tumor recurrence, secondary cancer, and stroke. Endocrine. 2017;56(2):267–78.
13. Chemaitilly W, Merchant TE, Li Z, Barnes N, Armstrong GT, Ness KK, et al. Central precocious puberty following the diagnosis and treatment of pediatric cancer and central nervous system tumors: presentation and long-term outcomes. Clin Endocrinol (Oxf). 2016;84(3):361–71.
14. Latronico AC, Brito VN, Carel J-C. Causes, diagnosis, and treatment of central precocious puberty. Lancet Diabetes Endocrinol. 2016;4(3):265–74.
15. van Santen HM, van den Heuvel-Eibrink MM, van de Wetering MD, Wallace WH. Hypogonadism in children with a previous history of cancer: endocrine management and follow-up. Horm Res Paediatr. 2019;91(2):93–103.
16. Biedka M, Kuźba-Kryszak T, Nowikiewicz T, Żyromska A. Fertility impairment in radiotherapy. Contemp Oncol. 2016;20(3):199–204.
17. Faw CA, Brannigan RE. Hypogonadism and cancer survivorship. Curr Opin Endocrinol Diabetes Obes. 2020;27(6):411–8.
18. Olivius C, Landin-Wilhelmsen K, Olsson DS, Johannsson G, Tivesten Å. Prevalence and treatment of central hypogonadism and hypoandrogenism in women with hypopituitarism. Pituitary. 2018;21(5):445–53.
19. Payne JB, Flowers CR, Allen PB. Supporting decision-making on fertility preservation among adolescent and young adult women with cancer. Oncol Williston Park N. 2020;34(11):494–9.
20. Poirot C, Brugieres L, Yakouben K, Prades-Borio M, Marzouk F, de Lambert G, et al. Ovarian tissue cryopreservation for fertility preservation in 418 girls and adolescents up to 15 years of age facing highly gonadotoxic treatment. Twenty years of experience at a single center. Acta Obstet Gynecol Scand. 2019;98(5):630–7.
21. Mauri D, Gazouli I, Zarkavelis G, Papadaki A, Mavroeidis L, Gkoura S, et al. Chemotherapy associated ovarian failure. Front Endocrinol. 2020;11:572388.
22. Wyns C, Kanbar M, Giudice MG, Poels J. Fertility preservation for prepubertal boys: lessons learned from the past and update on remaining challenges towards clinical translation. Hum Reprod Update. 2020;27(3):433.
23. Beck-Peccoz P, Rodari G, Giavoli C, Lania A. Central hypothyroidism—a neglected thyroid disorder. Nat Rev Endocrinol. 2017;13(10):588–98.
24. Chemaitilly W, Li Z, Huang S, Ness KK, Clark KL, Green DM, et al. Anterior hypopituitarism in adult survivors of childhood cancers treated with cranial radiotherapy: a report from the St Jude lifetime cohort study. J Clin Oncol. 2015;33(5):492–500.
25. Shulman DI, Palmert MR, Kemp SF. Adrenal insufficiency: still a cause of morbidity and death in childhood. Pediatrics. 2007;119(2):e484–94.
26. Jasim S, Alahdab F, Ahmed AT, Tamhane S, Prokop LJ, Nippoldt TB, et al. Mortality in adults with hypopituitarism: a systematic review and meta-analysis. Endocrine. 2017;56(1):33–42.
27. Verbalis JG. Acquired forms of central diabetes insipidus: mechanisms of disease. Best Pract Res Clin Endocrinol Metab. 2020;34(5):101449.
28. Kalra S, Zargar AH, Jain SM, Sethi B, Chowdhury S, Singh AK, et al. Diabetes insipidus: the other diabetes. Indian J Endocrinol Metab. 2016;20(1):9–21.
29. Fenske W, Refardt J, Chifu I, Schnyder I, Winzeler B, Drummond J, et al. A copeptin-based approach in the diagnosis of diabetes insipidus. N Engl J Med. 2018;379(5):428–39.
30. Rao AD, Ladra M, Dunn E, Kumar R, Rao SS, Sehgal S, et al. A road map for important centers of growth in the pediatric skeleton to consider during radiation therapy and associated clinical correlates of radiation-induced growth toxicity. Int J Radiat Oncol. 2019;103(3):669–79.

31. Ullah T, Patel H, Pena GM, Shah R, Fein AM. A contemporary review of radiation pneumonitis. Curr Opin Pulm Med. 2020;26(4):321–5.
32. Robison LL, Green DM, Hudson M, Meadows AT, Mertens AC, Packer RJ, et al. Long-term outcomes of adult survivors of childhood cancer. Cancer. 2005;104(11 Suppl):2557–64.
33. Inskip PD, Veiga LHS, Brenner AV, Sigurdson AJ, Ostroumova E, Chow EJ, et al. Hypothyroidism after radiation therapy for childhood cancer: a report from the childhood cancer survivor study. Radiat Res. 2018;190(2):117–32.
34. Brabant G, Toogood AA, Shalet SM, Frobisher C, Lancashire ER, Reulen RC, et al. Hypothyroidism following childhood cancer therapy-an under diagnosed complication. Int J Cancer. 2012;130(5):1145–50.
35. Behjati S, Gundem G, Wedge DC, Roberts ND, Tarpey PS, Cooke SL, et al. Mutational signatures of ionizing radiation in second malignancies. Nat Commun. 2016;7(1):12605.
36. Armenian SH, Robison LL. Childhood cancer survivorship: an update on evolving paradigms for understanding pathogenesis and screening for therapy-related late effects. Curr Opin Pediatr. 2013;25(1):16–22.
37. Dracham CB, Shankar A, Madan R. Radiation induced secondary malignancies: a review article. Radiat Oncol J. 2018;36(2):85–94.
38. Steinmeier T, Schulze Schleithoff S, Timmermann B. Evolving radiotherapy techniques in paediatric oncology. Clin Oncol (R Coll Radiol). 2019;31(3):142–50.
39. LaRiviere MJ, Santos PMG, Hill-Kayser CE, Metz JM. Proton therapy. Hematol Oncol Clin N Am. 2019;33(6):989–1009.
40. Park S, Jeon MJ, Song E, Oh H-S, Kim M, Kwon H, et al. Clinical features of early and late postoperative hypothyroidism after lobectomy. J Clin Endocrinol Metab. 2017;102(4):1317–24.
41. Volkin D, Yerram N, Ahmed F, Lankford D, Baccala A, Gupta GN, et al. Partial adrenalectomy minimizes the need for long-term hormone replacement in pediatric patients with pheochromocytoma and von hippel-lindau syndrome. J Pediatr Surg. 2012;47(11):2077; https://www.ncbi.nlm.nih.gov/pmc/articles/PMC3846393/. [cited 2021 Jan 31]
42. Neumann HPH, Tsoy U, Bancos I, Amodru V, Walz MK, Tirosh A, et al. Comparison of pheochromocytoma-specific morbidity and mortality among adults with bilateral pheochromocytomas undergoing total adrenalectomy vs cortical-sparing adrenalectomy. JAMA Netw Open. 2019;2(8):e198898.
43. Flitsch J, Müller HL, Burkhardt T. Surgical strategies in childhood craniopharyngioma. Front Endocrinol. 2011;2:96; [cited 2020 Nov 10]. https://www.ncbi.nlm.nih.gov/pmc/articles/PMC3355821/.
44. Hwangbo Y, Lee EK. Acute hyperglycemia associated with anti-cancer medication. Endocrinol Metab. 2017;32(1):23–9.
45. Vergès B, Cariou B. mTOR inhibitors and diabetes. Diabetes Res Clin Pract. 2015;110(2):101–8.
46. Higham CE, Olsson-Brown A, Carroll P, Cooksley T, Larkin J, Lorigan P, et al. Society for endocrinology endocrine emergency guidance: acute management of the endocrine complications of checkpoint inhibitor therapy. Endocr Connect. 2018;7(7):G1–7.
47. Cukier P, Santini FC, Scaranti M, Hoff AO. Endocrine side effects of cancer immunotherapy. Endocr Relat Cancer. 2017;24(12):T331–47.
48. Scott ES, Long GV, Guminski A, Clifton-Bligh RJ, Menzies AM, Tsang VH. The spectrum, incidence, kinetics and management of endocrinopathies with immune checkpoint inhibitors for metastatic melanoma. Eur J Endocrinol. 2018;178(2):173–80.
49. van As JW, van den Berg H, van Dalen EC. Platinum-induced hearing loss after treatment for childhood cancer. Cochrane Database Syst Rev. 2016;2016(8):CD010181; [cited 2021 Jan 31]. https://www.ncbi.nlm.nih.gov/pmc/articles/PMC6466671/.
50. Armenian SH, Hudson MM, Mulder RL, Chen MH, Constine LS, Dwyer M, et al. Recommendations for cardiomyopathy surveillance for survivors of childhood cancer: a report from the International late effects of childhood cancer guideline harmonization group. Lancet Oncol. 2015;16(3):e123–36.

51. McNerney ME, Godley LA, Le Beau MM. Therapy-related myeloid neoplasms: when genetics and environment collide. Nat Rev Cancer. 2017;17(9):513–27.
52. Blumenfeld Z. Chemotherapy and fertility. Best Pract Res Clin Obstet Gynaecol. 2012;26(3):379–90.
53. Pradhan KR, Chen Y, Moustoufi-Moab S, Krull K, Oeffinger KC, Sklar C, et al. Endocrine and metabolic disorders in survivors of childhood cancers and health-related quality of life and physical activity. J Clin Endocrinol Metab. 2019;104(11):5183–94.
54. Polgreen LE, Petryk A, Dietz AC, Sinaiko AR, Leisenring W, Goodman P, et al. Modifiable risk factors associated with bone deficits in childhood cancer survivors. BMC Pediatr. 2012;12(1):40.
55. Makale MT, McDonald CR, Hattangadi-Gluth J, Kesari S. Brain irradiation and long-term cognitive disability: Current concepts. Nat Rev Neurol. 2017;13(1):52–64.
56. PDQ Pediatric Treatment Editorial Board. Late effects of treatment for childhood cancer (PDQ®): health professional version. In: PDQ cancer information summaries. Bethesda, MD: National Cancer Institute (US); 2002; [cited 2021 Jan 31]. http://www.ncbi.nlm.nih.gov/books/NBK65832/.
57. Children's Oncology Group. [cited 2021 Jan 31]. http://www.survivorshipguidelines.org/.
58. Keegan THM, Tao L, DeRouen MC, Wu X-C, Prasad P, Lynch CF, et al. Medical care in adolescents and young adult cancer survivors: what are the biggest access-related barriers? J Cancer Surviv Res Pract. 2014;8(2):282–92.
59. King-Dowling S, Psihogios AM, Hill-Kayser C, Szalda D, O'Hagan B, Darabos K, et al. Acceptability and feasibility of survivorship care plans and an accompanying mobile health intervention for adolescent and young adult survivors of childhood cancer. Pediatr Blood Cancer. 2021;68(3):e28884.

Chapter 11
Metabolic Risk and Complications in the Treatment of Pediatric and Adolescent Neuroendocrine Neoplasms

Bader N. Alamri and Ivan George Fantus

Introduction

The incidence of neuroendocrine neoplasms or tumors (NETs) in the USA has increased from 1.09 per 100,000 in 1973 to 6.98 per 100,000 in 2012 [1]. Based on reports addressing NETs' prevalence among pediatric and adolescent patients, female dominance was observed [2, 3]. This was in keeping with the SEER (Surveillance, Epidemiology and End Results) database analysis and subsequent reports specifically investigating children and young adults [1, 4].

Although most NETs in children are benign or low-grade, about 10% present with metastasis [5]. Their slow growth and advancements in therapy mean there is a high survival rate and increased prevalence [5]. While midgut (especially the appendix) is the most common NET site, the typical carcinoid syndrome seen in adults is an uncommon presentation among the pediatric group. However, the late stage of bronchial NETs may present with symptoms, such as cough and wheezing, which can be misdiagnosed as asthma or reactive airway disease, delaying accurate diagnosis, and treatment [6].

While most NETs are sporadic, up to 30% are hereditary syndromes [7]. In multiple endocrine neoplasia type 1 (MEN1) syndromes, the mutation in the tumor suppressor gene, Menin, results in the clinical phenotype of primary hyperparathyroidism (PHPT), associated with pancreatic and pituitary NETs. An activating mutation in the RET tyrosine kinase proto-oncogene (MEN 2) manifests clinically as medullary thyroid cancer (MTC) and pheochromocytoma and classified as subtypes A and B. MEN 2B is characterized by neuromas and marfanoid habitus in up

B. N. Alamri · I. G. Fantus (✉)
Division of Endocrinology and Metabolism, Department of Medicine, McGill University, Montreal, QC, Canada

Research Institute, McGill University Health Centre (MUHC), Montreal, QC, Canada
e-mail: George.fantus@mcgill.ca

F. Hannah-Shmouni (ed.), *Familial Endocrine Cancer Syndromes*,
https://doi.org/10.1007/978-3-031-37275-9_11

177

to 95% of cases. Von Hippel-Lindau (VHL) syndrome is another cancer syndrome caused by an autosomal dominant gene mutation of the VHL tumor suppressor. This leads to the activation of HIF-1α (hypoxia inducible factor- 1α) and upregulation of targets such as erythropoietin and VEGF (vascular endothelial growth factor). It manifests as hemangioblastomas in the brain, pancreatic NETs, pheochromocytoma, and clear cell renal carcinoma. In neurofibromatosis type 1, the gene mutation in the Ras-GAP (GTPase activating protein), neurofibromin, leads to the clinical features of skin café au lait lesions, neurofibromas, optic gliomas, Lisch nodules, and pheochromocytomas. Pancreatic neuroendocrine tumors may occur more rarely and usually are somatostatinomas. Mutations in the succinate dehydrogenase genes (*SDHA, SDHB, SDHC, SDHD,* or *SDHAF2*) are known to cause hereditary pheochromocytoma-paraganglioma syndrome [7, 8]. NETs, whether sporadic or genetically-linked, appear to be significantly associated with short and long-term metabolic risks such as obesity and diabetes as reviewed below.

Obesity and the Metabolic Syndrome

Overview

Obesity has become widespread, not only among adults, but also in children. Indeed, over the last three decades, the prevalence of obesity in youth has increased almost eight-fold [9]. This rising trend has been associated with an increased occurrence of type 2 diabetes mellitus (T2DM) [10]. In addition to classical risk factors, e.g., increased calorie intake and sedentary lifestyle, treatment of childhood cancer appears to increase the likelihood of obesity and T2DM among survivors [11]. Metabolic syndrome (MetS) (obesity, insulin resistance, glucose intolerance, high blood pressure, and low HDL level), a precursor to the development of T2DM, is a documented late complication among childhood cancer survivors [12]. It is more prevalent among recipients of chemotherapy combined with cranial and abdominal radiation in comparison to those who only undergo chemotherapy [13]. In addition, among adult survivors of childhood acute lymphocytic leukemia (ALL) who were treated with total body irradiation (TBI), both insulin levels and pancreas volume were lower in comparison to a chemotherapy-only treatment group [14]. In the Childhood Cancer Survivors Study, the adult survivors were 1.8 times more likely to develop T2DM than their siblings (control group). Moreover, the survivors in the TBI group had the highest risk of T2DM in comparison to the survivors that underwent abdominal and cranial irradiation [15].

In a large cohort of childhood cancer survivors, patients who received pancreatic radiation at a dose of 10 Gy or higher had a higher risk of developing T2DM in adulthood. Interestingly, this risk was confined to pancreatic tail irradiation, where the beta cells are concentrated, but not to other parts of the pancreas [16] suggesting that β-cell functional impairment and/or loss plays a significant role. In a recent review, hypothalamic damage conferred the greatest risk for obesity and the MetS followed by cranial irradiation and therapy with glucocorticoids [17, 18]. In addition, those receiving HSCT (Hematopoietic stem cell transplant) had a high risk of developing insulin resistance (52%) and diabetes (5%) even in the absence of obesity, reflecting atypical body fat distribution and likely pancreatic β-cell impairment [18, 19]. In the obesity literature, the role of gut microbiota in insulin resistance and energy homeostasis has been a focus of research. Despite evidence that chemotherapy and radiation affect gut microbiota in children, the long-term effect and contribution of these changes is yet to be investigated [11, 20]. The frequent use of steroids in chemotherapy protocols, decreased physical activity, and poor dietary habits are other factors contributing to obesity and T2DM in cancer survivors [11, 19, 21].

The literature on long-term treatment consequences, specifically of pediatric neuroendocrine neoplasia, consists of studies of small cohorts. This is the case for MetS. Most of the endocrine-related treatment complications of childhood cancers come from research on pediatric solid and hematological malignancies. As described for these non-endocrine cancers, many of the long-term endocrine complications are related to the type of therapy rather than the actual tumor, especially if radiotherapy is used [18–22]. Here, we address the long-term complications after survival of NETs, with a specific focus on MetS.

Hypercortisolism

Upon review of survivors of childhood endocrine tumors, most research on obesity following treatment has been done on patients with Cushing's disease (CD); namely, ACTH-dependent hypercortisolism [23]. Although an uncommon tumor, it accounts for most functional pituitary adenomas among the pediatric age group [24, 25]. Wędrychowicz et al. reported four female cases of CD with a median age at diagnosis of 12 years and 8 months. All had obesity as one of their presenting signs [26]. Despite a successful cure after transsphenoidal surgery (TSS), all remained obese after a median follow-up of 16.5 months (range 12–78 months). In a larger study done by the NIH group, the records of 37 girls and 22 boys (mean age 14, range 4–12 years) with hypercortisolism (50 with CD, 6 with primary adrenal disease, and 3 with ectopic corticotropin secretion) were reviewed retrospectively [27]. All patients underwent surgical treatment ± pituitary irradiation (1 case) or ± mitotane (3 cases). The most common reported presenting symptom was weight gain (90%), followed by growth retardation (83%). After a mean follow-up period of 22 months (5–60 months), 56 patients out of the 59 had no recurrence. A significant weight loss was noted 1 year after surgery in the CD patients ($N = 50$) (mean SD of age- and sex-matched weights of normal controls: before surgery; +1.5 ± 1.8, 1 year after surgery; −0.2 ± 1.6; p-value <0.001). In the primary adrenal disease group, similar results were observed but with $n = 6$ did not reach statistical significance (SD of normal, before surgery +1.2 ± 1.7, after surgery −0.3 ± 1.2).

In a retrospective study of 73 pediatric and adolescent patients with hypercorti-solism, obesity (BMI ≥ 95th percentile) was observed in 52 patients [CD: 42 (72.4%); CS (ACTH- independent): 10 (66.6%)] and overweight (BMI ≥ 85th per-centile) was seen in 13 patients; CD group 11 (18.9%), CS group 2 (13.3%), before surgery [28]. After a median follow-up time of 22.4 ± 18.2 months post-treatment, the obesity rate decreased by ≥50% in both groups to 32.8% (19 cases) in the CD group, and 26.7% (4 cases) in the CS group. Notably, T2DM was diagnosed in four cases among the overweight and obese cases before surgery (two cases each). All these cases of T2DM resolved during the follow-up. Consistent with these data, Homeostatic Model Assessment for Insulin Resistance (HOMA-IR) showed an improvement in insulin resistance after treatment with a significant difference remaining between the obese and normal weight individuals as would be expected.

Taken together, these data suggest that the risk of obesity is present not only dur-ing active disease, but also, in spite of some improvement with therapy, remains increased after remission. The longest average follow-up study of CD and CS was about 2 years after surgery. It is unknown whether the risk of obesity and T2DM continues beyond this period. Therefore, longer follow-up studies addressing this risk are needed.

Craniopharyngioma

Craniopharyngioma is another tumor that can affect the pituitary. It is a childhood CNS tumor arising from Rathke's pouch remnants. The effect on pituitary function is due to the mass effect in up to 87% of cases [29]. Hyperphagia and hypothalamic obesity (HO) are among the presenting symptoms and signs of craniopharyngioma, occurring in 21% and 30% of cases, respectively [30]. In fact, the degree of obesity is related to the severity of hypothalamic damage. While damage to the appetite regulation center plays a major role in developing obesity, other hypothalamic dis-turbances, such as daytime sleepiness and lack of physical activity, are contributing factors [31]. Even after surgical resection, the prevalence of obesity and overweight among adults that had childhood craniopharyngioma are higher than in the general population, with a higher percentage of abdominal fat in relation to total body fat [32]. In a small retrospective cohort of 22 cases of childhood craniopharyngioma with a median follow-up of 18 years, 41% of the cohort were overweight (25 ≤ BMI < 30) in comparison to 28% of the control adult population. The obesity (30 ≤ BMI < 40) rate was also higher (36% vs. 24%). The rate of class 3 obesity (BMI ≥ 40) was not different among the two populations [33]. These rates appear to be influenced by the hypothalamic damage after surgical resection. Comparing extensive resection surgery (ERS) to hypothalamus-sparing surgery (HSS), the HSS group had lower body weight. Thus, Elowe-Gruau [29] et al. reported that while pre-operative weights were similar, 37 boys and 23 girls (median age, 8 years; median follow-up time 103 months) who underwent ERS, and 38 boys and 27 girls (median age, 9.3 years; median follow-up 33 months) who underwent HSS showed in the last follow-up that grade 2 obesity (BMI greater than +3 SD) was observed more often among the ERS cohort than the HSS cohort (54% vs. 28%, p-value = 0.05). Furthermore, the rate of return to a normal weight was also higher in the HSS group (38% vs. 17%, p-value = 0.01). Supporting these data, participants with Puget grade 2 had significantly higher BMI than those with grade 0 and grade 1 (grade 0 = no hypothalamic involvement, grade 1 = tumor displacing the hypothalamus, grade 2 = hypothalamic involvement of the tumor) [33].

In addition to obesity, insulin resistance, T2DM, and dyslipidemia are other metabolic complications observed among craniopharyngioma patients [34]. When comparing childhood craniopharyngioma post-treatment obese patients to controls with exogenous obesity, the former group had a higher MetS rate (73.3% vs. 20%, p-value = 0.03) despite matching BMI, age, gender, and pubertal status between the two groups. While fasting insulin levels were not different between the treated craniopharyngioma group and the controls, both the first and second phase insulin release after the oral glucose tolerance test (OGTT) were significantly higher in the craniopharyngioma cases, suggesting increased peripheral tissue insulin resistance. Measures of insulin sensitivity were considerably reduced in the craniopharyngioma group. While there was no difference in diastolic blood pressure or HDL cholesterol, other markers of MetS, systolic BP and triglyceride levels were higher among the craniopharyngioma cases [34]. Thus, tumors and/or therapy involving the hypothalamus, a major site of regulation of food intake and energy expenditure, are significant causes of long-term metabolic complications.

Hyperaldosteronism

Hyperaldosteronism, due to a mineralocorticoid-producing adenoma (Conn's syndrome), is rare in pediatric and adolescent age groups, with fewer than 20 reported cases in the literature [35]. Other etiologies, including autosomal dominant familial hyperaldosteronism syndromes (types I–IV), are reported more frequently, yet overall remain unusual [36].

Clinical data have shown an association between hyperaldosteronism and MetS. In the German Conn's registry, the frequency of T2DM and MetS was higher among primary aldosteronism (PA) cases in comparison to controls after adjusting for sex, age, and BMI (17.2% vs. 10.4%, p-value = 0.03; 56.8% vs. 44.8%, p-value = 0.02, respectively) [37]. In a meta-analysis comparing all essential hypertension to PA, the risks of T2DM and MetS among PA cases were 1.3 and 1.5 times higher, respectively [37]. Interestingly, even in the absence of autonomous hyperaldosteronism, a higher level of plasma aldosterone predicts new onset of T2DM and obesity in the general population [38, 39]. It should be noted that these studies were not specific to children or adolescents.

A number of studies have investigated the role of mineralocorticoids in energy homeostasis, namely in adipose tissue and pancreatic β cells [40–42]. While a primary function of white adipose tissue (WAT) is to store energy as lipids, the function of brown adipose tissue (BAT) is to promote thermogenesis by utilizing nutrient energy, including glucose. The excess accumulation of lipids in the WAT is associated with insulin resistance and obesity. BAT is associated with improved insulin sensitivity and protection against weight gain. Both tissues express mineralocorticoid receptors (MCRs). Thus, in human and rodent studies, blocking MCRs in BAT significantly improved insulin sensitivity and glucose uptake. In WAT, while MCR activation leads to adipogenesis and lipid accumulation, the use of MRC antagonists prevents these effects [41, 42].

In an animal study of pancreatic β-cells, excess aldosterone diminished glucose-stimulated insulin secretion and increased apoptosis [43]. However, these effects seem to be non-MCR mediated. In clonal β-cells, glucocorticoid receptor antagonists mitigated the impairment of insulin secretion induced by aldosterone. These data suggest that MCR's may affect insulin sensitivity more directly than insulin secretion [39, 43, 44].

Due to the low frequency of primary hyperaldosteronism among youths in comparison to adults, the data on aldosterone-induced metabolic abnormalities are limited. In a cohort of 15 children with idiopathic intracranial hypertension, a 12-year-old boy was reported to have MetS with obesity, systolic hypertension, and impaired glucose tolerance; he was later diagnosed with hyperaldosteronism [45]. Other case reports have not specifically reported glucose intolerance or MetS; however, most of the reported weights were low prior to diagnosis of PA [46–48]. Further studies focusing on metabolic parameters, before and after PA treatment, are needed.

Cranial Radiation

Cranial radiation therapy is a common modality of treatment of brain tumors. A targeted field for the pituitary is sometimes used for recurrent pituitary adenoma or unsuccessful surgical removal [49]. As with hypothalamic injury due to surgery or direct tumor invasion, cranial irradiation can cause hypothalamic obesity (HO) that can manifest more than a decade after the initial therapy. The risk of developing obesity is higher among young patients (<6 years), females, those receiving a high radiation dose (> 50 Gy), and those with a hypothalamic-pituitary axis (HPA) lesion, especially craniopharyngioma [21].

In a case-control study, Cooksey et al. compared 60 childhood cancer survivors who had been exposed to hypothalamic radiation with non-exposed controls [50]. After a mean survival time of 4.5 years (3.5–5.5 years), the MetS was significantly higher among the irradiated group (15% vs. 4.9%, P-value = 0.03). While glucose and HOMA-IR was high in the exposed cohort, there were no significant differences in HDL, triglycerides, or blood pressure between the groups. Although BMI and percentage of subcutaneous abdominal fat were similar between the two groups, higher visceral fat was observed in the cranial irradiated patients. In a childhood cancer survival study, the risk of developing T2DM after cranial irradiation was 1.6

times higher among the exposed cases in comparison to their siblings, even after adjusting for BMI [15]. MetS was significantly higher among women who received cranial radiation during childhood for ALL in comparison to the controls. While BMI, waist circumference, insulin level and HOMA-index were higher in female survivors, there were no significant differences detected in male survivors in comparison to the controls [51]. In another report of prophylactic cranial radiation for ALL, 1 year of growth hormone (GH) replacement therapy improved body composition in comparison to the untreated controls; however, hyperinsulinemia and impaired insulin sensitivity persisted [52]. These studies highlight the impact of cranial irradiation on the future risk of MetS among childhood cancer survivors and suggest the interesting possibility of a degree of sexual heterogeneity in the response.

Treatment

Weight gain and associated MetS, especially in HO, increase the risk of early cardiovascular morbidity and mortality [53]. As for the general population, the main treatment for obesity among childhood cancer survivors is diet and exercise. However, interventional studies of diet and exercise in this population show mostly insignificant weight loss [11].

HO treatment is challenging and usually unresponsive to such lifestyle therapy. Recent pharmacological interventions used to treat obesity and MetS in HO show mixed results. For instance, glucagon-like peptide-1 (GLP-1) agonists are approved for T2DM and obesity treatment. In a small cohort of nine adult patients with HO secondary to brain tumor treatment, GLP-1 agonist treatment resulted in significant weight loss and HgbA1c reduction in 8 patients [54]. A case series of five children with HO treated with exenatide for 1 year showed only a meaningful weight loss in 1 participant [55]. In a recent phase 3 randomized clinical trial, 42 participants with childhood-onset HO received either exenatide 2 mg once weekly ($n = 23$) or placebo ($n = 19$) for 36 weeks [56]. While changes in BMI, HgbA1c, glucose, and lipid levels were not observed, total body fat mass and waist circumference were significantly reduced in the intervention arm.

Metformin was also investigated as a potential treatment for insulin resistance in HO. Kalina et al. reported the use of metformin and fenofibrate in ten adolescents with MetS following craniopharyngioma treatment [57]. After 6 months of treatment, the decrease in triglyceride and HOMA-IR was significant in comparison to the control group; however, BMI gradually increased in both groups.

In craniopharyngioma patients with HO, there is a parasympathetic-predominant activation which leads, via the vagus nerve, to insulin hypersecretion [31]. With its anabolic effect, insulin can contribute to the weight gain observed in affected individuals. To investigate the result of mitigating hyperinsulinemia in HO, Lustig et al. conducted a double blind, placebo-controlled trial using octreotide in pediatric patients [58]. After 6 months of therapy, weight and BMI were significantly lower in the octreotide arm ($n = 9$). Moreover, the insulin response after the OGTT was lower in the octreotide arm in comparison to the control group ($n = 9$). While no changes were detected in psychological and social functions, the octreotide cohort reported improved physical functioning. This study's results suggest that hyperinsulinemia may contribute to weight gain and decreased quality of life of hypothalamic obese patients.

Diazoxide, used to suppress insulin secretion in the setting of insulinoma and neonatal hypoglycemia, has also been studied in HO [59, 60]. In a 2-month randomized trial, 30 of 40 subjects completed the study. While leptin levels were reduced and insulin levels tended to be lower ($p = $ NS), there was no significant weight reduction. However, the glucose levels were elevated in the diazoxide group suggesting that compensatory hyperinsulinemia in the face of insulin resistance was impaired [59]. In a second study of HO in patients with Prader–Willi syndrome, a new formulation, diazoxide choline controlled release tablet, was administered daily for 10 weeks in an open label phase. In the 11 subjects that completed the trial there was a dose-dependent decrease in hyperphagia. This was associated with significant improvements in body composition, a decrease in leptin concentrations, triglyceride levels and of interest, in aggressive behaviors [60]. However, similar to the previous report, there were marked increases in glucose levels manifested as hyperglycemia/impaired glucose tolerance (eight subjects) and 1 with overt diabetes. Thus, it is not clear whether the benefits of diazoxide therapy will outweigh long-term risks in the context of HO.

In July of 2021, a novel treatment for HO and Prader–Willi syndrome was granted orphan drug designation by the United States Food and Drug Administration [61]. Tesomet is a fixed-dose combination therapy of a triple monoamine reuptake inhibitor (tesofensine) and a beta-blocker (metoprolol). The data on adults with HO was recently released [62]. Twenty-one adults with hypopituitarism and HO were randomized to Tesomet or placebo (2:1) for 24 weeks. Tesomet resulted in a significant weight loss in comparison to the placebo (6.3% vs. –0.3%; p-value = 0.017); and a reduction in the waist circumference of 5.7 cm (p-value = 0.054). The treatment-induced weight loss was primarily due to the reduction in fat mass and to a small reduction in lean mass. Tesomet was generally well tolerated. In 2 cases randomized to Tesomet, adverse events due to anxiety and dry mouth resulted in discontinuation. The most frequently reported side effects included sleep disturbances, dry mouth, and dizziness. There were no reported side effects concerning QTc, heart rate, or blood pressure. A phase 2a study of Tesomet was recently completed in adolescents and adults with Prader–Willi syndrome, and a phase 2b study is planned. No longer term clinical data has yet been published [63].

Recently, a novel anti-obesity agent has been introduced. Setmelanotide, a MCR4 receptor agonist, has shown positive results in treating genetic obesity syndromes caused by POMC (proopiomelanocortin) and LEPR (leptin receptor) deficiency [64]. It has also shown efficacy in a few subjects with Bardet–Biedl syndrome [65]. It remains to be seen in further studies whether, and to what extent, HO following tumors, e.g., craniopharyngioma, and their treatments, cranial irradiation, will be responsive to this agent.

Finally, surgical treatment, namely bariatric surgery, is very effective in weight loss. Non-reversible methods (e.g., Roux-en-Y gastric bypass) showed great weight reduction in HO in comparison to reversible adjustable gastric banding [31]. However, these interventions have mainly been studied in adults. They are controversial in the pediatric population, due to ethical and legal concerns.

Growth

In addition to the medical treatment of CD, pituitary irradiation can be used in persistent disease after TSS [24]. Both surgical and radiotherapy treatments affect normal pituitary function; this effect can range from mild hormonal deficiency to panhypopituitarism. In hypercortisolism (either in ACTH-dependent or ACTH-independent), linear growth is slower than in normal subjects, mainly due to GH suppression. Even after achieving a cure, the catch-up growth is poor. In parallel to this observation, there is a high frequency of GH deficiency (GHD) after pituitary surgery ± irradiation [24, 66]. In a small cohort of adolescents, the target height was achieved with GH replacement after TSS or radiation therapy [67]. In a single-center report of pediatric and adolescents with CD, 14 out of 19 cases had GHD in the short-term assessment post-TSS ± pituitary irradiation (mean interval 0.5 years) [68]. In the long-term assessment (mean interval 8.5 years), 4 out of 9 investigated patients had persisting GHD. Most had achieved adult height after GH replacement. These limited studies indicate that linear growth among CD patients is impaired due to steroid-induced GH suppression before treatment or can be iatrogenic after pituitary surgery ± irradiation. Clinical guidelines for growth hormone treatment in survivors of childhood cancers have been published [69]. As alluded to above, growth hormone deficiency is associated with obesity and decreased lean body mass thus contributing to MetS and cardiovascular risk [69].

Puberty

In general, the data on hypothalamic-pituitary disorders among childhood NET survivors are limited. Pre-pubertal CD manifests differently from adult disease, particularly in linear growth and puberty [70]. A small number of studies reporting on pediatric and adolescent CD showed different presentations consistent with either precocious or delayed puberty. In a cohort of 27 pediatric and adolescent patients, Dupuis et al. reported 13 patients (11 male, 2 females; mean age 10.5 years; range 6·4–13·7) who had excessive virilization [71]. Despite advanced pubic hair growth, the patients had unmatched testicular volume (in males) and breast growth stage (in females), indicating delayed true puberty. Normalization of hypercortisolism, either medically or surgically, restored normal puberty in most children with CD [72]. After adjuvant pituitary radiotherapy for CD adenomas, at a follow-up interval of

1.4–12 years, Storr et al. reported seven patients with CD who had normalization of cortisol as well as gonadotropin secretion [73]. It should be noted that in most cases of children and adolescents with GHD post-treatment, gonadotropin analogue is used to delay puberty and to allow time for linear growth.

Other Hormonal Functions

Among CD patients, transient adrenal insufficiency (AI) after surgical resection of pituitary adenoma is a good indicator of cure. However, the recovery of the HPA axis is expected. In a case series of children and adolescents with CD treated with TSS, 75% achieved full recovery before 18 months post-TSS [74]. By changing the threshold to 10 μg/dL cortisol level after 250 μg ACTH (instead of >18 μg/dL), 21.5% of the participants showed suboptimal response indicating partial HPA axis recovery [74].

Data on HPA axis recovery in CD after radiotherapy in children are lacking. However, one can extrapolate outcomes based on data from cranial radiation for central nervous system (CNS) tumors. In a 1997 study conducted by Oberfield et al., 17 patients with a median age of 3.75 years at diagnosis of CNS tumor were investigated for AI after a median of 5-years after radiation therapy [75]. By administering corticotropin-releasing factor, all patients had lower cortisol peaks in comparison to the controls. However, no difference was observed in the ACTH level between groups.

Surgery is the only curative intervention in treating medullary thyroid carcinoma (MTC) (either sporadic or hereditary). Prophylactic total thyroidectomy is recommended for germline (e.g., RET gene) mutation-associated MTC. Although hypothyroidism requires thyroxine replacement, major surgical complications (e.g., recurrent laryngeal nerve palsy, hypoparathyroidism) are infrequent and mostly transient, unless there is significant local invasion [76, 77].

Long-term data on childhood pancreatic NETs are limited. In an international MEN1-related insulinoma cohort, 15 out of 96 cases were younger than 21 years at the time of surgical intervention [78]. Only two cases of the young subgroup developed recurrent disease after surgical resection. Pancreatic insufficiency and new onset diabetes among the total cohort were reported in 25 and 18 cases, respectively. The authors did not specify the age of the cases in which these complications developed and diabetes onset would be expected to be influenced by the extent of pancreatic resection [17].

Conclusion

Childhood and adolescent endocrine tumors and NET syndromes are relatively unusual. Many of the complications associated with these syndromes are treatment related. The long-term consequences of treatment vary based on the location of the primary tumor and the treatment modality used (e.g., surgical, medical, or radiation). The data available are limited due to the deficiency in prospective large cohorts of pediatric and adolescent populations. The most well-documented and studied NET is Cushing's (both the syndrome and the disease). However, most reports consist of a small number of cohorts and a brief follow-up time.

The treatment complications of endocrine tumors and NETs include HO, MetS, and T2DM. The pathophysiology of these consequences, namely hypothalamic injury and, in some cases, pancreatic radiation, is unique in patients with NET syndromes in comparison to the general population with obesity, MetS, and T2DM. Thus, the treatments approved for the general population may not necessarily be effective in survivors of these tumors. Further studies and international collaborations are needed to address this knowledge gap in order to improve prevention and therapy.

Acknowledgements Supported by grants from CIHR (Canadian Institutes of Health Research) and the Department of Medicine, MUHC.

References

1. Dasari A, Shen C, Halperin D, Zhao B, Zhou S, Xu Y, et al. Trends in the incidence, prevalence, and survival outcomes in patients with neuroendocrine tumors in the United States. JAMA Oncol. 2017;3(10):1335–42.
2. Dall'Igna P, Ferrari A, Luzzatto C, Bisogno G, Casanova M, Alaggio R, et al. Carcinoid tumor of the appendix in childhood: the experience of two Italian institutions. J Pediatr Gastroenterol Nutr. 2005;40(2):216–9.
3. Pawa N, Clift AK, Osmani H, Drymousis P, Cichocki A, Flora R, et al. Surgical management of patients with neuroendocrine neoplasms of the appendix: appendectomy or more. Neuroendocrinology. 2018;106(3):242–51.
4. Navalkele P, O'Dorisio MS, O'Dorisio TM, Zamba GK, Lynch CF. Incidence, survival, and prevalence of neuroendocrine tumors versus neuroblastoma in children and young adults: nine standard SEER registries, 1975–2006. Pediatr Blood Cancer. 2011;56(1):50–7.
5. Sarvida ME, O'Dorisio MS. Neuroendocrine tumors in children and young adults: rare or not so rare. Endocrinol Metab Clin N Am. 2011;40(1):65–80. vii
6. Farooqui ZA, Chauhan A. Neuroendocrine tumors in pediatrics. Glob Pediatr Health. 2019;6:2333794X19862712.
7. Gaal J, de Krijger RR. Neuroendocrine tumors and tumor syndromes in childhood. Pediatr Dev Pathol. 2010;13(6):427–41.
8. Gut P, Komarowska H, Czarnywojtek A, Waligorska-Stachura J, Baczyk M, Ziemnicka K, et al. Familial syndromes associated with neuroendocrine tumours. Contemp Oncol (Pozn). 2015;19(3):176–83.

9. Collaboration NCDRF. Worldwide trends in body-mass index, underweight, overweight, and obesity from 1975 to 2016: a pooled analysis of 2416 population-based measurement studies in 128.9 million children, adolescents, and adults. Lancet. 2017;390(10113):2627–42.

10. Buttermore E, Campanella V, Priefer R. The increasing trend of type 2 diabetes in youth: an overview. Diabetes Metab Syndr. 2021;15(5):102253.

11. Barnea D, Raghunathan N, Friedman DN, Tonorezos ES. Obesity and metabolic disease after childhood cancer. Oncology (Williston Park). 2015;29(11):849–55.

12. Talvensaari KK, Lanning M, Tapanainen P, Knip M. Long-term survivors of childhood cancer have an increased risk of manifesting the metabolic syndrome. J Clin Endocrinol Metab. 1996;81(8):3051–5.

13. de Haas EC, Oosting SF, Lefrandt JD, Wolffenbuttel BH, Sleijfer DT, Gietema JA. The metabolic syndrome in cancer survivors. Lancet Oncol. 2010;11(2):193–203.

14. Wei C, Thyagiarajan M, Hunt L, Cox R, Bradley K, Elson R, et al. Reduced beta-cell reserve and pancreatic volume in survivors of childhood acute lymphoblastic leukaemia treated with bone marrow transplantation and total body irradiation. Clin Endocrinol. 2015;82(1):59–67.

15. Meacham LR, Sklar CA, Li S, Liu Q, Gimpel N, Yasui Y, et al. Diabetes mellitus in long-term survivors of childhood cancer. Increased risk associated with radiation therapy: a report for the childhood cancer survivor study. Arch Intern Med. 2009;169(15):1381–8.

16. de Vathaire F, El-Fayech C, Ben Ayed FF, Haddy N, Guibout C, Winter D, et al. Radiation dose to the pancreas and risk of diabetes mellitus in childhood cancer survivors: a retrospective cohort study. Lancet Oncol. 2012;13(10):1002–10.

17. Tonorezos ES, Vega GL, Sklar CA, Chou JF, Moskowitz CS, Mo Q, et al. Adipokines, body fatness, and insulin resistance among survivors of childhood leukemia. Pediatr Blood Cancer. 2012;58(1):31–6.

18. Chemaitilly W, Cohen LE, Mostoufi-Moab S, Patterson BC, Simmons JH, Meacham LR, Van Santen HM, Sklar CA. Endocrine late effects in childhood cancer survivors. J Clin Oncol. 2018;36(21):2153–9.

19. Friedman DN, Tonorezos ES, Cohen P. Diabetes and metabolic syndrome in survivors of childhood cancer. Horm Res Paediatr. 2019;91(2):118–27.

20. Touchefeu Y, Montassier E, Nieman K, Gastinne T, Potel G, des Bruley Varannes S, et al. Systematic review: the role of the gut microbiota in chemotherapy- or radiation-induced gastrointestinal mucositis—current evidence and potential clinical applications. Aliment Pharmacol Ther. 2014;40(5):409–21.

21. Rose SR, Horne VE, Howell J, Lawson SA, Rutter MM, Trotman GE, et al. Late endocrine effects of childhood cancer. Nat Rev Endocrinol. 2016;12(6):319–36.

22. Oberfield SE, Garvin JH Jr. Thalamic and hypothalamic tumors of childhood: endocrine late effects. Pediatr Neurosurg. 2000;32(5):264–71.

23. Kanter AS, Diallo AO, Jane JA Jr, Sheehan JP, Asthagiri AR, Oskouian RJ, et al. Single-center experience with pediatric Cushing's disease. J Neurosurg. 2005;103(5 Suppl):413–20.

24. Savage MO, Lienhardt A, Lebrethon MC, Johnston LB, Huebner A, Grossman AB, et al. Cushing's disease in childhood: presentation, investigation, treatment and long-term outcome. Horm Res. 2001;55(Suppl 1):24–30.

25. Storr HL, Alexandraki KI, Martin L, Isidori AM, Kaltsas GA, Monson JP, et al. Comparisons in the epidemiology, diagnostic features and cure rate by transsphenoidal surgery between paediatric and adult-onset Cushing's disease. Eur J Endocrinol. 2011;164(5):667–74.

26. Wedrychowicz A, Hull B, Tyrawa K, Kalicka-Kasperczyk A, Zielinski G, Starzyk J. Cushing disease in children and adolescents—assessment of the clinical course, diagnostic process, and effects of the treatment—experience from a single paediatric centre. Pediatr Endocrinol Diabetes Metab. 2019;25(3):127–43.

27. Magiakou MA, Mastorakos G, Oldfield EH, Gomez MT, Doppman JL, Cutler GB Jr, et al. Cushing's syndrome in children and adolescents. Presentation, diagnosis, and therapy. N Engl J Med. 1994;331(10):629–36.

28. Valdes N, Tirosh A, Keil M, Stratakis CA, Lodish M. Pediatric Cushing's syndrome: greater risk of being overweight or obese after long-term remission and its predictive factors. Eur J Endocrinol. 2021;184(1):179–87.
29. Elowe-Gruau E, Beltrand J, Brauner R, Pinto G, Samara-Boustani D, Thalassinos C, et al. Childhood craniopharyngioma: hypothalamus-sparing surgery decreases the risk of obesity. J Clin Endocrinol Metab. 2013;98(6):2376–82.
30. Puget S, Garnett M, Wray A, Grill J, Habrand JL, Bodaert N, et al. Pediatric craniopharyngiomas: classification and treatment according to the degree of hypothalamic involvement. J Neurosurg. 2007;106(1 Suppl):3–12.
31. Muller HL. Craniopharyngioma and hypothalamic injury: latest insights into consequent eating disorders and obesity. Curr Opin Endocrinol Diabetes Obes. 2016;23(1):81–9.
32. Srinivasan S, Ogle GD, Garnett SP, Briody JN, Lee JW, Cowell CT. Features of the metabolic syndrome after childhood craniopharyngioma. J Clin Endocrinol Metab. 2004;89(1):81–6.
33. Hidalgo ET, Orillac C, Kvint S, McQuinn MW, Dastagirzada Y, Phillips S, et al. Quality of life, hypothalamic obesity, and sexual function in adulthood two decades after primary gross-total resection for childhood craniopharyngioma. Childs Nerv Syst. 2020;36(2):281–9.
34. Simoneau-Roy J, O'Gorman C, Pencharz P, Adeli K, Daneman D, Hamilton J. Insulin sensitivity and secretion in children and adolescents with hypothalamic obesity following treatment for craniopharyngioma. Clin Endocrinol. 2010;72(3):364–70.
35. Abdullah N, Khawaja K, Hale J, Barrett AM, Cheetham TD. Primary hyperaldosteronism with normokalaemia secondary to an adrenal adenoma (Conn's syndrome) in a 12 year-old boy. J Pediatr Endocrinol Metab. 2005;18(2):215–9.
36. Stowasser M, Gordon RD. Familial hyperaldosteronism. J Steroid Biochem Mol Biol. 2001;78(3):215–29.
37. Hanslik G, Wallaschofski H, Dietz A, Riester A, Reincke M, Allolio B, et al. Increased prevalence of diabetes mellitus and the metabolic syndrome in patients with primary aldosteronism of the German Conn's registry. Eur J Endocrinol. 2015;173(5):665–75.
38. Val Buglioni A, Cannone V, Sangaralingham SJ, Heublein DM, Scott CG, Bailey KR, et al. Aldosterone predicts cardiovascular, renal, and metabolic disease in the general community: a 4-year follow-up. J Am Heart Assoc. 2015;4(12):e002505.
39. Thuzar M, Stowasser M. The mineralocorticoid receptor-an emerging player in metabolic syndrome? J Hum Hypertens. 2021;35(2):117–23.
40. Valaiyapathi B, Calhoun DA. Role of mineralocorticoid receptors in obstructive sleep apnea and metabolic syndrome. Curr Hypertens Rep. 2018;20(3):23.
41. Tirosh A, Garg R, Adler GK. Mineralocorticoid receptor-an emerging player in metabolic syndrome? Curr Hypertens Rep. 2010;12(4):252–7.
42. Feraco A, Marzolla V, Scuteri A, Armani A, Caprio M. Mineralocorticoid receptors in metabolic syndrome: from physiology to disease. Trends Endocrinol Metab. 2020;31(3):205–17.
43. Luther JM, Luo P, Kreger MT, Brissova M, Dai C, Whitfield TT, et al. Aldosterone decreases glucose-stimulated insulin secretion in vivo in mice and in murine islets. Diabetologia. 2011;54(8):2152–63.
44. Chen F, Liu J, Wang Y, Wu T, Shan W, Zhu Y, et al. Aldosterone induces clonal beta-cell failure through glucocorticoid receptor. Sci Rep. 2015;5:13215.
45. Salpietro V, Mankad K, Kinali M, Adams A, Valenzise M, Tortorella G, et al. Pediatric idiopathic intracranial hypertension and the underlying endocrine-metabolic dysfunction: a pilot study. J Pediatr Endocrinol Metab. 2014;27(1–2):107–15.
46. Baranwal AK, Singhi SC, Narshimhan KL, Jayashree M, Singhi PD, Kakkar N. Aldosterone-producing adrenocortical adenoma in childhood: a case report. J Pediatr Surg. 1999;34(12):1878–80.
47. Pozzan GB, Armanini D, Cecchetto G, Opocher G, Rigon F, Fassina A, et al. Hypertensive cardiomegaly caused by an aldosterone-secreting adenoma in a newborn. J Endocrinol Investig. 1997;20(2):86–9.

48. Abasiyanik A, Oran B, Kaymakci A, Yasar C, Caliskan U, Erkul I. Conn syndrome in a child, caused by adrenal adenoma. J Pediatr Surg. 1996;31(3):430–2.
49. Mathieu D, Kotecha R, Sahgal A, De Salles A, Fariselli L, Pollock BE, et al. Stereotactic radiosurgery for secretory pituitary adenomas: systematic review and international stereotactic radiosurgery society practice recommendations. J Neurosurg. 2021;1-12:801.
50. Cooksey R, Wu SY, Klesse L, Oden JD, Bland RE, Hodges JC, et al. Metabolic syndrome is a sequela of radiation exposure in hypothalamic obesity among survivors of childhood brain tumors. J Investig Med. 2019;67(2):295–302.
51. Follin C, Gabery S, Petersen A, Sundgren PC, Bjorkman-Burtcher I, Latt J, et al. Associations between metabolic risk factors and the hypothalamic volume in childhood leukemia survivors treated with cranial radiotherapy. PLoS One. 2016;11(1):e0147575.
52. Bulow B, Link K, Ahren B, Nilsson AS, Erfurth EM. Survivors of childhood acute lymphoblastic leukaemia, with radiation-induced GH deficiency, exhibit hyperleptinaemia and impaired insulin sensitivity, unaffected by 12 months of GH treatment. Clin Endocrinol. 2004;61(6):683–91.
53. Deepak D, Furlong NJ, Wilding JP, MacFarlane IA. Cardiovascular disease, hypertension, dyslipidaemia and obesity in patients with hypothalamic-pituitary disease. Postgrad Med J. 2007;83(978):277–80.
54. Zoicas F, Droste M, Mayr B, Buchfelder M, Schofl C. GLP-1 analogues as a new treatment option for hypothalamic obesity in adults: report of nine cases. Eur J Endocrinol. 2013;168(5):699–706.
55. van Schaik J, Begijn DGA, van Iersel L, Vergeer Y, Hoving EW, Peeters B, et al. Experiences with glucagon-like Peptide-1 receptor agonist in children with acquired hypothalamic obesity. Obes Facts. 2020;13(4):361–70.
56. Roth CL, Perez FA, Whitlock KB, Elfers C, Yanovski JA, Shoemaker AH, et al. A phase 3 randomized clinical trial using a once-weekly glucagon-like peptide-1 receptor agonist in adolescents and young adults with hypothalamic obesity. Diabetes Obes Metab. 2021;23(2):363–73.
57. Kalina MA, Wilczek M, Kalina-Faska B, Skala-Zamorowska E, Mandera M, Malecka TE. Carbohydrate-lipid profile and use of metformin with micronized fenofibrate in reducing metabolic consequences of craniopharyngioma treatment in children: single institution experience. J Pediatr Endocrinol Metab. 2015;28(1–2):45–51.
58. Lustig RH, Hinds PS, Ringwald-Smith K, Christensen RK, Kaste SC, Schreiber RE, et al. Octreotide therapy of pediatric hypothalamic obesity: a double-blind, placebo-controlled trial. J Clin Endocrinol Metab. 2003;88(6):2586–92.
59. Brauner R, Serreau R, Souberbielle JC, Pouillot M, Grouazel S, Recasens C, Zerah M, Sainte-Rose C, Treluyer JM. Diazoxide in children with obesity after hypothalamic-pituitary lesions: a randomized, placebo-controlled trial. J Clin Endocrinol Metab. 2016;101:4825–33.
60. Kimonis V, Surampalli A, Wencel M, Gold JA, Coen NM. A randomized pilot efficacy and safety trial of diazoxide choline controlled-release in patients with Prader-Willi syndrome. PLoS One. 2019;14(9):e0221615.
61. Saniona Receives U.S. FDA Orphan Drug Designation for Tesomet in Hypothalamic Obesity [press release]. https://www.globenewswire.com/news-release/2021/07/26/2268298/0/en/Saniona-Receives-U-S-FDA-Orphan-Drug-Designation-for-Tesomet-in-Hypothalamic-Obesity.html2021.
62. Huynh KD, Klose MC, Krogsgaard K, Drejer J, Byberg S, Madsbad S, et al. Weight loss, improved body composition and fat distribution by Tesomet in acquired hypothalamic obesity. J Endocr Soc. 2021;5(Supplement_1):A64–A5.
63. Co-administration of Tesofensine/Metoprolol in Subjects With Prader-Willi Syndrome (PWS). https://ClinicalTrials.gov/show/NCT03149445.
64. Clement K, van den Akker E, Argente J, Bahm A, Chung WK, Conners H, DeWaele K, Farooqi IS, Gonneau-Lejeune J, Gordon G, Kohlsdorf K, Poitou C, Puder L, Swain J, Stewart M, Yuan G, Wabitscht M, Kuhnent P. Efficacy and safety of setmelanotide, an MC4R agonist,

in individuals with severe obesity due to LEPR or POMC deficiency: single-arm, open-label, multicentre, phase 3 trials. Lancet Diabetes Endocrinol. 2020;8:960–70.

65. Haws R, Brady S, Davis E, Fletty K, Yuan G, Gordon G, Stewart M, Yanovski J. Effect of set-melanotide, a melanocortin-4 receptor agonist, on obesity in Bardet-Biedl syndrome. Diabetes Obes Metab. 2020;22:2133–40.

66. Magiakou MA, Mastorakos G, Gomez MT, Rose SR, Chrousos GP. Suppressed spontaneous and stimulated growth hormone secretion in patients with Cushing's disease before and after surgical cure. J Clin Endocrinol Metab. 1994;78(1):131–7.

67. Lebrethon MC, Grossman AB, Afshar F, Plowman PN, Besser GM, Savage MO. Linear growth and final height after treatment for Cushing's disease in childhood. J Clin Endocrinol Metab. 2000;85(9):3262–5.

68. Yordanova G, Martin L, Afshar F, Sabin I, Alusi G, Plowman NP, et al. Long-term outcomes of children treated for Cushing's disease: a single center experience. Pituitary. 2016;19(6):612–24.

69. Sklar CA, Antal Z, Chemaitilly W, Cohen LE, Follin C, Meacham LR, Murad MH. Hypothalamic-pituitary and growth disorders in survivors of childhood cancer: an Endocrine Society clinical practice guideline. J Clin Endocrinol Metab. 2018;103(8):2761–84.

70. Storr HL, Savage MO. Management of endocrine disease: paediatric Cushing's disease. Eur J Endocrinol. 2015;173(1):R35–45.

71. Dupuis CC, Storr HL, Perry LA, Ho JT, Ahmed L, Ong KK, et al. Abnormal puberty in paediatric Cushing's disease: relationship with adrenal androgen, sex hormone binding globulin and gonadotrophin concentrations. Clin Endocrinol. 2007;66(6):838–43.

72. Motte E, Rothenbuhler A, Gaillard S, Lahlou N, Teinturier C, Coutant R, et al. Mitotane (op'DDD') restores growth and puberty in nine children with Cushing's disease. Endocr Connect. 2018;7(12):1280–73.

73. Storr HL, Plowman PN, Carroll PV, Francois I, Krassas GE, Afshar F, et al. Clinical and endocrine responses to pituitary radiotherapy in pediatric Cushing's disease: an effective second-line treatment. J Clin Endocrinol Metab. 2003;88(1):34–7.

74. Lodish M, Dunn SV, Sinaii N, Keil MF, Stratakis CA. Recovery of the hypothalamic-pituitary-adrenal axis in children and adolescents after surgical cure of Cushing's disease. J Clin Endocrinol Metab. 2012;97(5):1483–91.

75. Oberfield SE, Nirenberg A, Allen JC, Cohen H, Donahue B, Prasad V, et al. Hypothalamic-pituitary-adrenal function following cranial irradiation. Horm Res. 1997;47(1):9–16.

76. Matsushita R, Nagasaki K, Ayabe T, Miyoshi Y, Kinjo S, Haruna H, et al. Present status of prophylactic thyroidectomy in pediatric multiple endocrine neoplasia 2: a nationwide survey in Japan 1997-2017. J Pediatr Endocrinol Metab. 2019;32(6):585–95.

77. Machens A, Dralle H. Long-term outcome after DNA-based prophylactic neck surgery in children at risk of hereditary medullary thyroid cancer. Best Pract Res Clin Endocrinol Metab. 2019;33(4):101274.

78. van Beek DJ, Nell S, Verkooijen HM, Borel Rinkes IHM, Valk GD, Vriens MR, et al. Surgery for multiple endocrine neoplasia type 1-related insulinoma: long-term outcomes in a large international cohort. Br J Surg. 2020;107(11):1489–99.

Chapter 12
Fertility in Cancer Survivors

Grace Whiteley, Alan DeCherney, and Jennifer Chae-Kim

Introduction

Individuals undergoing treatment for cancer may be at risk of treatment-related infertility depending on their type of cancer and treatment modalities utilized. Cancer treatments can damage gonadal tissue, gametes or sex hormones [1, 2]. Ovarian tissue is susceptible to damage during chemotherapy, radiation or surgery. Ovarian damage from chemotherapy is drug and dose dependent and related to the age at the time of cancer treatment. There is a higher risk of infertility and premature ovarian insufficiency in older women who receive, for instance, alkylating agents with a high CED. By one estimate, the typical chemotherapy protocol can result in depletion of 10 years' worth of ovarian reserve [3].

Risk of Chemotherapy and Radiation on Fertility

There are three proposed mechanisms by which chemotherapy agents are thought to lead to ovarian insufficiency or infertility. First, chemotherapeutic agents have been shown to accelerate recruitment of primordial follicles, by activating the PI3K/PTEN/Akt pathway. This leads to early activation of follicles, then a "burn out effect" of the ovarian follicle deposit [3–5]. Secondly, chemotherapeutic agents can directly damage quiescent follicles by way of DNA damage; particularly, alkylating agents and doxorubicin, both of which cross-link with DNA leading to cellular apoptosis. DNA damage-induced follicle death appears to be mediated by TAp63, a

G. Whiteley · A. DeCherney (✉) · J. Chae-Kim
National Institute of Child Health and Human Development, NIH, Bethesda, MD, USA
e-mail: jennifer.chae-kim@nih.gov

F. Hannah-Shmouni (ed.), *Familial Endocrine Cancer Syndromes*,
https://doi.org/10.1007/978-3-031-37275-9_12

193

transcription factor in the p53 family [6]. Finally, chemotherapeutic agents are thought to indirectly injure the ovary by disrupting vascularization in the ovary, and lead to fibrosis of the ovarian cortex. The pre-pubertal ovary appears to be more resistant to gonadotoxic chemotherapeutic agents, which may be due to the presence of more follicles of the absence of active folliculogenesis in this patient population [7]. The testis, and specifically primordial sperm cells, are also extremely susceptible to the toxic effects of both radiation and chemotherapy and treatment can result in oligospermia or azoospermia.

Several risk stratifying calculators have classified the gonadotoxic risk of cancer treatment into several categories: no risk, low risk (<20%), intermediate risk (21–80%), and high risk (80%) [8]. The LIVESTRONG/American Society of Clinical Oncology (ASCO) fertility risk calculator, in particular, describes the risk of amenorrhea in women. Criteria used for this risk calculator include cancer type, treatment dose and duration, age, and pubertal status. Although fertility risk calculators are frequently utilized in clinical decision-making, there are some issues to keep in mind. Risk calculators that describe the risk of amenorrhea may not accurately reflect the risk of infertility. Women who undergo chemotherapy may resume regular menstrual cycles despite significantly diminished ovarian reserve [3]. Secondly, the wide range of risk in the intermediate category (ranging from 21% to 80%) makes counseling regarding actual risk and recommendations for fertility sparing treatment more challenging. Furthermore, the LIVESTRONG risk calculator is based on cancer treatment protocols in the USA and Europe, and may not be applicable to different demographics [9].

Other risk stratification systems include the alkylating agent dose (AAD) and cyclophosphamide equivalent dose (CED). Both systems quantify the exposure to an alkylating agent such as cyclophosphamide. The AAD is based on the drug dose distribution of patients from the Childhood Cancer Survivor Study; the CED, on the other hand, is independent of this study population. A classification chart reported by Anderson et al., based on pretreatment AMH levels of women with early stage breast cancer, is meant to predict loss of ovarian function, characterized as ongoing menses or treatment-induced amenorrhea [10]. Per this chart, the resumption of spontaneous menses was seen at AMH above 20.3 pmol/L, and amenorrhea following AMH below 3.8 pmol/L. For AMH values between 3.8 and 20.3 pmol/L, an age threshold of 38.6 years predicted menses or amenorrhea. A recent study also reported on a standardized risk assessment for adolescent and young adult patients [11]. Depending on the CED, the type of chemotherapy, or radiation exposure measured in Gy, treatment-related infertility or gonadal insufficiency is categorized into "minimally increased," "significantly increased" or "high level of increased" risk [11].

Certain chemotherapeutic agents have been associated with various impacts on gonadal tissue. Alkylating agents such as cyclophosphamide or chlorambucil, known to be highly gonadotoxic, function as metabolites that cross-link with DNA, leading to inhibition of DNA synthesis and function, and subsequent apoptotic death of primordial follicles [3, 12]. Alkylating agents have an intermediate to high chance of causing infertility based on the cumulative dose that is prescribed [1].

Platinum agents, such as cisplatin and carboplatin, act by platination of DNA which is similar to alkylation and also acts to induce apoptosis [13]. Platinum-based compounds are considered to entail an "intermediate" risk of gonadotoxicity. Additionally, higher doses of chemotherapy that are used for priming for hematopoietic stem cell transplant are associated with high risk of infertility, which can often be permanent [14]. Other intermediate risk agents include anthracyclines and taxanes [1]. Another "intermediate" gonadotoxic agent is doxorubicin, which inhibits the topoisomerase II enzyme and intercalates into DNA, to impair DNA replication. This has multiple effects, including the accumulation of DNA fragments leading to cell death, as well as the production of oxygen-free radicals [3, 15]. Agents including methotrexate, 6-mercaptopurine, 5-fluorouracil, vincristine, bleomycin, and actinomycin have little or no risk of causing infertility.

Radiation to the abdomen and pelvis, in addition to total body irradiation or cranio-spinal radiation that can impact the hypothalamic pituitary gonadal axis, is associated with a high risk of infertility. Whole abdominal/pelvic radiation >15 Gy in pre-pubertal females, >10 Gy in post-pubertal females, and > 6 Gy in adults has been associated with infertility [1]. The impact of radiation on future fertility is additionally related to fractionation schedule and age at the time of radiation treatment [16].

Workup Prior to Fertility Preservation

The gonadotoxic effects of cancer treatment has raised the need for a marker that assesses ovarian reserve and can predict ovarian function after treatment. A biomarker that accomplishes both tasks is key to patient counseling regarding fertility preservation treatment options. There are a number of markers of ovarian reserve, including FSH, E2, AMH, inhibin B, ovarian volume and total AFC; of these, AMH appears to have the most potential as a biomarker to track ovarian reserve and function prior to and after cancer treatment. AMH is produced by granulosa cells of growing preantral and small antral follicles. Its value remains relatively constant over the menstrual cycle. It can also be used as a marker in adolescent patients, for whom FSH and inhibin B levels are not useful in measuring ovarian reserve. Pretreatment AMH informs the clinician about the responsiveness of the functional ovarian reserve in women planning for ovarian stimulation for gamete cryopreservation [10]. While AMH level does not reliably predict clinical outcomes such as pregnancy or live birth rate, it has been used to help determine the stimulation dose of FSH in ovarian stimulation [4].

AMH also has been shown to predict ovarian function after cancer treatment, depending on the woman's age. Studies have shown that post-treatment AMH is reduced compared to pretreatment baseline, however, the trajectory of AMH recovery after cancer treatment depends on the pretreatment level, as well as type of chemotherapy received and the woman's age [3, 10]. Specifically, cancer survivors older than 30 years of age the time of diagnosis had lower post-treatment AMH trajectories, compared to patients under the age of 30. Pretreatment AMH has been used as part of an infertility risk calculus, as explained above [17].

There are a few caveats to keep in mind regarding the interpretation of AMH. Pretreatment AMH levels may be decreased in women with lymphoma, as well as women with *BRCA1* mutations [18, 19]. For women who receive GnRH agonist therapy during chemotherapy, post-treatment AMH levels may be suppressed as a result [20]. Further, interpretation of AMH values can be challenging in puberty, when AMH levels tend to decline in the peri-pubertal stage. Lastly, there is no standardization of commercially available assays measuring AMH, each with varying reference ranges, and inter-assay differences make direct comparisons difficult [20].

When counseling patients on fertility preservation options, it is important to discuss infertility risks and predicted post-treatment ovarian function, whether by way of risk calculators (as discussed above) or biomarkers such as AMH. Modifiable risk factors to infertility, such as tobacco or alcohol use, environmental toxin exposure and high body mass index, should also be taken into consideration. A previous history of infertility should also be noted.

Importantly, reproductive-age cancer patients should be assessed for hereditary or familial cancer syndromes, given their relatively early onset of cancer. They should be referred for genetic counseling and testing. Identification of a hereditary or familial cancer syndrome changes not only fertility preservation but also the cancer treatment regimen. For women with BRCA 1/2 or Lynch Syndrome, for instance, the recommendation for risk-reducing bilateral salpingo-oophorectomy narrows the fertility preservation options and affects the timeline for treatment. As noted above, women with BRCA mutations have been found to have lower AMH levels; it is unclear whether this suggests decreased ovarian reserve or fertility in the context of a germline mutation, however, patients should be counseled appropriately. Patients with hereditary cancer syndromes should be offered sperm or oocyte/embryo cryopreservation as the first line. This is particularly helpful because preimplantation genetic diagnosis (PGD) can be undertaken after IVF. PGD is a procedure that tests the blastomere biopsy for aneuploidy or genetic disorders, before embryo transfer. This genetic testing is particularly valuable for patients with hereditary cancer syndromes, such as BRCA1 and 2, Lynch Syndrome, familial adenomatous polyposis (FAP), Von Hippel-Lindau disease (VHL), Li-Fraumeni syndrome, multiple endocrine neoplasia (MEN) syndromes or retinoblastoma. Other techniques of prenatal diagnosis, such as chorionic villus sampling and amniocentesis, can be discussed as well.

Fertility Preservation Options in Females

If it is possible to delay cancer treatment after diagnosis, established fertility preservation procedures should be considered prior to treatment, which include oocyte cryopreservation and embryo cryopreservation (Fig. 12.1). Both procedures involve approximately 10–14 days of controlled ovarian stimulation with gonadotropins prior to retrieval of oocytes, followed by cryopreservation of mature oocytes via slow freezing or vitrification techniques [21]. Ovarian stimulation is not feasible prior to puberty, given the inactive HPO axis in pre-pubertal girls. Since conventional ovarian stimulation is associated with high serum estrogen levels, treatment with selective estrogen receptor modulators like tamoxifen or aromatase inhibitors

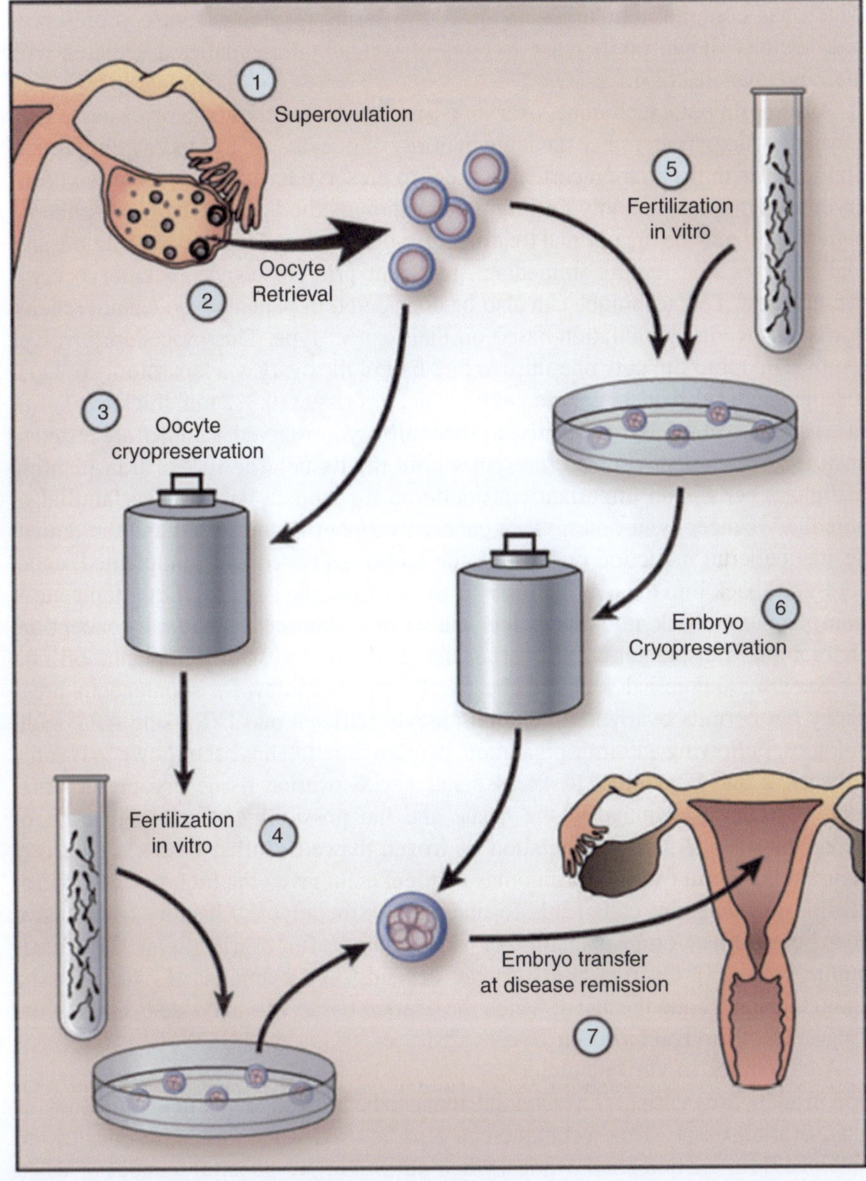

Fig. 12.1 Established fertility preservation technologies

such as letrozole, may be beneficial to keep estrogen levels low during stimulation in estrogen-sensitive cancers such as breast and endometrial cancer [22]. After oocyte retrieval, embryo cryopreservation involves fertilization of harvested oocytes with sperm via in vitro fertilization or intracytoplasmic sperm injection. Single women who are not partnered, decline sperm donation, or are opposed to embryo creation, may opt to cryopreserve oocytes as opposed to creating embryos for cryopreservation. The Italian Registry of Assisted Reproductive Technology (ART), which has compiled outcomes on 2152 live births resulting from cryopreserved oocytes, has shown no increase in rates of congenital anomalies associated with these pregnancies [23].

An experimental technique, ovarian tissue cryopreservation, involves harvesting ovarian cortical tissue, since the large majority of oocytes are located within primordial follicles in the ovarian cortex, in order to preserve fertility [24]. Ovarian tissue cryopreservation is the only fertility preservation method available for pre-pubertal patients and may be the optimal treatment for post-pubertal patients with aggressive malignancies that require immediate treatment prior to oocyte or embryo cryopreservation. This technique can also be considered in patients who cannot receive hormonal ovarian stimulation based on their cancer type. This procedure involves removal of approximately one-third to one-half of the ovary, via laparotomy or laparoscopy, with subsequent creation of thin slices of tissue (0.3–2 mm thickness) prior to cryopreservation. Before the tissue slices are cryopreserved, samples are tested to ensure no malignant cells are present within the tissue. The risk of transplanting malignant cells is an important consideration for women with known familial or hereditary cancer syndromes. Once cancer treatment is completed and the patient desires pubertal induction or fertility, the tissue is thawed and reimplanted, as an auto-graft back into the ovarian fossa or to a heterotopic site [25]. Orthotopic auto-transplantation back into the pelvis allows for attempts at natural conception. Heterotopic transplantation of ovarian tissue, performed with reimplantation into the forearm, abdominal wall and chest wall, does not allow for spontaneous pregnancy but permits ovarian stimulation, oocyte retrieval and IVF using ART technologies. Following autotransplantation, ovarian function has been shown to resume between 2 and 9 months. Risks associated with ovarian tissue cryopreservation include ischemic damage to the tissue and the possibility of reimplantation of malignant cells. Autotransplantation of frozen-thawed ovarian tissue is currently contraindicated in ovarian carcinomas and leukemia given the high risk of reintroduction of malignant cells [26]. To date, approximately 120 healthy babies have been born from autotransplantation of ovarian tissue after ovarian tissue slow freezing/thawing [27]. Ovarian graft survival depends on the amount of ovarian tissue autotransplanted and the age at which the ovarian tissue was harvested. To date, the longest graft survival has been 7 years [28].

Additionally, in vitro maturation, a process by which oocytes undergo maturation in an in vitro setting, is a technique that can be utilized to obtain mature oocytes from ovarian tissue. This technique can also be used when immature oocytes are obtained from unstimulated ovaries, when utilized in pre-pubertal females or when stimulatory cycles cannot be performed due to time limiting factors or treatment limiting factors [29, 30]. Immature oocytes are cultured for 24–48 h in order to mature into metaphase (II) oocytes that can be used for IVF or be frozen through slow freeze or vitrification processes. In vitro maturation is a promising method for patients who cannot delay gonadotoxic therapy or for whom ovarian stimulation is contraindicated [31]. Studies have demonstrated that the number of mature oocytes achieved through IVM has been shown to be associated with AMH [32]. This suggests that a patient with lower pretreatment AMH level may not achieve a sufficient number of mature oocytes after IVM.

For patients undergoing cancer treatment that has been associated with complete ovarian failure, whole ovary cryopreservation prior to treatment with subsequent slow freezing or vitrification, is an experimental technique that has been performed in both animal and human models. A fresh whole ovary transplant between a living donor and recipient has resulted in live birth, but no live births have been documented after transplantation of previously cryopreserved autologous ovaries [33]. While the majority of whole ovary cryopreservation cases have been associated with high follicular loss due to cryoinjury and vascular complications post-transplant, the inclusion of a large vascular pedicle with the removed ovary can salvage blood supply to the ovarian graft [34].

Other current experimental studies in animals have looked at utilization of the "artificial ovary," a multi-step ex-vivo process of sequential in-vitro culture of ovarian tissue, follicles and oocytes to produce mature oocytes for IVF. In a study using a murine model, preantral follicles were grown in a fibrin scaffold which functioned as the artificial ovary; the follicles were later transplanted and found to be viable in vivo [35].

Ovarian tissue culture research and stem cell research to produce oocytes are other topics of active research for fertility preservation. Recent findings have challenged the dogma that the number of oocytes in the human ovary is finite. Studies have reported the isolation of oogonial stem cells, in human ovaries as well as murine models [36, 37]. However, the role of oogonial stem cells in the lifespan of ovarian function is yet to be fully elucidated, and how stem cells can improve reproductive function remains unclear. There is currently no therapy involving oogonial stem cells in the development of human gametes.

New research has explored the use of "ferto-protectant" pharmaceutical agents that protect against chemotherapy-induced ovarian insufficiency or infertility, in the preclinical setting. A recent study showed that recombinant AMH decreased primordial follicle loss after administration of cyclophosphamide, cisplatin or doxorubicin [38]. Other pharmaceutical agents that have been studied include: sphingosine-1-phosphate (S1P), shown to help resist radiation-induced follicular apoptosis in murine models; imatinib, which blocks apoptotic pathways in primordial follicles exposed to cisplatin; AS101, shown to decrease activation of the PI3K/PTEN/Akt pathway thereby limiting early activation of primordial follicles and the "burn out effect" in rodents after cyclophosphamide treatment; G-CSF, which promotes vascularization and can counteract chemotherapy-induced ovarian vascular ischemia; tamoxifen, which may help preserve the ovarian follicle deposit, although data are conflicting; and nanoparticles to encapsulate chemotherapeutic agents to improve delivery and limit exposure of surrounding tissue [39–43]. Other agents under investigation include crocetin, mTORC inhibitors, LH, ghrelin, and antioxidants [15].

Currently there is conflicting data on the utility of GnRH agonists in preventing primary ovarian insufficiency in cancer patients undergoing treatment by suppressing folliculogenesis [12, 22]. It has been postulated that the administration of GnRH agonists before and during chemotherapy suppresses the number of primordial follicles entering the growing pool of follicles, making them less sensitive to gonadotoxic chemotherapy. Other theories suggest that GnRH agonists may upregulate intra-ovarian anti-apoptotic molecules and protect ovarian germline stem cells [44–46]. For women with known hereditary cancer syndromes requiring risk-reducing salpingo-oophorectomy after cancer treatment, the provider may consider the use of GnRH agonists for ovarian suppression during chemotherapy [46]. Currently the National Comprehensive Cancer Network (NCCN) guidelines acknowledge use of GnRH agonists in preventing chemotherapy-induced ovarian failure in estrogen receptor negative tumors (National Comprehensive Cancer Network), however, the American Society of Clinical Oncology (ASCO) does not have recommendations regarding GnRH agonists for this indication. Additional neoadjuvant cytoprotective pharmacotherapies are currently being investigated.

To preserve fertility in patients undergoing radiation, techniques such as gonadal shielding and oophoropexy can be utilized to shield the ovaries from the detrimental effects of abdominal/pelvic radiation. Oophoropexy involves surgical transposition of the ovaries, either laterally toward the pelvic sidewall or medially behind the uterus, to move the ovaries away from the field of pelvic irradiation. The success of oophoropexy has been related to the dose, type and site of pelvic radiation, patient age and coadministration of chemotherapy [47].

Advancements in cancer treatment have additionally allowed for fertility sparing treatments that avoid surgery that would otherwise render a patient infertile. Such advancements include the hormonal management of early endometrial cancer, radical trachelectomy for cervical cancer and uterine-sparing surgery for early stage ovarian cancers.

Fertility Preservation Options in Males

The gold standard for fertility preservation in post-pubertal males involves sperm cryopreservation. Previous studies have demonstrated fertility success rates in young men (14–30 years old) utilizing previously frozen sperm is 36% for intrauterine insemination and 50% when utilizing IVF/ISCI [48]. If certain underlying medical comorbidities preclude patients from successful ejaculation, electro-ejaculation can be utilized for microsurgical testicular sperm extraction (TESE), which extracts spermatozoa from testicular tissue [49, 50]. In children, who cannot ejaculate, epididymal or testicular sperm extraction can be considered. Limited options remain available for pre-pubertal males undergoing cancer treatment, since the pre-pubertal testis does not produce mature spermatozoa. Experimental procedures currently available include maturation of spermatogonia from testicular tissue biopsy which has been shown to be successful in animal models [51].

Ethical/Legal Considerations

There are a number of ethical issues related to fertility preservation for cancer patients. Reproductive-age cancer patients should receive counseling, even if they express no interest in future children, as many fertility preservation options also preserve ovarian endocrine function. First and foremost is the question of informed consent. Patients should be counseled thoroughly on the various fertility preservation options, as well as associated pregnancy and live birth rates. Importantly, some methods of fertility preservation are experimental or not as well established, and patients should be informed that fertility preservation aims to preserve future reproductive potential but does not ensure it [52]. Providers should also ascertain whether patients are psychologically, intellectually and emotionally competent to consent or assent to treatment. When minors are faced with cancer diagnoses, they often make decisions with their family and parents have decision-making capability when it comes to preserving their child's fertility, if the intervention is likely to provide benefit. If and when possible, it is recommended to obtain child consent. There is a consensus for a two-stage consent process: at diagnosis, then after treatment when the patient is at a developmentally appropriate age [52]. If minors openly object to treatment, fertility preservation treatments should not be performed.

Particularly for patients with known familial or hereditary cancer syndromes, they should be counseled on the importance of preimplantation genetic testing (PGT). The benefits of avoiding transfer of an affected embryo, and passing on the mutated gene, is critical for the patient's decision-making process. However, patients and their families may have religious, cultural or personal objections to PGT or embryo cryopreservation, so these issues should be addressed prior to cancer treatment if possible.

Another area of ethical concern is the disposition or posthumous use of cryopreserved gametes. Unless otherwise specified, gametes should be discarded if the child does not survive to adulthood, however, when possible, instructions regarding the disposition of gametes should be made at the time of fertility preservation [53]. The provider should also address how potential disagreements between family members regarding the posthumous use of gametes should be adjudicated. It is also helpful to ascertain the patient's wishes to donate his or her gametes or gonadal tissue to scientific research. Often a multi-disciplinary approach is taken to address potential conflicts of interest in the event of the patient's death.

Any medical decision made with an adolescent patient should be navigated carefully and with the patient's best interests in mind. The provider should determine whether the patient is an appropriate candidate for enrollment in available clinical trials, and discuss this with the patient and family. Participation in a clinical trial may provide new opportunities for fertility preservation, however research on children and adolescent patients is strictly regulated and will require informed consent or assent. Children are a vulnerable population, and their decision-making can be easily influenced by their parents' or families' wishes [54]. The provider should advocate for the patient, and try to ensure that any decision regarding fertility preservation reflects patient autonomy and respects the opportunity for future family building, if desired. In short, all decisions should be made with the goal of providing "an open future" for the patient [53]. Lastly, all ethical considerations should be made within the legal framework.

Post-Treatment Follow-Up for Cancer Patients

Compared to healthy controls without cancer, reproductive-age cancer survivors have lower rates of post-treatment pregnancies [55]. The chances of post-treatment pregnancy depend heavily on the female patient's age at time of diagnosis, cancer treatment as well as cancer type. Post-treatment counseling may include measures of ovarian failure, which can be objectively measured through follicle-stimulating hormone, FSH, the most common biochemical marker used to assess ovarian damage or failure. Additionally, anti-mullerian hormone (AMH) and antral follicle count can be used to assess ovarian reserve post-treatment. Post-treatment AMH, compared to pretreatment baseline, may predict return of ovarian function, as discussed above.

Optimal timing for pregnancy following cancer treatment is currently unknown and largely depends on the patient's current medical status, prognosis, and possible harmful effects of therapy. The timing of attempting pregnancy should be based on shared decision-making and involve the oncologist as well as reproductive endocrinologist. Some patients attempt pregnancy 2–3 years after finishing cancer treatment, and after monitoring for possible cancer recurrence. Other patients, such as those with hormone receptor positive breast cancer, require long-term hormonal therapy after treatment. The data on the timing of pregnancy for these women, as well as the safety of pregnancy, is very limited but encouraging [55]. Planning for pregnancy should take into account the "wash-out" period needed for patients on adjuvant endocrine therapies (i.e., 3 months after discontinuing tamoxifen). The data on the safety of ART in women with hormone receptor positive cancer is also very limited; this subset of fertility preservation patients often require the use of third-party reproduction. Studies evaluating pregnancy outcomes in cancer survivors have found no increase in congenital malformations in offspring, primarily in women who have conceived spontaneously after chemotherapy [56]. However, some studies have suggested increased obstetric complications in post-treatment pregnancies, such as increased risk of premature birth, low birth weight, and need for cesarean delivery [55].

References

1. Levine J, Canada A, Stern CJ. Fertility preservation in adolescents and young adults with cancer. J Clin Oncol. 2010;28(32):4831–41.
2. Stern C, Conyers R, Orme L, Barak S, Agresta F, Seymour J. Reproductive concerns of children and adolescents with cancer: challenges and potential solutions. Clin Oncol Adolesc Young Adult. 2013;3:63–78.
3. Bedoschi G, Navarro PA, Oktay K. Chemotherapy-induced damage to ovary: mechanisms and clinical impact. Future Oncol. 2016;12(20):2333–44.
4. Sonigo C, Beau I, Binart N, Grynberg M. Anti-Mullerian hormone in fertility preservation: clinical and therapeutic applications. Clin Med Insights Reprod Health. 2019;13:1–7.
5. Mauri D, Gazouli I, Zarkavelis G, Papadaki A, et al. Chemotherapy associated ovarian failure. Front Endocrinol. 2020;11:572388.
6. Tuppi M, Kehrloesser S, Coutandin D, Rossi V, Luh LM, et al. Oocyte DNA damage quality control requires consecutive interplay of CHK2 and CKI to activate p63. Nat Struct Mol Biol. 2018;25:261–9.
7. Byrne J, Fears TR, Gail MH, et al. Early menopause in long-term survivors of cancer during adolescence. Am J Obstet Gynecol. 1992;166:788–93.
8. Cyclophosphamide Equivalent Dose Calculator. https://fertilitypreservationpittsburgh.org/fertility-resources/fertility-risk-calculator/.
9. Roo SF, Rashedi A, Beerendunk C, Anazodo A. Global infertility index-data gap slows progress. Biol Reprod. 2017;96(6):1124–8.
10. Anderson R, Su HI. The clinical value and interpretation of Anti-Mullerian hormone in women with cancer. Front Endocrinol. 2020;11:574263.
11. Meacham L, Burns K, Orwig KE, Levine J. Standardizing risk assessment for treatment-related gonadal insufficiency and infertility in childhood adolescent and young adult cancer: the pediatric initiative network risk stratification system. J Adolesc Young Adult Oncol. 2020;9(6):662.
12. Blumenfeld Z, et al. Chemotherapy and fertility. Best Pract Res Clin Obstet Gynecol. 2012;26:379–90.
13. Balis FM, Hocenberg JS, Blaney SM. General principles of chemotherapy. In: Principles and practices of pediatric oncology. 4th ed. Philadelphia, PA: Lippincott, Williams & Wilkins; 2002. p. 237–308.
14. Meistrich ML. Effects of chemotherapy and radiotherapy on spermatogenesis. Eur Urol. 1993;23(1):136–41.
15. Spears N, Lopes F, Stefansdottir A, Rossi V. Ovarian damage from chemotherapy and current approaches to its protection. Hum Reprod Update. 2019;25(6):673–93.
16. Critchley HO, Bath LE, Wallace WH. Radiation damage to the uterus—review of the effects of treatment of childhood cancer. Hum Fertil (Camb). 2002;5:61–6.
17. Anderson R, Rosendahl M, Kelsey T, Cameron D. Pretreatment Anti-Mullerian hormone predicts for loss of ovarian function after chemotherapy for early breast cancer. Eur J Cancer. 2013;49(6):3404–11.
18. Lekovich J, Lobel AL, Stewart J, Pereira N. Female patients with lymphoma demonstrate diminished ovarian reserve even before initiation of chemoterahpy when compared with healthy controls and patients with other malignancies. J Assist Reprod Genet. 2016;33(5):657–62.
19. Phillips K, Collins IM, Milne RL, McLachlan SA. Anti-Mullerian hormone serum concentrations of women with germline BRCA1 or BRCA2 mutations. Hum Reprod. 2016;31(5):1126–32.
20. Dunlop C, Anderson RA. Uses of Anti-Mullerian hormone (AMH) measurement before and after cancer treatment in women. Maturitas. 2015;80:245–50.
21. Gosden R. Cryopreservation: a cold look at technology for fertility preservation. Fertil Steril. 2011;96(2):264–8.

22. Oktay K, Buyuk E, Libertella N, Akar M. Fertility preservation in breast cancer patients: a prospective controlled comparison of ovarian stimulation with tamoxifen and letrozole for embryo cryopreservation. J Clin Oncol. 2005;23(19):4347–53.
23. Levi-Setti PE, Borini A, Patrizio P, Bolli S, Vigilian V, De Luca R, Scaravelli G. ART results from frozen oocytes: data from the Italian ART registry (2005–2013). J Assist Reprod Genet. 2016;33:123–8.
24. Armstrong AG, Kimler BF, Smith BM, Woodruff TK, Pavone ME, Duncan FE. Ovarian tissue cryopreservation in young females through the oncofertility consortium's National Physicians Cooperative. Future Oncol. 2018;14(4):363–78.
25. Meirow D, Roness H, Kristensen SG, Andersen CY. Optimizing outcomes from ovarian tissue cryopreservation and transplantation; activation versus preservation. Hum Reprod. 2015;30(11):2453–6.
26. Imbert R, Moffa F, Tsepelidis S, Simon P, et al. Safety and usefulness of cryopreservation of ovarian tissue to preserve fertility: a 12-year retrospective analysis. Hum Reprod. 2014;29(9):1931–40.
27. Van der Ven H, Liebenthron J, Beckmann M, Toth B, et al. Ninety-five orthotopic transplantations in 74 women of ovarian tissue after cytotoxic treatment in a fertility preservation network: tissue activity, pregnancy and delivery rates. Hum Reprod. 2016;31(9):2031–41.
28. Andersen CY, Silber SJ, Bergholdt SH, Jorgensen JS, Ernst E. Long-term duration of function of ovarian tissue transplants: case reports. Reprod Biomed Online. 2012;25(2):128–32.
29. Abir R, Ben-Aharon I, Garor R, Yaniv I, et al. Cryopreservation of in vitro matured oocytes in addition to ovarian tissue freezing for fertility preservation in paediatric female cancer patients before and after cancer therapy. Hum Reprod. 2016;31(4):750–62.
30. Wang X, Gook DA, Walters KA, Anazodo A, Ledger WL, Gilchrist RB. Improving fertility preservation for girls and women by coupling oocyte in vitro maturation with existing strategies. Womens Health (Lond). 2016;12(3):275–8.
31. Pfeifer S. ASRM Committee opinion. In vitro Matur. 2013;99(3):P663–6.
32. Sermondade N, Sonigo C, Sifer C, Valtat S. Serum anti-Mullerian hormone is associated with the number of oocytes matured in vitro and with primordial follicle density in candidates for fertility preservation. Fertil Steril. 2019;111:357–62.
33. Silber SJ, Grudzinskas G, Gosden RG. Successful pregnancy after microsurgical transplantation of an intact ovary. N Engl J Med. 2008;359(24):2617–8.
34. Bedaiwy MA, Falcone T. Whole ovary transplantation. Clin Obstet Gynecol. 2010;53(4):797–803.
35. Luyckx V, Dolmans MM, Vanacker J, Legat C, et al. A new step toward the artificial ovary: survival and proliferation of isolated murine follicles after autologous transplantation in a fibrin scaffold. Fertil Steril. 2014;101(4):1149–56.
36. White YA, Woods DC, Takai Y, Ishihara O, et al. Oocyte formation by mitotically active germ cells purified from ovaries of reproductive-age women. Nat Med. 2012;18(3):413–21. https://doi.org/10.1038/nm.2669; Published 2012 Feb 26.
37. Grieve KM, McLaughlin M, Dunlop CE, Telfer EE, et al. The controversial existence and functional potential of oogonial stem cells. Maturitas. 2015;82(3):278–81.
38. Kano M, Sosulski AE, Zhang L, Saatcioglu HD, et al. AMH/MIS as a contraceptive that protects the ovarian reserve during chemotherapy. Proc Natl Acad Sci U S A. 2017;114(9):E1688–97.
39. Morita Y, Perez GI, Paris F, Miranda SR, et al. Oocyte apoptosis is suppressed by disruption of the acid sphingomyelinase gene or by sphingosine-1-phosphate therapy. Nat Med. 2000;6(10):1109–14.
40. Gonfloni S, Di Tella L, Caldarola S, Cannata SM, et al. Inhibition of the c-Abl-TAp63 pathway protects mouse oocytes from chemotherapy-induced death. Nat Med. 2009;15(10):1179–85.
41. Kalich-Philosoph L, Roness H, Carmely A, Fishel-Bartal M. Cyclophosphamide triggers follicle activation and "burnout"; AS101 prevents follicle loss and preserves fertility. Sci Transl Med. 2013;5(185):185ra62.

42. Skaznik-Wikiel ME, McGuire MM, Sukhwani M, Donohue J, et al. Granulocyte colony-stimulating factor with or without stem cell factor extends time to premature ovarian insufficiency in female mice treated with alkylating chemotherapy. Fertil Steril. 2013;99(7):2045–54.
43. Ahn R, Barrett SL, Raja MR, Jozefík JK. Nano-encapsulation of arsenic trioxide enhances efficacy against murine lymphoma model while minimizing its impact on ovarian reserve in vitro and in vivo. PLoS One. 2013;8:e58491.
44. Blumenfeld Z, Eckman A. Preservation of fertility and ovarian function and minimization of chemotherapy-induced gonadotoxicity in young women by GnRH-a. J Natl Cancer Inst Monogr. 2005;34:40–3.
45. Blumenfeld Z. How to preserve fertility in young women exposed to chemotherapy? The role of GnRH agonist cotreatment in addition to cryopreservation of embrya, oocytes, or ovaries. Oncologist. 2007;12(9):1044–54.
46. Lambertini M, Horicks F, Del Mastro L, Partridge AH, et al. Ovarian protection with gonadotropin-releasing hormone agonists during chemotherapy in cancer patients: from biological evidence to clinical application. Cancer Treat Rev. 2019;72:65–77.
47. Lee SJ, Schover LR, Partridge AH, Patrizio P, et al. American Society of Clinical Oncology. American Society of Clinical Oncology recommendations on fertility preservation in cancer patients. J Clin Oncol. 2006;24(18):2917–31.
48. Neal MS, Nagel K, Duckworth J, Bissessar H, et al. Effectiveness of sperm banking in adolescents and young adults with cancer: a regional experience. Cancer. 2007;110(5):1125–9.
49. Gat I, Toren A, Hourvitz A, Raviv G. Sperm preservation by ejaculation in adolescent cancer patients. Pediatr Blood Cancer. 2014;61:256–90.
50. Meseguer M, Garrido N, Remohí J, Pellicer A, et al. Testicular sperm extraction (TESE) and ICSI in patients with permanent azoospermia after chemotherapy. Hum Reprod. 2003;18(6):1281–5.
51. Harlev A, Abofoul-Azab M, Har-Vardi I, Levitas E, et al. Fertility preservation by cryopreservation of testicular tissue from pre-pubertal boys undergoing GONADOTOXIC treatment—preliminary results. Harefuah. 2016;155(2):102–4; 131-2.
52. Mulder RL, Font-Gonzalez A, van Dulmen-den Broeder E, Quinn GP, PanCareLIFE Consortium, et al. Communication and ethical considerations for fertility preservation for patients with childhood, adolescent, and young adult cancer: recommendations from the PanCareLIFE consortium and the international late effects of childhood cancer guideline harmonization group. Lancet Oncol. 2021;22(2):e68–80.
53. Klipstein S, Fallat ME, Savelli S, Committee on Bioethics; Section on Hematology/Oncology; Section On Surgery. Fertility preservation for pediatric and adolescent patients with cancer: medical and ethical considerations. Pediatrics. 2020;145(3):e20193994.
54. Patrizio P, Caplan AL. Ethical issues surrounding fertility preservation in cancer patients. Clin Obstet Gynecol. 2010;53(4):717–26.
55. Lambertini M, Peccatori FA, Demeestere I, Amant F, ESMO Guidelines Committee, et al. Fertility preservation and post-treatment pregnancies in post-pubertal cancer patients: ESMO clinical practice guidelines†. Ann Oncol. 2020;31(12):1664–78.
56. Hudson MM. Reproductive outcomes for survivors of childhood cancer. Obstet Gynecol. 2010;116(5):1171–83.

Chapter 13
Home Care and Resources for Cancer Survivors

Vipan Nikore and Varona Nikore

Introduction

Due to advancements in treatment, cancer survivors are living longer than ever before. Survivorship is now a key stage in the cancer care continuum (see Fig. 13.1). Physical health and mental health have unfortunately both shown to be adversely affected in cancer survivors [1]. For this reason, how to improve Quality of Life (QOL) in cancer survivors needs more attention than ever.

A variety of interventions may increase the quality of life in cancer survivors. For example, 12-week home-based exercise programs have demonstrated promise in improving quality of life and psychological health in colorectal cancer survivors [2], and improving employment opportunities appears to enhance QOL in young cancer survivors [3].

Often overlooked in the continuum of care for cancer survivors is the delivery of care and support services to allow people to live safely in their home, otherwise known as home care, as well as the procurement of such services. Understanding this important topic is important since finding appropriate and timely home care services can lead to improvements in quality of life. Furthermore, the procurement of home care services is often a frustrating experience and thus an understanding of how to navigate the home care system can be useful for cancer survivors and their families. Lastly, recent innovations in health and home care services have enabled

V. Nikore (✉)
Department of Medicine, Trillium Health Partners, University of Toronto Faculty of Medicine, Toronto, ON, Canada

Department of Medicine, Cleveland Clinic Foundation, Cleveland, OH, USA
e-mail: vipan.nikore@homecarehub.com

V. Nikore
Department of Pediatrics, Homecare Hub, Los Angeles, CA, USA

F. Hannah-Shmouni (ed.), *Familial Endocrine Cancer Syndromes*,
https://doi.org/10.1007/978-3-031-37275-9_13

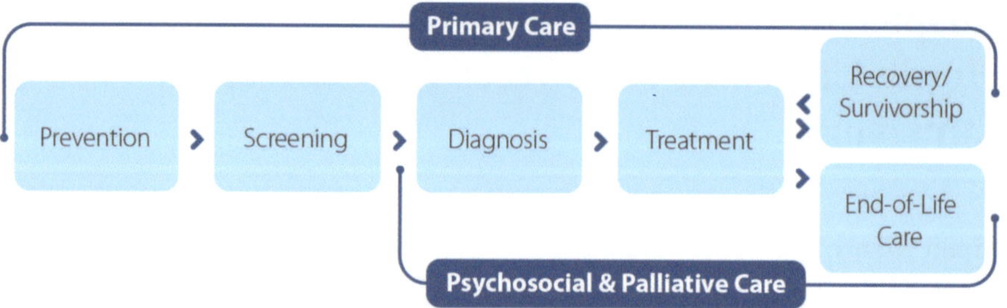

Fig. 13.1 Flow chart showing the cancer care continuum. (Source: Cancer Care Ontario. https://www.cancercareontario.ca/en/cancerplan)

many survivors to live more comfortably at home, in ways that were not previously possible.

Each country, state, province, and city typically have unique home care delivery systems, and therefore providing a standard prescriptive roadmap explaining payment models, navigation barriers, and specific resources available is unfeasible. However, there are many aspects of home care related to quality of care, procurement, and access that are universal in nature. Therefore, an understanding of these principles as well as what home care is, the benefits of home care, the home care procurement process, and new innovations in the home care can be beneficial regardless of the jurisdiction one receives home care in.

Home Care Services Available

When discussing home care, a first place to start is to understand in detail what services may be offered at home. In many countries, there has been a shift toward delivering more services and care into the home for patients. Patients often want to stay in the home instead of living a facility, and more services can be delivered into the home now than ever before. Most countries have a slightly different nomenclature for services provided in the home, though in many areas of the world when one speaks of "home health" services, one typically refers to the regulated, clinical, professional medical services that are delivered into the home, such as registered nursing, physiotherapy, or physician services. Home health services are continuing to expand in scope, and hospital at home programs are beginning to emerge as we find new ways to care for acute patients in the home. With the advancement of telehealth, remote patient monitoring, and technology in general there are also opportunities for care that were previously not available. When speaking of "home care," one commonly refers to non-clinical or less clinically heavy services such as personal support services, companionship, and meal preparation. The range of home health care and home care services that are commonly delivered to cancer survivors include:

Nursing Care

Many cancer survivors suffer from chronic pain, require routine monitoring of various blood markers, need routine IV medications, or continuous monitoring. In home nursing can help with many of these tasks.

Nurses can complete a wide variety of complex nursing tasks. Some examples include monitoring vitals, intravenous therapy, injections, tube feeding and care, catheter changes, dressing changes, advanced wound care, medication management and administration, tracheostomy care, lab draws, ventilator care, chronic disease management, pain management, patient education, administering immunizations, peritoneal dialysis, and other advanced care.

There are typically different designations of nurses in various countries, some which suggest more skills and credentials to carry out advanced tasks, and some which suggest an ability to carry less advanced tasks. Furthermore, nurses often specialize in certain tasks or specific patient diseases or populations.

More recently, many advanced IV medications that would typically require monitoring in a supervised clinic or hospital setting can now be administered at home by nurses. This shift in administration has allowed more complex conditions to be treated at home.

Home Health Aide and Personal Support Care Services

The designation for these caregivers varies by region, and may be referred to as Home Health Aides, Personal Support Workers, Health Care Assistants, Certified Nursing Assistants, and more. Regardless of their designation they are one of the most common caregiver positions in the home care system, and these caregivers can help with various tasks such as bathing, washing, toileting, dressing, grooming, personal hygiene, feeding/eating, lifts and transfers, mobility, skin care, and more.

Companions and Homemakers

Companion caregivers typically don't have a skilled training or formal designation, but may support with social interaction, help with recreational activities, or accompany patients to appointments, shopping, events, etc. Homemakers may help with light housework, meal preparation, dishes, laundry, ironing, grocery shopping, trash removal, picking up medications, and other errands. While such caregivers don't provide typical health services, they can be tremendously valuable as they help ease the burden faced by cancer survivors and their families, and can help from a mental health perspective as well.

Physiotherapy

Physiotherapists help restore movement, function and improve quality of life when someone is affected by injury, illness or disability. They help strengthen weakened muscles, improve range of motion, and treat specific musculoskeletal injuries. Physiotherapists can be particularly helpful in the early recovery period for cancer survivors, but also continuously throughout for those who face continued injury or disability.

Occupational Therapy

Occupational therapists work to assist and train individuals to complete everyday activities. Typically, patients have been impacted due to illness, disability, and injury. Depending on the functional impairment resulting from their illness, cancer survivors may benefit significantly from occupation therapy. Everyday activities that can be restored with occupational therapy include self-care activities such as getting dressed, eating, moving around the house, and leisurely tasks. This itself can improve quality of life, but further, occupational therapists may be able to help in transitioning to work or school or help with specialized equipment if needed as well.

Speech and Language Therapy

Speech and language therapists can help treat a broad range of issues including communication and swallowing. Custom plans can be created for an individual to resolve common issues such as speech sounds, voice, fluency, language, and feeding/swallowing.

Social Workers and Care Coordination

Social workers have many diverse skills that provide tremendous benefit to cancer survivors and many patients. Navigating complex healthcare systems can be challenging and social workers can serve as case managers to help coordinate care and find resources in the community. They can help find financial help, can counsel patients, helping them cope with their conflicts and challenges patients face.

Others Healthcare and Professional Services

Many professional services may come into the home to provide care. While many of these are somewhat limited and less common, such service providers may include dentists who are skilled in assessing and treating conditions related to teeth and gums, optometrists who can assess and treat vision changes for people of all ages, audiologists who assess and treat everything related to hearing for individuals of all ages, and physician services by a licensed medical professional. Additional available services are pharmacy services to help with medication, dieticians to help with nutrition, podiatrists to assist with foot care, lab services to draw blood, and even yoga therapy to help with pain and mobility.

Non-Health Care Services

Additionally, many ancillary non-health care services can be tremendously valuable for those requiring care at home. Transportation services, meal delivery services, and home salon services are just a few examples. Educational services can be tremendously valuable for children and adolescents.

Benefits of Home Care

Home care services are often underutilized. Appropriate and timely care can help cancer survivors and their families in many ways. Consider the following benefits:

Improved Mental Well-Being

Following a new diagnosis, illness, or disability one may experience depression, anxiety, loneliness, stress, or isolation. Engaging with home care service providers may allow for needed social interaction and may even bring a sense of meaning to life for some.

Improved Health

There are many ways home care services may allow cancer survivors to achieve improved health. Some may benefit from medication management or other nursing tasks to carry our plans by healthcare providers. Preventative health tasks and visits may also be able to be performed at home leading to improved health. Others may experience improved nutrition through a dietician, meal preparation, or by receiving help to carry out tasks required when cooking. Of course, improved health through skilled professionals such as physiotherapists may also lead to improved health. As noted above, one's mental well-being may improve, which also contributes to over-all health.

Daily Activities and Hobbies

After a malignancy, many individuals are less capable of performing the activities of daily living that they used to be able to perform. Personal caregivers may help perform various tasks such as gardening or putting the dishes away, but they may even be able to have one engage in his or her favorite hobby that they otherwise were not able to experience routinely.

Respite for Families

It may be unsustainable for a family member or friend to single-handedly care for a cancer survivor. By acquiring additional support, one will hopefully be able to con-tinue to support their loved one, refreshed, patient, and energetic.

Safety

In-home care provides a level of supervision that keeps people safe while providing necessary peace of mind. Many people can live longer in their own homes because they have periods of care. Living alone 24 h a day makes accidents or sickness at home more likely for those who may be at risk.

Comfort

When compared to living in an institution, many prefer to stay at home in their com-munity. Staying at home for as long as possible typically provides a level of comfort and familiarity that cannot be replicated outside of the home. Home care services support the desire of many to stay at home.

Costs and Considerations When Finding Home Care

Finding home care can be a daunting task as there are many organizations and caregivers in each region that provide care. It is far more complicated than deciding between a typical consumer product, such as deciding between an Apple IOS and Android phone. Furthermore, finding a trusted provider is important since caring for a loved one or oneself is of utmost importance.

Providers may be non-profit organizations, for profit organizations, or individual caregivers who are essentially solo practitioners on their own. These home care companies can often be found by discussing with your doctor, hospitals, community and social service organizations, local government websites, online websites, through word of mouth from friends and family, or traditional outlets such as newspapers and classifieds.

Here are a few things to consider when finding a caregiver or home care agency to suit one's needs:

Caregiving Expertise

As with most things in life, experience and training are always valuable assets. Who is the main point of contact when receiving care? Do they genuinely care, and do they have the depth of knowledge and capability to create a personalized care plan for patients? If there is an emergency or decline in function, can they be trusted to make the best choices regarding care decisions? How does the company select caregivers? Do they provide extra education to help their caregivers continue to learn? For the pediatric patient population, do they provide adequate training for caregivers who have the skills to care for children?

Reliability and Continuity of Care

Developing a system to provide care from the same providers is a complicated process. Having continuity of care with caregivers is important, and how well is the home care agency able to assure this and prevent fragmentation of care? How reliable are they? What is the agency's track record of showing up on time? What hours are the agency available? Typically, a company with multiple caregivers will be able to offer more care and better backup coverage than an individual providing care on their own. This may be less important for a patient requiring only a handful of visits from a licensed professional such as a speech language pathologist, however, this becomes a much more heavily weighted criteria for a patient who is at an extreme risk of falls and is unable to function without a caregiver.

References, Credentials, Privacy

References and credentials are important in choosing a caregiver or home care agency. Top home care workers and agencies will not hesitate to provide these documents. Be sure appropriate background checks or vulnerable sector screening are completed for caregivers. Health data security and privacy is important as well so verify that the provider follows national privacy standards, such as PHIPA in Canada or HIPAA in the US.

Philosophy of Care

Finding someone who relates well to the patient is a unique challenge for every family.

Each agency has a unique philosophy of care which will attract staff with particular backgrounds and personality types. Depending on the personality and needs of your loved one, various cultures of care will be appropriate. For example, what are your loved one's expectations? Are their needs primarily medical or social? Would they benefit from service in a certain language or from a particular community?

Safety, Infection Control, and Quality of Care

If selecting a home care company, it is important to know their policies around infection and safety. Many companies list this on their website. Do they provide Personal Protective Equipment (PPE) for their staff such as masks, gloves, and sanitizer? What protocols do they have in place for staff inside and outside of working hours? Are they incentivizing staff to stay home if they are unwell? What measures are in place to replace these workers with minimal disruption to your loved one's care?

Cost

Funding or insurance coverage may or not be available to offset home care expenses. Home care services are often paid for by a mix of public and private funds. Some health systems provide excellent public coverage of services, other regions are much less comprehensive. When funding is unavailable this can be a real constraint for patients and their families. It is important to understand what funding is available in the public system and through insurance in the region one is seeking care.

Reaching out to one's physician or local cancer association are two avenues to learn of this information. When seeking private care, often home care agencies don't list their pricing in a transparent manner, so it is important to seek the actual pricing.

Client Reviews

Client reviews are an important element in choosing home care. Reviews can be found online or from friends who have dealt with similar care services.

Challenges in Procuring Home Care

There are many challenges and barriers to procuring home care. Some of these challenges include the following:

- **Quality and Reliability**—Quality and reliability of care being delivered in the home may vary significantly. Most home care systems are built on caregivers from unregulated professions, such as home health aides. In more recent times, there has been a push to regulate caregivers more though. Furthermore, quality can vary since the metrics and standards of providing longer term, chronic care at home to patients are not well established. Thus, having fewer quality targets to hold care delivery companies accountable for may lead to a higher variability in quality of care and less transparency in the industry.
- **Cost**—Cost of care can be challenging. Providing care at home is often a difficult job, and in a system where home care is largely driven by private care, the cost to patients may be prohibitive for someone with high care needs. Additionally, while more complex tasks can be delivered at home, these complex tasks and innovations may drive up the cost of care as well.
- **Shortages**—the supply of home care providers can vary significantly across countries and the same region may also experience either an undersupply or oversupply of providers depending on the time period. Currently in most places in the world, there are not enough home care providers in most home care professions to meet an ever-increasing demand of patients who require care at home. The recent COVID-19 pandemic has further exacerbated this problem in many areas, as the pandemic caused an increased demand for many services such as nursing.
- **Location**—Depending on the region where care needs to be delivered, location may prove to be a significant barrier. For example, the shortages in caregiver supply are often exacerbated in rural or remote areas.
- **Patient Limitations**—Those who need care the most, are often those who have the most disability and most difficulty in procuring care. Whether it be due to

mobility, vision, hearing loss, these challenges can make it difficult for certain individuals to find and procure care on their own.

- **Poorly Coordinated and Integrated Systems**—One major challenge in home care is that very few systems around the world have done a formidable job integrating community home care systems into traditional healthcare delivery systems such as outpatient clinics and inpatient hospitals. Particularly, health information technology systems are often siloed with little integration between these systems. This makes providing complete, coordinated, holistic care for the patient challenging.
- **Poor Caregiver Matching**—In an increasingly specialized and diverse world, when a caregiver is placed, too often the match between patient and caregiver is poor. There may be a poor fit based on disease process and skill set, for example, a caregiver who has an expertise in physical rehabilitation care may end up caring for a patient with specialized dementia care needs. Complex pediatric care is particularly challenging, with parents and professionals having cited a lack of well-trained pediatrics caregivers as a barrier to safe home care [4]. The poor fit may also manifest itself with respect to language, as a patient may face a significant language barrier with the caregiver.
- **Social Isolation**—Even if a great home care provider is obtained, those receiving home care may still be at risk for social isolation given the tendency to stay in a home environment. This makes it even more important to work to provide social interaction through family, friends, or other community programming such as a day program. The caregiver may provide some form of companionship, but this is still minimal compared to some shared communities that provide care.
- **Backup Care**—Occasionally an individual caregiver is procured for a patient outside of a company or organization, and if the caregiver gets sick or is unable to make attend their caregiving shift in the home, there is nobody to provide backup care to the patient. This may leave the patient in a vulnerable crisis depending on the needs of the patient.

Emerging Innovations in Home Care

Broadly speaking, healthcare has struggled to bring inventions to bedside and into clinical practice at a rapid pace. To some extent, this is understandable given the nature of healthcare and the fact that a failed solution in healthcare can lead to loss of human life. Having said that, healthcare is facing innumerable complex challenges, and failing to innovate leads to a failure to fix problems that affect human life. Incremental improvements in our health system can result in improved morbidity and mortality in millions of people. Therefore, there has been an increased focus on increasing the speed of innovation across healthcare in recent years. Within healthcare, home care is one area that is beginning to see advancement in innovation.

The term healthcare innovation typically causes one to think about the development of new diagnostics, therapeutics, or even digital health. These are certainly important, but innovation does not need to be biomedical or technology driven—one can innovate in an innumerable number of ways such as around service delivery, customer service, culture, brand, education, physical infrastructure, or even patient experience. Some of the innovations in or related to home care that we have seen in recent years that will continue to play a role in home health delivery include:

- **Traditional Pharmaceuticals**—not to be overlooked, advancements that we make in the general treatment of disease help patients live longer and manage disease better. Of course, when we look at the outstanding innovations in areas such as oncology, a downstream outcome is that more people can live and manage their disease at home.
- **Diagnostics**—healthcare diagnostics continues to advance. Diagnostic devices continue to become smaller and more portable. Tests are becoming processed in a more rapid manner, and the breadth of diseases that can be monitored and diagnosed at home continues to advance. Whether a portable handheld ultrasound to monitor a pleural effusion, a pulse oximeter to monitor oxygen levels, or a home blood test to monitor various indicators of disease recurrence, innovations in diagnostics are helping transform care monitored and delivered at home.
- **Sensors, Wearables, and Remote Monitoring**—sensor technology has improved and in healthcare we are finding more ways to embed sensors into our solutions. Sensors have helped lead to an improvement in wearable products which can be particularly helpful for cancer survivors at home. These wearables allow for remote patient monitoring to help monitor anything from falls monitoring to the monitoring of vitals for patients.
- **Telehealth and Virtual Care**—telehealth, or virtual care, is the provision of remote medical care, and dates back to Dutch physician Willem Einthoven's long-distance transfer of electrocardiograms in 1906 [5]. After decades of advancements in telehealth, finally in the past several years, largely due to technological advancements and societal shifts such as increased broadband availability and usage as well as a surge in video communication, virtual care is starting to increase dramatically. Health innovations such as those advancements noted in remote monitoring and diagnostics have also driven the adoption of virtual care, and certainly the COVID-19 pandemic has accelerated this process as well. As telehealth becomes ubiquitous in the years ahead, it will increase access to care for those living at home and drive further improvements in quality of care. We will see more care delivered remotely from physicians as well for some nursing tasks, physical therapy, occupational therapy, speech therapy, and many other services.
- **Smart Home Monitoring**—the uptake of smart home technology that monitors surroundings with video, regulates temperature, and activates tasks based on voice will serve to benefit patients requiring assistance in the home. Specific healthcare smart home applications that exist can advance patient care as well, such as technology applications that help monitor falls, and ones that help homebound patients manage medications in the home.

- **Virtual Reality**—Virtual reality has begun to make its way into healthcare through areas such as healthcare education, pediatric vaccinations, and phobia desensitization to name a few. Virtual reality may provide homebound patients unique experiences to improve quality of life, among other potential applications for cancer survivors.
- **Digital Health**—there have been many software advancements beyond virtual health technologies. Several home care and caregiving online marketplaces to help procure home care with integrated payments and quality of care measures have sprouted up. Artificial intelligence is being embedded into many clinical applications and back-office applications. In addition we have seen the emergence of care navigation services, improved backend software platforms for home care agencies, and improved integration with traditional health system electronic health records. Digital healthcare communication platforms to help coordinate care in a secure manner have also emerged.
- **Autonomous Cars**—while not typically thought to be directly health related, the adoption of autonomous cars will increase access to transportation and can subsequently increase the independence of homebound patients who are unable to drive.
- **Robotics**—we are beginning to see the adoption of robotic technologies in operating rooms, and in supply chain management in hospitals among other places in healthcare. In home care, robots may play a role in the completion of tasks for homebound patients.
- **Home Medical Equipment and Supplies**—often overlooked, we continue to see advancements in home equipment and supplies. From hospital beds for the home, to incontinence products, to mobility aids, these devices benefit patients and help them remain in the home.
- **Residential Care/Group Homes**—Shared Living Houses as alternatives to institutional facilities are popular in various areas of Europe, some areas of North America, and many other areas in the world, and becoming more popular in other regions. Many of these small care homes can deliver care at a lower price than a traditional facility and at a lower price than one would pay in an individual home care situation. The quality of care when these smaller homes are implemented well may be better compared to nursing homes [6]. Families are often more satisfied with the care delivered to their loved one as well [7]. Such arrangements provide a more home like environment relative to institutional facilities and provide much needed social interaction to decrease the likelihood of social isolation.
- **Day Programs for Patients**—Day Programs that provide 9 am–5 pm daily care, companionship, activity programming, and physical exercise are often underutilized but can be great resources for cancer survivors who meet program requirements. Virtual day programs have also emerged, which again can be helpful for a certain subset of the population.
- **Hospital at Home**—while the terms home care and home healthcare traditionally conjure up long term or chronic disease care, there has been an increased interest in caring for acute care patients in the home. These emerging hospital at home programs have been driven by the advancements in caring for patients at

home, cost savings in caring for patients at home, and an increased desire for patients to be cared for in the comfort of their own home. In the years ahead, cancer survivors who experience medical concerns related to their illness that traditionally would require an inpatient hospital stay, may find that they are able to remain at home with hospital level care in certain situations.

References

1. Firkins J, Hansen L, Driessnack M, Dieckmann N. Quality of life in "chronic" cancer survivors: a meta-analysis. J Cancer Surviv. 2020;14(4):504–17.
2. Kim JY, Lee MK, Lee DH, Kang DW, Min JH, Lee JW, Chu SH, Cho MS, Kim NK, Jeon JY. Effects of a 12-week home-based exercise program on quality of life, psychological health, and the level of physical activity in colorectal cancer survivors: a randomized controlled trial. Support Care Cancer. 2019;27(8):2933–40.
3. Stone DS, Ganz PA, Pavlish C, Robbins WA. Young adult cancer survivors and work: a systematic review. J Cancer Surviv. 2017;11(6):765–81.
4. Fratantoni K, Raisanen JC, Boss RD, Miller J, Detwiler K, Huff SM, Neubauer K, Donohue PK. The pediatric home health care process: perspectives of prescribers, providers, and recipients. Pediatrics. 2019;144(3):e20190897.
5. Strehle EM, Shabde N. One hundred years of telemedicine: does this new technology have a place in paediatrics? Arch Dis Child. 2006;91(12):956–9.
6. Kane RA, Lum TY, Cutler LJ, Degenholtz HB, Yu TC. Resident outcomes in small-house nursing homes: a longitudinal evaluation of the initial green house program. J Am Geriatr Soc. 2007;55(6):832–9. https://doi.org/10.1111/j.1532-5415.2007.01169.x.
7. Lum TY, Kane RA, Cutler LJ, Yu TC. Effects of green house nursing homes on residents' families. Health Care Financ Rev. 2008;30(2):35–51.

Index